Fundamentals of Neuropathology

Fundamentals of Neuropathology

Haruo Okazaki, M.D.

Professor of Pathology
Mayo Medical School

Consultant in Neuropathology and Anatomic Pathology
Mayo Clinic and Mayo Foundation
Rochester, Minnesota

IGAKU-SHOIN   New York • Tokyo

Published and distributed by

IGAKU-SHOIN Ltd.,
5-24-3 Hongo, Bunkyo-ku, Tokyo

IGAKU-SHOIN Medical Publishers, Inc.,
1140 Avenue of the Americas, New York, N.Y. 10036

Library of Congress Cataloging in Publication Data

Okazaki, Haruo.
  Fundamentals of neuropathology.

  Bibliography: p.
  Includes index.
  1. Nervous system—Diseases—Outlines, syllabi, etc.
I. Title. [DNLM: 1. Nervous system—Pathology. WL 100
041f]
RC347.038 1983   616.8   83-224
ISBN 0-89640-086-7

Printed and bound in the United States of America

10 9 8 7 6 5 4

To my wife *Bikhar*

Foreword

For a multitude of reasons, the publication of this text is a fulfilling event: it meets a compelling need for an understandable, reliable, and comprehensive coverage of the morphology of central nervous system disease; it represents, in its author, a rare conjunction of focused talent and disciplined experience; and its appearance heralds the culmination of the professional labors of a dear friend and colleague, Haruo Okazaki.

The pages that follow reflect Dr. Okazaki's critical distillation of almost 30 years of direct observations of nervous system tissues, normal and diseased, seen and recorded while he was at the State University of New York, Downstate Medical Center; at Columbia University, College of Physicians and Surgeons; and now at the Mayo Clinic and Mayo Medical School.

I doubt that there is another neuropathologist in practice today with the accumulated dissection-table experience equal to that of Haruo Okazaki. Trained in the related fields of neuropathology, anatomic pathology, and clinical neurology (and self-trained as a neuroradiologist), while blessed with both patience and ability to suspend judgment, he is uniquely qualified to perceive and record diseases in terms of their altered spatial and histologic structures.

Haruo Okazaki has an extraordinary ability to generate and maintain precise records of his own autopsy room observations, as well as to make careful notation of the observations of others, and this skill has contributed much to reinforce his deserved reputation as a major archivist of nervous system disease. His office, whether in New York or Rochester, Minnesota, has always borne an uncanny resemblance to a curator's workroom at the British Museum. Walls originally designed for other purposes became progressively covered with packed bookcases, and when no further wall space was available, new bookcases projected into the room like mitochondrial septa. Floor space yielded progressively to proliferating filing cabinets filled with accumulated observations, photographs, and autopsy protocols from institutions near and far; and desktops served as intermediate stations in the passage of photographs, reprints, and autopsy observations to their ultimate archival destination, but only after careful cross-filing notations had been undertaken.

This monograph on the fundamentals of neuropathology has its modest origins in a mimeographed syllabus that Dr. Okazaki had previously prepared for Mayo Clinic resident physicians. During this past decade the syllabus underwent repeated scrutiny and unsparing revision. Although it makes no pretense at comprehensive coverage of abnormal neurophysiology or neurochemistry, it does represent, in my judgment, a superb outline of the fundamentals of neuropathology.

There are few people as qualified as Haruo Okazaki to provide our professional community with a working text in practical neuropathology, based almost exclusively on primary observation and free of the mythologies that color many of our texts. I happily commend these pages to the thoughtful reader who wishes to learn the rudiments of nervous system pathology.

Stanley M. Aronson, M.D.

Preface

Despite the fact that the discipline of neuroscience has seen an explosive expansion of knowledge in recent years, that portion of the clinical and pathologic residency training which is devoted to neuropathology has probably, if it has changed at all, decreased in proportion. Rarely do clinical neurology or neurosurgical training programs in the United States still include a 6- or 12-month rotation in neuropathology, as was my experience more than 20 years ago. This change is largely due to increased competition for available time from other, more "clinically useful" courses such as electroencephalography and electromyography. Yet the recent rapid advances in clinical imaging techniques have reminded us that familiarity with structural features of various neurologic disorders is still essential, or indeed is even more essential than before, in clinical practice.

This monograph is offered as a review book on neuropathology for residents in various specialties that deal, primarily or secondarily, with neurologic diseases. The book takes its origin in a syllabus I prepared earlier for the benefit of Mayo Clinic residents who take a 3-month rotation in neuropathology, as a guide to a collection of color transparencies numbering more than 3,000. This combination was designed to provide a self-study set (although aided by twice-weekly tutorial sessions) and to amplify and organize the residents' actual experiences in the autopsy room and during brain-cutting sessions. To stress practicality, conciseness, and orderliness, I have retained a syllabus-style presentation in this book. Special efforts were made to remedy some of the conceptual or factual deficiencies I have found to be common to generations of residents from diverse medical school backgrounds.

Ideally, teaching of neuropathology should incorporate recent knowledge in ultrastructural alterations, biochemistry, molecular biology, immunology, and so on, as it relates to neurologic disorders. However, neither my 3-month course nor this book was intended to be a comprehensive, up-to-date treatise on all aspects of neuropathology. In fact, its contents may be said to constitute the bare minimum of knowledge in neuropathology, particularly those basic morphologic aspects that neurology, neurosurgery, and pathology residents should acquire before they enter the practice of their respective disciplines. This restriction reflects mainly my own limitations in experience and knowledge with regard to those more specialized areas, since my own day-to-day activities are confined largely to a rather pedestrian "general practice" of neuropathology. Fortunately, I have colleagues who are well-versed in some of these other areas and to whom I can turn for advice. It is my hope that this limitation might work in the reader's favor, in that he or she can get through the book from cover to cover within a relatively short time while nevertheless acquiring a broad practical overview of the subject. To this end, I have intentionally chosen to oversimplify when practicality and clarity seemed more important than completeness, and so I have omitted from consideration many relatively rare or obscure disorders, particularly those that are not associated with visible tissue reactions. References have also been kept to a minimum. The majority of the readers undoubtedly have ready access to computerized telecommunication devices that can generate on command a list of recent articles on any subject; accordingly, no effort was made to duplicate such a service in this book. For those who wish to study further, a short list of general reading references follows the text.

The selection of photographs posed special problems for me, for their numbers had to be drastically reduced from what I would routinely utilize in teaching, and they had to be converted from living color to a drab monochromatic spectrum of gray in order to contain the cost of the book. I very much regret that the strong visual impact of some of the pathologic alterations cannot therefore be effectively conveyed to the reader. Nevertheless, the emphasis is placed on the gross morphologic features of the disorders which can now be indirectly visualized by computed tomography or by some other modern imaging techniques. The few computed tomographs included are regrettably not of the latest machine generation because of the time involved in the preparation of this book. Only essential microscopic features have been reproduced; the innumerable variations that practicing pathologists have to be familiar with in their daily diagnostic work have had to be ignored. I believe that the task of training pathologists in these details is outside the scope of this book. Electron micrographs were not included, since I did not consider them essential for the main thrust of the book; had they been included and in the size needed for sufficient clarity, they would have taken up an inordinately large amount of space.

In acknowledging the contributions to this book by others, I owe a special debt of gratitude first and foremost to my long-time teacher and friend, Dr. Stanley M. Aronson, who first taught me the joy of neuropathology and got me hooked on the subject, and who, in fact, is largely responsible for what I am professionally today. Other teachers to whom I owe a great deal are Dr. Abraham Rabiner of Downstate Medical Center, for his patient guidance in my early years of neurology training in the United States, and Drs. Abner Wolf and David Cowen of Columbia University, for allowing me a glimpse of academic neuropathology.

Among the many colleagues who materially helped me in enriching my teaching material, I am especially grateful to Dr. Joanna Sher for allowing the use of many photographs of cases I encountered at Kings County Hospital in Brooklyn, New York, and Dr. Juan Olvera-Rabiela, of Mexico City, for his generous supply of those cases that are difficult to obtain in this country.

Here in this institution, my special thanks are due to Mrs. Connie L. McDonough for her faithful and capable services as my secretary for the past 15 years, Dr. Werner Heidel for his valuable editorial and other advice, Mrs. Roberta J. Flood for her editorial services, Mr. Thomas F. Flood for his help in photography, and Mr. Robert C. Benassi for his artwork. I would also like to thank my colleagues in the Department of Pathology, Section of Medical Pathology, par-

ticularly the former chairman, Dr. Keith E. Holley, for their very willing cooperation and encouragement, and my clinical colleagues and residents in neurology and neurosurgery for their help in making my practice of neuropathology a very enjoyable one for me over the years by keeping it from becoming an exercise in a vacuum. Finally, the books in the list that follows were very valuable to me in my formulation of the teaching syllabus and this monograph:

Adams RD, Sidman RL: *Introduction to Neuropathology.* New York, McGraw-Hill Book Company, 1968.

Blackwood W, Dodds TC, Sommerville JC: *Atlas of Neuropathology.* Second edition. Baltimore, Williams & Wilkins Company, 1964.

Courville CB: *Pathology of the Central Nervous System: A Study Based Upon a Survey of Lesions Found in a Series of Forty Thousand Autopsies.* Third edition. Mountain View, California, Pacific Press Publishing Association, 1950.

Escourolle R, Poirier J: *Manual of Basic Neuropathology.* Second edition. (Translated by LJ Rubinstein.) Philadelphia, WB Saunders Company, 1978.

Lewis AJ: *Mechanisms of Neurological Disease.* Boston, Little, Brown & Company, 1976.

Minckler J (ed): *Pathology of the Nervous System.* 3 Vols. New York, McGraw-Hill Book Company, 1968–1972.

Peters G: *Klinische Neuropathologie: Spezielle Pathologie der Krankheiten des zentralen und peripheren Nervensystems.* Second edition, Stuttgart, Georg Thieme Verlag, 1970.

Tedeschi CG (ed): *Neuropathology: Methods and Diagnosis.* Boston, Little, Brown & Company, 1970.

Zülch KJ: *Brain Tumors: Their Biology and Pathology.* Second edition. (Translated by AB Rothballer, J Olszewski.) New York, Springer Publishing Company, 1965.

Haruo Okazaki, M.D.

Contents

Introduction: General Methodology and Pathologic Cellular Reactions

Methodology in Neuropathology   1
    Gross Examination of the Brain and Spinal Cord   1
    Fixation   1
    Processing of Tissue for Microscopy   1
    Staining of Histologic Sections for Microscopic Examination   1
Neurocellular Reactions to Disease: General Discussion   7
Alterations of Neurons, Axons, and Myelin Sheaths   9
    Alterations of the Neuron   9
    Alterations of the Axon   13
    Alterations of the Myelin Sheath   14
Alterations of Oligodendroglia, Astrocytes, Ependymal Cells, and Choroid
    Plexus   15
    Alterations of Oligodendroglia   15
    Alterations of Astrocytes   16
    Alterations of Ependymal Cells   18
    Alterations of Choroid Plexus   18
Alterations of Microglia, Blood Vessel-Connective Tissue, Leptomeninges,
    and Dura   19
    Alterations of Microglia   19
    Alterations of Blood Vessel-Connective Tissue   20
    Alterations of the Leptomeninges   20
    Alterations of the Dura   23
Alterations of the Pineal Gland   23

1.   Cerebrovascular Disease

Ischemic/Anoxic Conditions of the CNS   25
Arterial Infarction   25
    Causes of Arterial Infarction   25
    Pathomorphology of Cerebral Infarction (Softening, Encephaloma-
        lacia)   30
    Morphologic Evolution   32
    Topographic Features   36
    Natural History of Ischemic Cerebral Vascular Disease   46
Central Nervous System Damage due to Systemic Circulatory Factors (Anoxic
    or Hypoxic Encephalopathy)   51
    Types of Conditions that Lead to Hypoxic Encephalopathy   51
    Morphologic Changes Seen in Hypoxic Encephalopathy   52
    The "Respirator Brain"   55

Hypertensive Vascular Disease of the CNS   55
　Hypertensive Lesions of the Arteries   55
　Effects of Arteriolar (and Arterial) Sclerosis on Brain Parenchyma   57
Malformative Vascular Lesions   62
Noninfectious Vasculitides or Inflammatory Angiitis ("Connective Tissue Disease")   72
Venous Diseases: Vein and Dural Sinus Thrombosis   76
Blood Dyscrasia   79
Cerebral Edema   79
Cerebral Herniations and Their Secondary Vascular Effects   81

2. Traumatic Lesions of the Nervous System

Mechanisms and Types of Cranial Injury   87
Skull Fractures   87
Meningeal Hemorrhage   89
　Epidural or Extradural Hemorrhage   89
　Subdural Hemorrhage   89
　Subarachnoid Hemorrhage   90
Focal Cerebral Parenchymal Damage   93
　Contusions   93
　Lacerations   96
　Hemorrhages   96
　Cerebral Concussion   98
Deep Penetrating Wounds of the Brain   98
　Missile Factors   98
　Traumatic Effects of a Bullet on the Brain   98
Delayed Vascular Complications   99
　Traumatic Cerebral Edema   99
　Rebleeding Following Evacuation of Epidural, Subdural, and Intracerebral Hemorrhage   100
　Development of True or False (or Dissecting) Aneurysm or Thrombotic Occlusion   100
　Fat Embolism   100
Spinal Cord Injuries   100
　Indirect (Closed) Injuries   100
　Direct, Penetrating Injuries   101
　Traumatic Hematomyelia   102
　Subarachnoid Hemorrhage   104
　Subdural and Epidural Hemorrhages   104
Chronic or Subacute Compressive Myelopathies   104
Peripheral Nerve Injuries   105

3. Infectious Disease

Suppurative Bacterial Infections of the Intracranial and Intraspinal Contents   107
　Suppurative Dural Lesions   107
　Suppurative (or Purulent) Leptomeningitis   107
　Brain Abscess   109
　Septic Embolism   111
Tuberculous and Syphilitic Infections and Sarcoidosis   113
　Tuberculous Infection of the Nervous System   113

    Sarcoidosis   118
    Syphilis (Lues) (*Treponema pallidum* Infection)   118
  Fungal Infections   123
  Viral Infections   130
    Dissemination, Morphology, and Histopathology   130
    Principal Forms of CNS Viral Infection   130
      Picorna Viruses   130
      Arboviruses   131
      Myxovirus   132
      Rhabdovirus   134
      Herpes   134
      Suspected Viral Disease in Which the Etiologic Agent has Escaped
        Detection   137
      Transmissible Encephalopathies Suspected of Being Slow Virus Infections
        in Man   137
  Rickettsial Infections   138
  Parasitic Infections   138
    Protozoal Infection   138
    Metazoal infections   140

4. Demyelinating Disease

  Introduction   141
  Myelinoclastic Diseases   141
    Pattern of Disseminated Perivascular Demyelination   141
    Pattern of Irregular Patches of Demyelination
    (Multiple Sclerosis)   143
    Diffuse Continuous Pattern of Demyelination
    (Schilder's Disease)   146
    Combined Patchy and Diffuse Pattern of Demyelination   146
  Dysmyelinating Diseases (Leukodystrophies)   146
    Metachromatic Leukodystrophy   147
    Globoid Cell Leukodystrophy (Krabbe's Disease)   148
    Sudanophilic (Orthochromatic) Leukodystrophies   149
    Leukodystrophy with Rosenthal Fibers (Alexander's Disease)   150
    Spongy Degeneration of the Nervous System (Van Bogaert-Bertrand Dis-
      ease, Formerly Canavan's Spongy Sclerosis)   151

5. Degenerative Diseases

  Senile and Presenile Dementias (with Predominant Cerebral Cortical In-
    volvement)   153
    Simple (Senile or Presenile Cerebral) Atrophy   153
    Alzheimer's Disease (Senile or Presenile Onset)   153
    Pick's Disease or Lobar Atrophy   155
    Creutzfeldt-Jakob Disease   156
    Conditions Other than Primary Neuronal Degeneration Associated with
      Dementia of Presenile and Senile Periods   156
  Conditions with Predominant Involvement of the Extrapyramidal System   158
    Huntington's Chorea   158
    Dystonia Musculorum Deformans   158
    Parkinson's Disease (Paralysis Agitans)   158
    Postencephalitic Parkinsonism   159

Parkinson-Dementia Complex of Guam   **159**
Progressive Supranuclear Palsy (Steele-Richardson-Olszewski Syndrome); Heterogeneous System Degeneration   **159**
Hallervorden-Spatz Disease   **159**
Spinocerebellar Degeneration   **160**
Predominantly Spinal Forms   **162**
Predominantly Cerebellar Forms   **162**
Predominantly Cerebellar and Spinal Forms   **162**
Multiple System Atrophy   **162**
Cerebellar Ataxias Associated with Systemic Metabolic Disorders   **162**
Myoclonus Epilepsy   **162**
Retinal and Optic Degeneration in Association with Heredofamilial Neurologic Disorders   **163**
Pigmentary Retinal Degeneration ("Retinitis Pigmentosa")   **163**
Optic Atrophies   **163**
Conditions with Predominant Involvement of the Motor System (Progressive Nuclear Myelopathies, Nuclear Amyotrophies, or Motor Neuron Disease)   **163**
Amyotrophic Lateral Sclerosis (ALS; Charcot's Disease)   **163**
Infantile Spinal Muscular Atrophy (Werdnig-Hoffmann Disease)   **164**
Peroneal Muscular Atrophy (Charcot-Marie-Tooth Disease)   **165**
Hypertrophic Interstitial Neuritis (or Neuropathy) (Dejerine-Sottas Disease)   **165**

6. Metabolic and Toxic Diseases

Storage Diseases   **167**
Disorders of Lipid Metabolism   **167**
Gangliosidoses   **167**
Cerebrosidoses   **167**
Sulfatidoses   **169**
Sphingolipidoses   **170**
Disorders of Mucopolysaccharide (Glycosaminoglycan) Metabolism   **170**
Disorders of Carbohydrate Metabolism   **171**
Disorders of Amino Acid Metabolism   **172**
Disorders of Metal Metabolism   **172**
Disorders of Pigment Metabolism—Porphyria   **173**
Chronic Alcoholism and Thiamine- and Other Vitamin-Deficiency States   **173**
Nutritional Polyneuropathy   **173**
Wernicke's Encephalopathy   **174**
Korsakoff's Disease   **174**
Alcoholic Cerebral Atrophy   **174**
Alcoholic Cerebellar Degeneration (or Atrophy)   **174**
Marchiafava-Bignami Disease   **174**
Central Pontine Myelinolysis   **174**
Pellagra   **174**
Subacute Combined Degeneration of the Spinal Cord   **174**
Somatic Metabolic Diseases Affecting the Nervous System   **175**
Hepatic Encephalopathy   **175**
Uremia   **176**
Diabetes Mellitus   **177**

Somatic Malignancies   178
Amyloidosis   179
Reye's Syndrome   179
Anoxic Poisons   179
Anesthetics and Hypnotics   179
Carbon Monoxide Poisoning   179
Other Poisons   180
Lead Poisoning   180
Organic Mercury Poisoning   180
Nervous System Damage by Physical Agents: Radiation Necrosis of the CNS   182

7. **Neoplastic and Related Lesions**

General Discussion   183
Intracranial Tumors   183
Spinal Tumors   184
Tumors of Neuroglial Cells (Gliomas)   185
Astrocytomas   185
Oligodendroglioma   196
Ependymoma   196
Papilloma of the Choroid Plexus   200
Colloid Cyst of the Third Ventricle   201
Tumors of Primitive Bipotential Precursors and Nerve Cells   202
Medulloblastoma   202
Ganglioneuroma and Ganglioglioma (Gangliocytoma, Neuroastrocytoma)   206
Other, Rare, Primitive (Embryonal) (and Malignant) Central Neuroectodermal Tumors Occurring in Early Life   206
Tumors of the Pineal Parenchyma   207
Nerve Sheath Tumors   208
Schwannoma (Neurinoma, Neurilemoma)   208
Neurofibroma   208
Malignancy in Nerve Sheath Tumors   214
Tumors of Mesenchymal Tissue   214
Meningioma   214
Xanthomatous Tumors   221
(Capillary) Hemangioblastoma (Capillary Hemangioendothelioma)   221
Sarcomas   221
Tumors of the Lymphoreticular System and Leukemia   225
Hodgkin's Disease   225
Lymphosarcoma (Lymphocytic Lymphoma)   226
Reticulum Cell Sarcoma (Histiocytic Lymphoma, Immunoblastic Sarcoma)   226
Multiple Myeloma   228
Histiocytosis X   228
Leukemia   228
Tumors of Maldevelopmental Origin   229
Primary Intracranial (and Spinal) Germ Cell Neoplasms and Tumors   229
Dermoid and Epidermoid (or Dermoid Cyst and Epidermoid Cyst)   232
Lipoma   234
Neuroepithelial Ectopic Tumors and Hamartomas   234

Phakomatoses   235
  Tuberous Sclerosis (Tuberous Sclerosis Complex; Bourneville's Disease)   235
  Multiple Neurofibromatosis (Recklinghausen's Disease)   237
  Sturge-Weber Disease (Sturge-Weber-Dimitri Disease, Encephalo-Trigeminal or Meningofacial Angiomatosis)   241
  Von Hippel-Lindau Disease   241
  Neurocutaneous Melanoma and Primary Meningeal Melanoma   241
Secondary Neoplasms of the CNS—Direct Extension of Local Tumors Affecting the Cranium and Spine   242
  Pituitary Adenoma   242
  Chemodectoma (Paraganglioma) of the Glomus Jugulare   246
  Chordoma   247
  Carcinoma Arising in the Ear, Mastoid Cavity, and Nasopharynx   247
Metastatic Neoplasms   247
  Metastatic Neoplasms in the Skull, Spine, and Dura Mater   248
  Direct Hematogenous Metastases to the CNS and Its Coverings   250

8. Perinatal Nervous System Damage and Malformations

Congenital Malformation   253
  Disorders of Closure: Dysraphic States   253
    Major Forms of Dysraphism   253
    More Limited Forms of Dysraphism   253
    Aqueductal Malformations   257
    Hydromyelia   259
    Syringomyelia   259
  Disorders of Diverticulation: Failure of Cleavage   261
    Holoprosencephaly (Holotelencephaly)   261
    Chiari (Arnold-Chiari) Malformations   262
    Dandy-Walker Syndrome   264
  Disorders of Migration and Sulcation   264
    Neuronal Heterotopia   265
    Lissencephaly (Agyria)and Pachygyria   265
    Micropolygyria (Synonym, Polymicrogyria)   266
    Cerebellar Microgyria   266
  Disorders of Proliferation (Disorders of Size)   266
    Megalencephaly   266
    Micrencephaly   266
    Restricted Forms of Abnormal Proliferation   268
    Schizencephaly   268
  Disorders of Commissuration   268
  Agenesis of the Corpus Callosum   268
  Agenesis or Hypoplasia of the Septum Pellucidum   268
  Cavum Septi Pellucidi ("Fifth Ventricle")   268
  Other Malformations: Down's Syndrome (21 Trisomy)   270
Perinatal Encephaloclastic Lesions   271
  Anoxic-Ischemic Lesions   271
    Infarct-Like Lesions   271
    Hemorrhagic Lesions   275
  Other Forms of CNS Damage During the Perinatal Period   275
    Focal Circulatory Disorders of the Brain   275

Traumatic Lesions Due to Molding and Other Forceful Cranial Distortion
During Delivery: Subdural Hemorrhage   **275**
Perinatal Infections   **275**
Toxic Metabolic Conditions   **276**
Special Note on Hydrocephalus   **279**

General Reading References   **281**

Index   283

Introduction: General Methodology and Pathologic Cellular Reactions

0.1 METHODOLOGY IN NEUROPATHOLOGY

Diagnosis in neuropathology is based on gross and microscopic study of the nervous tissue. The three consecutive steps that are involved and that are closely interrelated are (1) a morphologic analysis of the lesions, (2) a topographic analysis of the lesions, and (3) a correlation of the findings with the clinical and laboratory data and general autopsy findings. This will permit an etiologic diagnosis to be made in most instances.

A. Gross examination of the brain and spinal cord
1. External

Our autopsy procedures involved in removal of the brain, spinal cord, and peripheral nerves are described in chapter 6 of Ludwig's *Current Methods of Autopsy Practice,* 2nd edition, 1979. These structures should be carefully examined during and immediately after their removal from the body, even though further dissection may be deferred until after adequate fixation.

2. Internal

The specimens may be cut to suitable size, pieces, or slices in the "fresh" (unfixed) state, or they may be left in a fixative for 7 to 10 days or longer before sectioning. However, there is no need to wait for 6 to 7 weeks as suggested by some.

The advantages and disadvantages of each method of dissection are listed in Table 0–1.

B. Fixation

Formalin (40% formaldehyde) in 10 to 20% strength is the most universal fixative, and it permits a wide variety of histologic examinations.

C. Processing of tissue for microscopy

Various ways by which nerve tissue is prepared for microscopic examination are outlined in Figure 0–1, and their advantages and disadvantages are tabulated in Table 0–2.

In the United States, most laboratories use the paraffin method for routine diagnostic study, with very satisfactory results, particularly because this requires no additional instrumentation or training of personnel other than those employed in any pathology laboratory. Minor artifacts inherent to the method constitute no significant problems, either diagnostically or esthetically. The nervous or somatic tissues can be simultaneously processed and examined by the same methods, and histologic changes are easily compared (see the next section on stains). In fact, traditional insistence on the celloidin method by some European neuropathologists has acted as a stumbling block for general pathologists in becoming familiar with neuropathology. The usefulness of the celloidin method is largely confined to topographic demonstration of the extent of lesions and their secondary effects, such as edema, herniations, and so on, or when the tissue shrinkage has to be minimized for a meticulous cell count or precise morphometry.

D. Staining of histologic sections for microscopic examination

Demonstration of various cellular elements that constitute the nervous system may be facilitated by the use of a relatively large number of specialized staining methods, each of which often shows only one structure preferentially. Even with these special stains, complete demonstration of an entire cell structure, such as a neuron and all its branches, in one section is usually not possible.

It must be realized that what any of these staining methods is capable of demonstrating represents, at best, carefully controlled artifacts rather than a picture that is equivalent to the living state of cellular structures ("Equivalentbild"), in suspended animation, as it were, as was once hoped by the insistence on a certain method of tissue processing (e.g., alcohol fixation and Nissl stain).

Furthermore, most of these stains are not entirely specific for the intended structures, and certain degrees of cross staining may occur, either by the fault of the techniques

TABLE 0–1. Advantages and Disadvantages of Unfixed (Fresh) or Fixed Brain Cutting

Fresh Section	*Postfixation Cutting*
Advantages	
• It is possible with this method to determine immediately the nature of changes (grossly or with fresh-frozen sections for microscopy).	• This method permits more precise topographic study of lesions because of the minimal tissue distortion upon dissection.
• This method permits histochemical and chemical studies or microbiologic examinations that are not possible after fixation.	• It is possible to produce the very thin slices necessary in demonstrating small lesions.
• It often permits adequate fixation for electron microscopy, despite a time lapse between death and the processing.	
Disadvantages	
• Subsequent fixation discolors and distorts slices. This makes their surface features irregular, and therefore adequate representation of small lesions on histologic sections is difficult or impossible. This in turn makes a precise topographic analysis difficult.	• This method causes delay in diagnosis. It may be realized later, with chagrin, that certain structures have not been removed which are necessary for a complete understanding of neuropathologic lesions discovered at brain cutting at a later date.
• This method allows already necrotic tissue or blood clot to run out of the tissue.	

themselves or by faulty execution of them. In the final analysis, the judgment of the microscopist, based on his knowledge of the peculiarity of the stains in question and on his familiarity with the normal and abnormal structures to be demonstrated, should prevail.

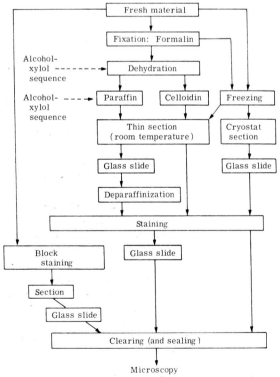

Figure 0–1. Flow sheet illustrating various routine methods of tissue preparation for light microscopy. Paraffin is a wax. Celloidin is a purified form of colloidin or nitrocellulose.

In practice, it is far better to have a few reliable and thoroughly familiar methods at one's disposal than to have a large battery of poorly controlled or unfamiliar methods. This holds true both for laboratory technicians and for pathologists.

Thus, of many methods available, our discussions will be focused on the most frequently employed methods in the routine diagnostic (light microscopic) practice of neuropathology (Fig. 0–2 and Table 0–3).

The same recipe might result in either successful or poor staining, even though it is executed precisely according to the instructions. Apparently such intangible or subtle factors as local water quality, the amount of sunlight, and the like, can markedly influence the results. Therefore, it is imperative that the best method or modifications thereof be found for each laboratory.

1. Overview (or survey) stain

The *hematoxylin and eosin* (H&E) stain is the most practical method, employed in most, if not all, pathologic laboratories, at least in the United States. It is suitable for any tissue virtually without exception, and it is familiar to every student of histology. In the context of neuropathologic practice, it has largely replaced the traditional Nissl methods, which are excellent for demonstration of the Nissl substance of the neuron and nuclei in general but fail to bring out the background neural tissue, cell bodies, or vascular and connective tissues in the manner that the H&E stain is capable of. In many instances, this is the only stain necessary for the establishment of a tissue diagnosis. With the addition of a small quantity of phloxine B to the eosin solution, myelin sheaths, astroglial fibers, and collagen fibers take on different hues of red, and this facilitates separate recognition of these structures more easily than with regular H&E.

TABLE 0–2. Relative Merits of Various Processing Methods

Paraffin Embedding	Celloidin Embedding	Frozen Sections
Advantages		
• Rapid processing is possible. Stained preparations can be made in less than 24 hours.	• This method permits embedding and sectioning of very large pieces, such as entire brain slices.	• The tissue is not processed through fat solvents; thus, staining of lipids and use of other special techniques are permitted which are not possible with embedded material.
• Very thin (3 to 8 µm) in addition to serial sections are possible at the same time.	• It results in relatively little development of shrinkage artifacts, in part because of room-temperature processing.	
• Although standard sections are usually less than 3 by 3 cm in size, considerably larger sections, up to coronal sections of the cerebral hemispheres, are also possible.		• The completed preparation can be examined within a matter of minutes.
Disadvantages		
• Lipids are removed during preliminary treatment with alcohol and xylol and therefore are not demonstrable in the tissue.	• This method usually takes several weeks to complete. Even with the help of an ultrasound vibrator, the procedure takes 10 days for infiltration and an additional 30 days for adequate sectioning.	• Sections are thicker than those obtained by paraffin embedding, and cellular details are difficult to make out.
• Some degree of shrinkage artifact is inevitable because of the need to subject the tissue to moderate heat (ca 50°C) to melt paraffin (which allows it to penetrate into the tissue).	• It is impossible to obtain sections as thin as those achieved by paraffin embedding.	• Larger sections are difficult to obtain because of the lack of support for the tissue.
	• The method removes lipids during preliminary treatment with alcohol and xylol	
	• The material is more expensive, and the personnel time is also costly.	

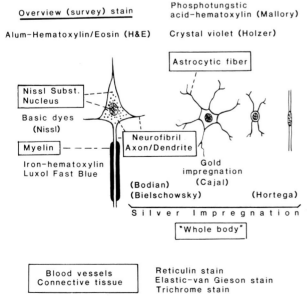

Figure 0–2. Diagrammatic representation of major tissue elements and more commonly used methods for staining them. See text for explanation.

2. Nissl stains (Fig. 0–3 *A*)

Nissl stains were the main methods of traditional neuropathology. As discussed above, they have little merit by themselves. Heavy reliance on these as a routine stain can result in serious diagnostic errors, such as missing ischemic neuronal changes or eosinophilic intranuclear inclusion bodies. One of its variants, cresyl violet, however, is one of the most important reagents as a counterstain for the Luxol Fast Blue method of myelin staining, to be discussed below.

3. Myelin stains (Fig. 0–3 *B*)

Traditional methods employing hematoxylin which stain myelin sheaths deep blue-black have more recently (in the last 2 to 3 decades) given way to *Luxol Fast Blue* (LFB), a copper-containing dye, which stains myelin sheaths a brilliant blue. The dye is usually used in conjunction with *cresyl violet* (CV), a type of Nissl stain dye (see above), as Klüver-Barrera stain (Fig. 0–3 *C*).

Most traditional hematoxylin methods (e.g., Weigert or Spielmeyer) are used for frozen or celloidin sections and are generally not suited for nuclear counterstains (with some exceptions). The once popular Weil method, a paraffin modification, suffers from the same disadvantage.

LFB-CV stain, in contrast, is capable of staining myelin

TABLE 0–3. Some of the Common Staining Reagents Used in Neuropathology*

General overview stain			
Hematoxylin and eosin		Alum-hematoxylin and eosin	

Nissl stains		(Stain)	(Differentiator)‡
		Thionin (P)	Alcohol
		Toluidine blue (P)	Alcohol
		Cresyl violet (P)	Alcohol
		Gallocyanine-chrome alum (P)	

Myelin stains	(Mordant)†	(Stain)	(Differentiator)‡
Weigert (C)	Potassium dichromate	Hematoxylin (H)	Borax ferricyanide
	Cupric acetate	+ ferric chloride	
Pal (C)	K dichromate	H + lithium carbonate	Potassium permanganate
			Sulfite-oxalic acid
Loyez (C)	Iron alum	H + lithium carbonate	Alcohol
			Borax ferricyanide
Spielmeyer (F)	Iron alum	Hematoxylin	Iron alum
Weil (P)		H + iron alum	Borax ferricyanide
Marchi (F)	K dichromate	Osmium tetroxide	
Klüver-Barrera (P)		Luxol Fast Blue	Lithium carbonate
		(Copper phthalocyanin)	Alcohol
		(Cresyl violet counterstain)	

Axon stains	(Metal)	(Reducing agent)	
Bielschowsky (F)	Ammoniacal silver nitrate	Formalin	
Bodian (P)	Protargol	Hydroquinone	
		Sodium sulfite	
Von Braunmühl (F)	Silver nitrate	Formalin	

Glial metallic impregnation methods	(Metal)	(Reducing agent)	
Cajal (F)	Gold chloride sublimate		for astrocytes
Del Rio Hortega (F)	Ammoniacal silver nitrate	Formalin	variants for astrocytes
			oligodendroglia
			microglia

Glial fiber stains	(Mordant)	(Stain)	(Differentiator)
Mallory's phosphotungstic acid-hematoxylin (P)	Mercuric chloride	Phosphotungstic acid-hematoxylin	Alcohol
Holzer (P)	Phosphomolybdic acid	Crystal violet	Aniline oil

* (C) = celloidin embedding; (P) = paraffin embedding; (F) = frozen section.

† Mordant = Substance capable of intensifying the reaction of a specimen to a stain.

‡ Differentiator = Reagent that removes stains from structures not intended for demonstration and leaves only the intended structures strongly bound with the dye used. Acid alcohol in the acid-fast stain for tubercle bacilli is an example.

sheaths, nuclei, and Nissl substance simultaneously. Thus, this stain allows side-by-side demonstration of myelinated fiber tracts and neuronal nuclear groups and, as such, is indispensable for anatomic studies. It is equally adaptable to large celloidin and to routine paraffin sections. The addition of CV to LFB gives a "deep sea blue" hue to myelin sheaths. Other stains, such as silver impregnation for axons, phosphotungstic acid-hematoxylin, and periodic acid-Schiff (see below), have been successfully adapted to LFB stain (Fig. 0–3 D).

Some laboratories use an LFB-H&E combination method routinely for the neural tissues. But in our hands, this lacks the clarity and crispness of LFB-periodic acid-Schiff-hematoxylin.

Marchi stain has been used to demonstrate certain stages of myelin breakdown. Although extensively employed in an-atomic studies for tracing fiber tracts after the placement of lesions in animals, it is of limited use in human diagnostic practice.

4. Neurofibrillary and axon stains

The *Bielschowsky* method and its modifications on frozen sections have been favorites of neuropathologists for many years. Paraffin-adapted methods are also devised with varying ease and success (or rather, difficulty and failure).

Bodian stain (Fig. 0–3 E), a paraffin method with relative simplicity of use and consistency of results, appears to be the favorite of laboratories in the United States, including ours. This stain is not a particularly good stain for demonstration of fine neurofibrillary bundles in the neuronal cell bodies. This is a relatively minor drawback, for these structures rarely provide important diagnostic features in light microscopy except when one is dealing with Alzheimer's

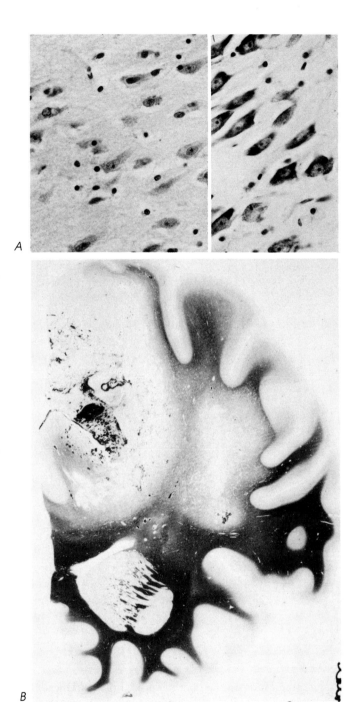

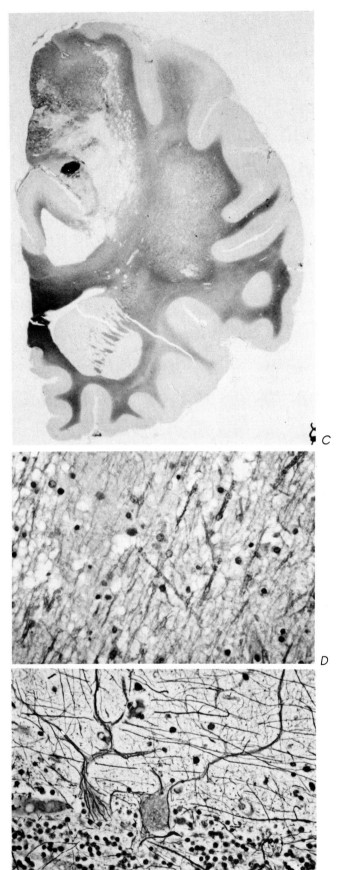

Figure 0–3. Some routine histologic methods. *A*, Nissl stain of pyramidal neurons of the hippocampi, ischemic area on right and uninvolved side on left. Affected neurons show reduced staining of Nissl substance. H&E stain would have shown them more distinctly eosinophilic and therefore more readily discernible. *B*, Right frontal lobe with infiltrating astrocytoma as demonstrated by hematoxylin type of myelin stain (Loyez). The affected areas appear "negatively" as those of "demyelination." Collections of red cells (hemorrhages) appear "positively." *C*, Same area as in *B* stained with LFB/CV (Kluver-Barrera). Concentration of tumor cell nuclei is stained "positively" in purplish by this method. *D*, LFB/PAS/H stain of edematous white matter adjacent to metastatic melanoma. Edema fluid in background is stained pink by this method. Compare this with Figure 1–51 *B* (LFB/CV), which fails to show edema fluid. *E*, Portion of cerebellar cortex stained with axonal stain (Bodian).

neurofibrillary tangles. For these, a relatively simple frozen-section method such as the *von Braunmühl* stain is preferred, with which only abnormal tangles are demonstrable against the pale background. With the other methods described above, staining of the normal neurofibrillary and axonal structures interferes with easy recognition of the target abnormalities (see section 5.1).

5. Stains for astrocytes (Fig. 0–4)

One or more of the following stains should be available for use. Since astrocytes are easily recognized as such by H&E stain, in both their normal and abnormal states, the application of these methods is largely for didactic purposes or for more graphic or colorful demonstration.

Problems often arise, however, when excessive fibrous gliosis has to be differentiated from similarly exuberant proliferation of collagen fibers. This applies both to scar tissue and to neoplastic tissue.

a. *Mallory's phosphotungstic acid-hematoxylin* (PTAH) stain

The PTAH stain is widely used in general pathology, mainly for differentiating muscle fibers (blue) from collagen fibers (brown). It stains astroglial fibers (and cell bodies when these are not overly swollen) blue against brown-stained collagen fibers. Other connective tissue stains or reticulin stains (see below) are similarly useful in this situation. Being a hematoxylin method, PTAH

stain also brings out myelin sheaths. Although in some ways this is a definite disadvantage, it may be a blessing in disguise. This is particularly true with peripheral nerves, which contain enough collagen connective tissue to present a bothersome problem when LFB-CV is applied. Here connective tissue may not be sufficiently differentiated in color from myelin sheaths. PTAH, on the other hand, will allow clear differentiation of myelin sheaths (blue) from collagen fibers (brown), and any quantitative imbalance between those two elements is more readily appreciated than with LFB-CV.

b. *Holzer* stain

This stain is designed for preferential staining of delicately fibrous astrocytic processes against a relatively clear background. As such, it is excellent for macroscopic (topographic) demonstration of subtle gliosis on a large slide. Unfortunately, collagen connective tissue, blood vessels, and even myelin sheaths can be stained by this method, and precipitates are often bothersome. In contrast to PTAH stain, this method offers little in microscopy.

c. *Cajal's gold sublimate* (CGS) method

As with all other so-called metallic impregnation methods for frozen sections, the CGS method tends to be capricious and to give inconsistent results. Although it can give an exquisite picture of hypertrophied astro-

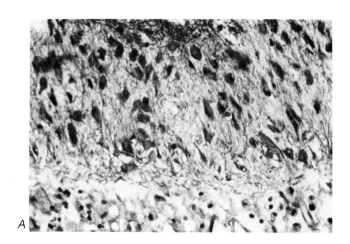

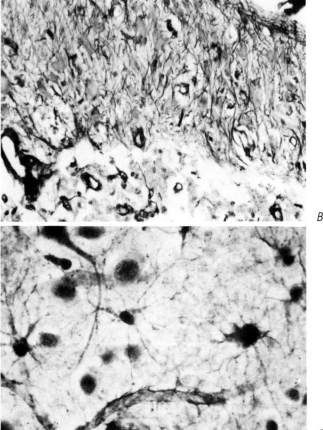

Figure 0–4. Variety of stains for astrocytes and their processes. *A,* Mallory's PTAH. *B,* Holzer. *C,* Cajal's gold sublimate.

cytes "in entirety," the main value of CGS appears to lie in esthetics rather than practicality. Identification of the astrocytic nature of a cell and of fiber proliferation is accomplished more readily by other methods.

6. Silver impregnation methods for other glial elements

Numerous modifications of the *Del Rio Hortega* method are available for astrocytes, oligodendroglial cells, and microglial cells. Because of their technical cumbersomeness, the inconsistency of results, and the relatively little need, in day-to-day practice, to stain these elements preferentially, these methods are rarely required.

7. Connective tissue stains

Normally, only a small amount of connective tissue is present in the central nervous system. Under certain circumstances, however, there is excessive growth of reticulin or collagen fibers, often with an admixture of astrocytic proliferation. In such instances, some of the connective tissue stains routinely used in general pathology are helpful. One of these, namely the PTAH stain, has already been discussed under stains for astrocytes. *Trichrome* stains are the second choice. The *Masson* method stains astrocytic fibers (and muscles and myelin sheaths) reddish brown and collagen bluish green, whereas *Heidenhain's* modification stains the former red and the latter blue.

8. Reticulin stains

Reticulin stains, such as *Wilder's* and *Gomori's,* are extremely useful in tumor pathology. Differentiation of carcinomas from sarcomas is often based on this stain in general pathology. In neuropathology, it is used primarily to differentiate glial tissue from the connective tissue, be it reactive or neoplastic. Examples are given in the chapter dealing with neoplasia (Chapter 7). A reticulin stain also preferentially demonstrates increased vascularity, particularly of capillaries, because of its ability to stain the basement membrane of capillaries.

9. Vascular stain

Connective tissue stains in general are useful in demonstrating arteries and veins differentially, as is necessary in cases of vascular malformation. However, *elastic-van Gieson* (EvG, or VvG for Verhoeff-van Gieson) is the best stain for this task because of its clear staining of the internal elastic lamina of arteries. It is also of great help in assessing the degree and extent of arterial lesions such as atherosclerosis or arteritides. For demonstration of capillaries, however, a reticulin stain or periodic acid-Schiff stain is more helpful.

10. Other important stains in neuropathology
    a. Fat stains

    Because "fat" is not a normal constituent of the nervous tissue (except for perineural fat tissue of the peripheral nervous system), any stainable fat may be considered abnormal. It usually occurs in the cytoplasm of macrophages as a result of digestion and degradation of lipid material liberated by tissue necrosis, as in an infarct. *Sudan IV* and *Oil Red O* are among the more commonly employed dyes. The materials that stain a brilliant red with these stains are triglycerides and cholesterol esters, so-called neural fat. These are soluble in

alcohol and xylol, and therefore frozen sections are a prerequisite in order to avoid subjecting the tissue to these soluents (see section 0.1, C). Counterstaining with hematoxylin brings out nuclei and myelin sheaths. In fact, one of the hematoxylin myelin stains, Spielmeyer's, for example, can be combined with a fat stain.
    b. *Periodic acid-Schiff* (PAS)

    The commonly used PAS stain has a long history in histochemistry. It depends on the oxidation of 1,2 glycol groups (CHOH-CHOH) by periodic acid. The resultant dialdehydes react with Schiff reagent (fuchsin sulfurous acid) to produce a reddish purple stain. A number of compounds, including glycogen, mucopolysaccharides, mucoproteins and glycoproteins, glycolipids, and some unsaturated lipids and phospholipids, are stained with this reaction. Hematoxylin is the usual nuclear counterstain (PAS-H). This stain demonstrates certain stages of lipid breakdown products in macrophages even in paraffin section (after treatment with alcohol and xylol), and so it is conveniently and nearly routinely used for the nervous system as LFB-PAS-H stain (Fig. 0–3 *D*). Lipofuscin, capillary walls, amyloid (as in senile plaques), and edema fluid are among the tissues stained by this method in the nervous system. Because only peripheral myelin sheaths are stained by PAS, LFB-PAS serves to differentiate these from central myelin sheaths.

In summary, for routine diagnostic studies, a complete technical control of the following "special" stains and a thorough familiarity with various tinctorial features of the normal structures and abnormal products should make a student of neuropathology quite competent in most situations:

> LFB-CV or LFB-PAS-H
> Bodian stain
> PTAH or trichrome; reticulin
> Fat stain

Naturally, bacterial or fungal stains are essential when an infection is suspected, although only microbiologic investigations can provide a definitive answer (when positive under suitable conditions). With the steady increase in the number of aged persons coming to autopsy, the von Braunmühl and thioflavin S (to be viewed with ultraviolet light) stains are additional, relatively simple methods for identifying senile plaques, Alzheimer's neurofibrillary tangles, and cerebral amyloid angiopathy prevalent in the aged (see section 5.1).

0.2 NEUROCELLULAR REACTIONS TO DISEASE: GENERAL DISCUSSION

In some instances, a noxious condition that affects the nervous tissue results in biochemical and subsequent morphologic alterations, primarily in one of its constituents. However, because of their close functional and structural interdependence, a series of changes will almost invariably follow in other elements. In many other instances, a number of constituent cells are simultaneously affected by a single noxious condition, although individual modes of reaction may differ from one cell type to another. Therefore, it is probable that no pathologic process limits itself to a single cellular element, and the pathology of nervous diseases should be studied in terms of constellations of cellular reactions.

Many of these individual alterations are not diagnostic by themselves. However, constellations of cellular reactions considered in their totality will often permit etiologic diagnoses to be made.

For didactic purposes, however, it is convenient at first to evaluate separately the changes demonstrable in neurons, glia, and the connective tissue and vascular structures. Table 0–4 summarizes the limitedness or richness of histopathologic alterations (or expressions) of these elements. For convenience, the reaction types are categorized into two groups: regressive/degenerative and progressive/hypertrophic-hyperplastic. The former type is envisioned as the expressions of deteriorating ("diseased") conditions of the cells concerned, which may lead to their death, and the latter as those of defensive, constructive, or reparative ("healthy") efforts on the part of cells that have escaped the damage. This latter type is sometimes referred to simply as "reactive," although the former is also reactive to adverse conditions. Although this distinction can apply to many alterations that we encounter, it must be realized that some changes are difficult to fit into either of these categories, because of the limitations in our understanding of their basic nature. Table 0–4 summarizes these differences in cellular response.

It is apparent from the table that *neurons*, being probably the most easily damaged nerve elements, are diverse in their morphologic expressions of diseased states, but for all practical purposes they show no capacity to regenerate or to constitute reparative processes after the damage has been done. Many neuronal alterations, however, are nonspecific etiologically.

Oligodendroglial cells, ependymal cells, and epithelial cells of the choroid plexus are also damaged relatively easily but show few distinctive features to give clues as to etiologic factors involved. Their regenerative or hypertrophic capacities can be considered nil or of little significance.

Astrocytes appear to be more resistant to various noxious stimuli, and when they degenerate or die, few distinctive features are displayed. Astrocytes are most prominent in their reparative, reconstructive activities, which are manifested mainly by their increase in size and number in response to damage to other elements. Blood vessels and connective tissue cells also participate in the reparative process as seen elsewhere in the body, and their reactions can be quite exuberant. However, such reactions are seen in a relatively limited number of pathologic processes within the central nervous system. Microglial cells take part in inflammatory reactions and phagocytosis along with hematogenous cells. No distinctive features are noted in their regressive phase.

As useful as these morphologic alterations are in the diagnosis of nervous system disorders, students of neuro-

TABLE 0–4. Patterns of Cellular Response to Injuries Within the Central Nervous System

Cell Types	Types of Reaction		
	Regressive/Degenerative	Progressive/Hypertrophic-Hyperplastic (excluding neoplasia)	
Functional			
Neuron	Many specific and nonspecific alterations	None	
Interstitial ("Glia")			
Oligodendroglia (Schwann cell)	Limited	None (limited)	
Astrocyte	Limited	Scar formation (astrocytosis)	Neoplasia
Ependymal cell			
Epithelial cell of choroid plexus	Limited	None	
Microglia*	Limited	Inflammatory reactions, phagocytosis	
Mesodermal (mesenchymal) connective tissue			
Hematogenous cells (leukocytes)		Inflammatory reactions, phagocytosis	
Blood vessel and connective tissue	Limited (edema)	Scar formation (limited)	

*Microglia also have mesodermal features.

pathology must be aware of numerous artifacts and regional peculiarities of cellular morphology, which often lead to unwarranted diagnoses.

In general, any pathologic process that is manifested only by changes in nerve cells, their axons, or their myelin sheaths, unattended by any alterations of other elements, should be viewed with suspicion. Exceptions include rapidly fatal processes and extremely chronic disease accompanied only by a minimal, poorly cellular gliosis.

On the other hand, many fatal conditions that affect the nervous system are without clear-cut morphologic changes, particularly if they are acute in nature. Needs for various techniques from other disciplines such as toxicology, microbiology, and so on, must always be kept in mind in trying to establish a neuropathologic diagnosis. Accurate diagnoses can be expected only when one is fully aware of the limitations of the conventional methods described in this review.

More detailed accounts of pathologic alterations of these individual cell components and tissues of the nervous system will be given in the following sections. Some of these changes are clearly in reaction to more or less well-defined noxious stimuli—e.g., trauma, invasion of microorganisms—whereas others betray no etiologic factors. Some are due to subtle metabolic abnormalities of intrinsic or extrinsic origin. So-called physiologic changes of aging may be included in this group.

0.3 ALTERATIONS OF NEURONS, AXONS, AND MYELIN SHEATHS

A. Alterations of the neuron

As stated earlier, neurons are rich in morphologic expressions of their diseased states in comparison with other elements. However, relatively few of these expressions are diagnostic by themselves. Some of the more important or commonly encountered ones are listed below.

General Categories (Fig. 0–5)	Individual Types
1. Reactions to axonal damage (chromatolytic changes)	a. Central chromatolysis
	b. Peripheral chromatolysis
2. Acute necrosis	a. Ischemic nerve cell change
	b. Liquefaction or severe cell change
	c. "Acute swelling"
	d. Conglutination
3. Atrophic changes	a. Cell sclerosis; simple atrophy
	b. Retrograde degeneration
	c. Transsynaptic degeneration
4. Destruction and disappearance of neurons	a. Neuronal loss ("dropping out")
5. Abnormal accumulations (Fig. 0–6)	a. Lipofuscin excess
	b. Alzheimer's neurofibrillary degeneration
	c. Pick's argentophilic inclusion and ballooned cell
	d. Simchowicz's granular vacuolar degeneration
	e. Eosinophilic rodlike structure
	f. Intracytoplasmic hyalin body
	g. Bunina body
	h. Lewy body
	i. Marinesco body
	j. Lafora's amyloid inclusion
	k. Abnormal accumulation of "storage diseases"
	l. Inclusion bodies (cytoplasmic and/or nuclear) of viral diseases
6. Deposition of extraneous pigment	a. Hematin pigment
	b. Ferrugination or iron incrustation
7. Hypertrophic changes	a. Bi- or multi-nucleated neuron
	b. Monster neuron

The following explanations and comments pertain to individual neuronal alterations.

1.a. Central chromatolysis (= primary irritation, axonal reaction)

Best seen in large lower motor neurons whose axons have been severed distally, central chromatolysis represents a reaction whereby the cell attempts to restore the integrity of its axons. Once the axon regenerates, the cell body resumes its normal appearance.

Evidence of the restorative process includes prominence of the nucleolus, basophilic rim around the nuclear membrane (increased nucleoprotein synthesis), and appearance of definite Nissl bodies that migrate to the periphery of the cell.

Note: 1. When the axon is damaged too proximally, the neurons may degenerate completely.

2. The upper motor neuron with its axon severed, instead of showing central chromatolysis, may undergo atrophy and then degenerate (Gudden's simple atrophy) or survive (often presumably because of surviving axonal branches present proximal to the lesions).

3. Indistinguishable changes may be present in cortical neurons in cases of pellagra (without known axonal damages).

4. Balloon cells of Pick's disease also resemble this change, but their pathogenesis and significance have not been determined.

1.b. Peripheral chromatolysis

This change is rare and its significance is unclear. It

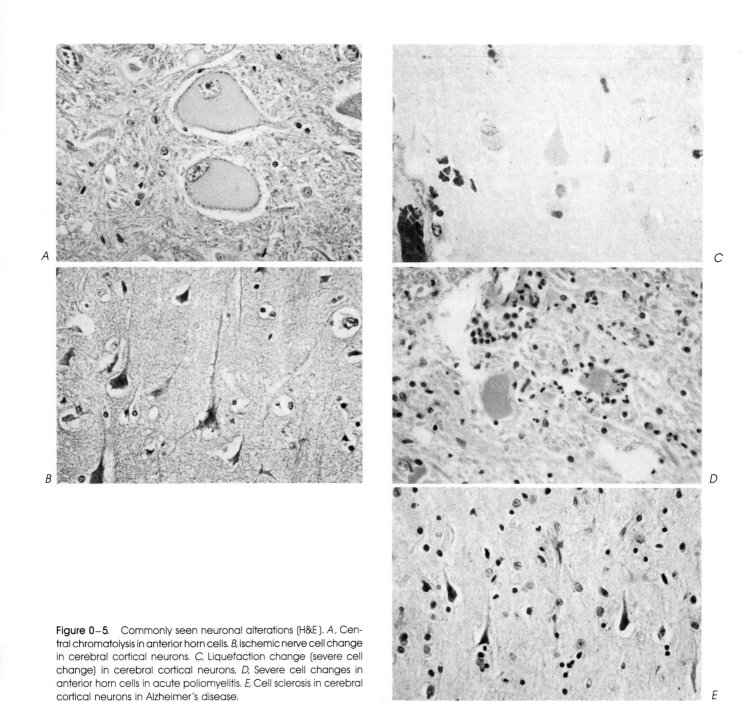

Figure 0–5. Commonly seen neuronal alterations (H&E). *A,* Central chromatolysis in anterior horn cells. *B,* Ischemic nerve cell change in cerebral cortical neurons. *C,* Liquefaction change (severe cell change) in cerebral cortical neurons. *D,* Severe cell changes in anterior horn cells in acute poliomyelitis. *E,* Cell sclerosis in cerebral cortical neurons in Alzheimer's disease.

Figure 0–6. Various neuronal changes characterized by abnormal intracytoplasmic structures. *A,* Lipochrome (lipofuscin) excess in thalamic neurons (H&E). *B,* Pigmentary atrophy in cerebral cortical neurons in Alzheimer's disease (H&E). *C,* Alzheimer's neurofibrillary tangles in cerebral cortical neurons (von Braunmühl). *D,* Pick's argentophilic inclusions in pyramidal neurons of the hippo-campus (Bodian). *E,* Pick's "ballooned" (globose) cells in cerebral cortical neurons (H&E). *F,* Simchowicz's granulovascular degeneration in pyramidal neurons of the hippocampus (H&E). *G,* Lewy bodies in pigmented neurons of the substantia nigra (H&E). *H,* Lafora bodies in cerebral cortical neurons (CV).

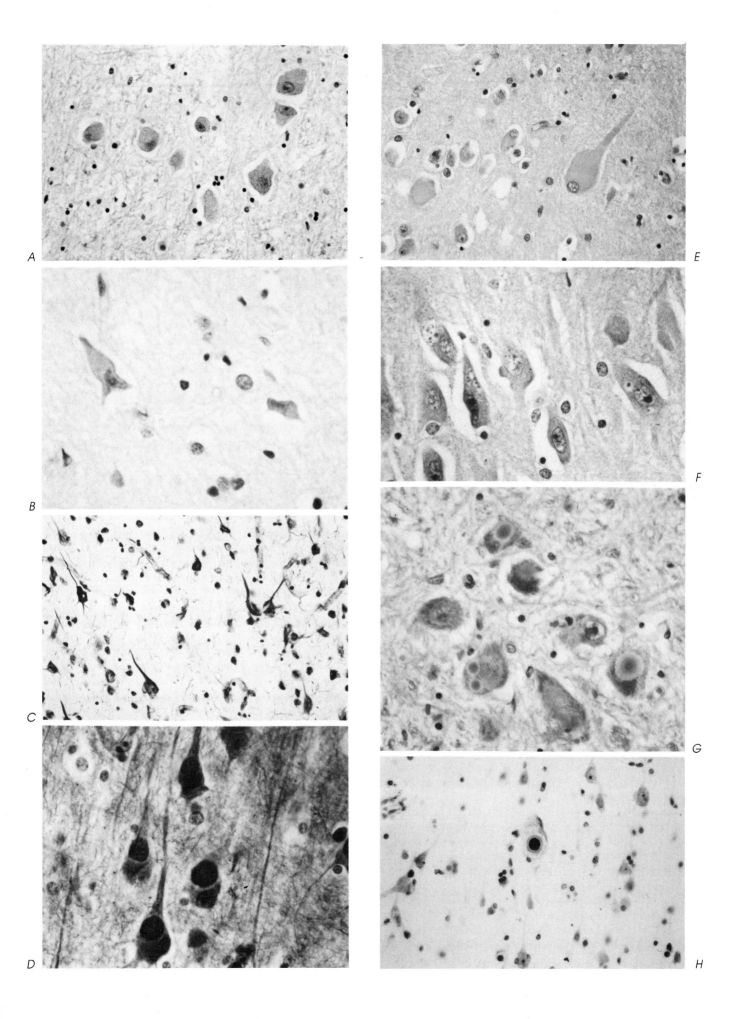

A

B

C

D

E

F

G

H

is said to represent a late stage of recovery from central chromatolysis.

2.a. Ischemic nerve cell change (= coagulation cell change, eosinophilic degeneration)

This change is seen in acute ischemic/anoxic tissue damage or in hypoglycemia. As such, it is probably the commonest neuronal change encountered in routine autopsies. It is followed by a pale-staining, ghost-like appearance and then eventually by dissolution of the cell. Occasionally, dying neurons are attended by neuronophagia if phagocytic elements escape injury. A condition described as homogenizing disorder (Spielmeyer) of Purkinje cells is probably the same process. At the edge of an acute cerebral infarct containing eosinophilic degenerating neurons, dark and shrunken neurons are often encountered. These appear to represent a milder or earlier change of the condition under discussion (see 3.a. below).

2.b. Liquefaction or severe cell change

This is a less specific change and has been described in classic terms as being at the margin of any destructive lesion of the cortex and within the area undergoing degenerative changes. In part, it corresponds to the irreversible phase of the ischemic/anoxic change described above. Ghost cells also appear in other severe nervous injuries, including poliomyelitis and severe contusion. Rapid destruction and resolution of the affected cell will follow.

2.c. Acute cell disease ("acute swelling")

This was described by classic authors as a mild or early change leading to the change described above (liquefaction). Today, it is regarded as being largely related to preagonal or terminal events or as autolytic change (artifact). No pathognomonic significance is to be attached.

2.d. Conglutination

This is the description given to the appearance of melting away of cells, as typically seen in granular cells of the cerebellar cortex. Today, this change is considered to be due largely to postmortem autolysis.

3.a. Cell sclerosis (chronic cell disease); simple atrophy

This change is regarded as evidence of physiologic or premature aging or dying of neurons due to subtle enzymatic failure. The cell eventually disappears without a trace. Neurons undergoing this type of change are often seen at the edge of an acute infarct, and this is regarded as an early and transient phase of ischemic degeneration (see 2.a. above).

Similar change is seen in Creutzfeldt-Jakob disease, a presumed slow viral infection. This fact makes it evident that caution is required in interpreting this sclerotic type of neuronal alteration.

Another very similar change is often seen in small biopsy specimens; it is thought to be due to mechanical artifact (spiky cell artifact). Identical changes are seen at postmortem due to handling of the brain before fixation; they can be prevented by perfusion fixation (with sufficient passage of time) before the brain is handled.

3.b. Retrograde degeneration

A change similar to that just described is characteristically seen in central nervous system (CNS) neurons (except lower motor neurons) and is the equivalent of the central chromatolysis described above. Examples are best noted in the thalamic nuclei and the lateral geniculate nucleus.

3.c. Transsynaptic degeneration

This change again is similar to "cell sclerosis" and is best seen in the lateral geniculate body (from optic nerve lesions) and inferior olive (from pontinetegmental tract lesions). In the latter, it is often associated with cytoplasmic vacuolation and hypertrophic appearance of neurons in the inferior olive. Elsewhere, the significance of vacuolar change is doubtful.

4.a. Neuronal loss ("dropping out")

This change may be preceded by any of the above-described acute and chronic alterations and is often attended by changes in other cellular elements. In acute processes, reaction of other elements is either "regressive" or "progressive," depending on the nature and severity of the insult. In slowly progressive conditions, a mild loss (even up to an estimated 30%) of neurons may be very difficult to detect by neuronal or overview staining alone. Its presence is suspected or assumed by demonstration of fibrous astrocytosis (gliosis) with appropriate glial stains (e.g., Cajal or Holzer).

5.a. Lipofuscin (lipochrome) excess

No clear line of demarcation can be drawn between normal (or physiologic) and abnormal amounts of lipofuscin, for lipofuscin content increases with age, apparently at a rate that varies from individual to individual. When pathologic, it is often associated with cell sclerosis. The combination of these two features is called "pigmentary atrophy." Some neurons are physiologically rich in lipofuscin (they are lipophilic), for example the thalamus, lateral geniculate body, and dentate nucleus. Others are poor even in the face of increase elsewhere (lipophobic), for example the Purkinje cells.

5.b. Alzheimer's neurofibrillary degeneration

This change is manifested by thick "argentophilic" tangles of various configurations in the cytoplasm which appear to persist in the tissue even after death of affected neurons. Earlier, it was thought to represent abnormal increase and coalescence of neurofibrils (which themselves proved to be a fixation artifact probably derived from microtubules and neurofilaments)—hence the term "neurofibrillary degeneration." These have been found to be composed of abnormal double helical structures (after they were briefly believed to be "twisted tubules"). Identical material is seen in focally swollen axons and dendrites, which contribute to the formation of senile plaques (see section 5.1). Contrary to the previously held view, they are probably not simply a consequence of physiologic aging, for they are seen in other conditions.

Major disorders that are characterized by the presence of Alzheimer's neurofibrillary tangles include the following:

- Alzheimer's disease (section 5.1)
- Progressive supranuclear palsy (heterogeneous system degeneration, Steele-Richardson-Olszewski syndrome) (section 5.2)
- Parkinsonism-dementia complex of Guam (section 5.2)
- Postencephalitic parkinsonism (section 5.2)

• Subacute sclerosing panencephalitis (protracted cases) (section 3.4)

5.c. Pick's argentophilic inclusion and ballooned cell

Spherical intracytoplasmic inclusion bodies with a strong affinity for silver impregnation (argentophilic inclusions) are the hallmark of a rare "degenerative" condition called Pick's disease or lobar atrophy (see section 5.1). These bodies, however, are often confined to the hippocampal region and are missing in many cases. Ultrastructurally, these bodies are composed of many neurofilaments (10 nm in diameter) and a few neurotubules (240 nm in diameter). Vesicles and complex lipid bodies are also prominent in them.

Neurons with pale swollen cytoplasm (by H&E or Nissl stains) with a peripherally displaced nucleus (ballooned, globose, or Pick cells) are more widespread in the affected cortex and at times in the basal ganglia and substantia nigra of this disease. These neurons, which resemble those showing central chromatolysis, contain less intensely argentophilic mass in the cytoplasm. Ultrastructurally, neurotubules outnumber neurofilaments, and vesicles and lipid bodies are sparse in contrast to the argentophilic inclusions described above.

5.d. Simchowicz's granular vacuolar degeneration

This change is also almost restricted to pyramidal neurons of the hippocampus and is often seen in association with Alzheimer's tangles in an older age group.

5.e. Eosinophilic rodlike structure (Hirano body)

This short, rod-shaped eosinophilic material often appears free in the tissue but is seen electron microscopically within the processes or at times in the cytoplasm of neurons. It is seen exclusively in Sommer's sector of the hippocampus in senility, Alzheimer's and Pick's diseases, dementia-parkinsonism complex of Guam, and other conditions and has no diagnostic significance.

5.f. Intracytoplasmic hyalin (colloid) body

This material is found in large motor neurons such as in the dorsal vagal nuclei and anterior horns of elderly persons. No pathognomonic significance is attached.

5.g. Bunina body

This minute (1 to 2 μm) eosinophilic intracytoplasmic inclusion, often seen in multiplicity, is reported in anterior horn cells in amyotrophic lateral sclerosis. Its significance is unknown.

5.h. Lewy body or eosinophilic intracytoplasmic inclusion

These are single or multiple round acidophilic intracytoplasmic bodies surrounded by a paler zone, some with concentric configuration with a deeper-staining center, which are found primarily in the pigment brainstem nuclei, particularly in the substantia nigra, at times in multiplicity. They are most numerous in Parkinson's disease but are also seen in small numbers in normal older persons.

5.i. Marinesco body

This paranucleolar amphophilic body, which is usually single, is found in the substantia nigra mainly and appears to increase with age. It is of unknown significance.

5.j. Lafora's amyloid inclusion

These concentric, rounded intracytoplasmic inclusions, a few to 30 μm in size, give staining reactions that are similar to those of corpora amylacea. They are widespread in myoclonic epilepsy.

5.k. Storage disease

This change is discussed in Chapter 6.

5.l. Inclusion bodies of viral diseases

These are discussed in Chapter 3 (see section 3.4).

6.a. Hematin pigment

These black to dark-brown pigment granules, derived from hemoglobin but negative for iron stain (unless treated with a strong acid), are found in the cytoplasm of neurons, for example in hemorrhagic areas. Neurons that contain this pigment are not necessarily degenerating. The presence of these granules suggests phagocytic activity of the neuron. However, the circumstances make it appear more like a case of "forced feeding."

6.b. Ferrugination or iron incrustation

This change represents heavy deposition of basophilic granules (positive for Prussian blue and therefore largely composed of iron) in the cytoplasm of apparently dead neurons (mostly as a result of ischemia). This phenomenon is found occasionally at the margins of old vascular lesions or contusions under exceptional and poorly understood conditions, either by precipitation of an iron salt from ferritin of the blood or from diffusion of iron from an adjacent hemorrhage.

7.a. Bi- or multi-nucleated neuron

Two or more nuclei can be seen in a single cell body that shows no evidence of impending cell division. These neurons are found in many CNS disorders of childhood, especially those of congenital origin (e.g., idiocy, megalencephaly, tuberous sclerosis, Werdnig-Hoffmann disease). They are also seen in some acquired diseases, such as infections (general paresis, meningovascular syphilis, postencephalitic parkinsonism) and trauma (at the edge of cerebral wounds, several days to years after injury).

7.b. Monster neuron

This change is characterized by abnormally large overall size, with numerous thick processes but otherwise normal appearance. Other neurons are distorted, vacuolated, or fenestrated and may be bi- or multinucleated. They are seen in tuberous sclerosis as an expression of a genetically determined hamartomatous process (phakomatosis).

B. Alterations of the axon (Fig. 0–7)

Although both CNS and peripheral nervous system axons undergo common, relatively limited forms of degeneration and breakdown, the presence of Schwann cells in the peripheral nerves is largely responsible for the differences that exist between the behaviors of these two systems.

1. Wallerian degeneration

The prototype of this alteration was produced by Waller (1850) by sectioning peripheral nerves of frogs. Both the axons and the myelin sheaths distal to the cut become fragmented and eventually disappear. The same change proceeds proximally for a short distance. The debris is removed by macrophages. This pattern of breakdown is seen in many other peripheral nerve lesions of diverse etiologies—vascular, inflammatory, toxic-metabolic, and so on. Death of the

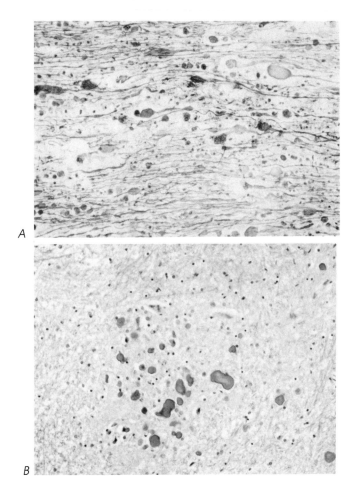

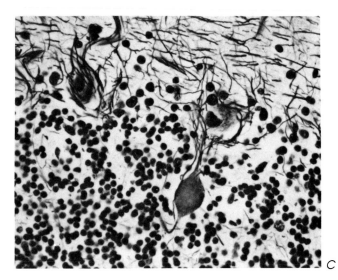

Figure 0–7. *A*, Wallerian degeneration in the thoracic spinal cord distal to traumatic injury (Bodian). *B*, Neuroaxonal dystrophy in the nucleus cuneatus of an elderly person (H&E). *C*, Torpedo formation of Purkinje cells of the cerebellar cortex (Bodian).

nerve cell body is also followed by Wallerian degeneration of its nerve fibers. Collectively, this type of alteration is known as axonal neuropathy, in contrast to another form of nerve fiber degeneration, i.e., segmental. During the recovery phase, vigorous sprouting at the proximal axonal stumps takes place. If there is good approximation, the sprouts will quickly make contact with the distal segment. Schwann cells in the distal segment proliferate to form a long cylindric aggregate, along which the newly formed axons grow. Subsequent remyelination of these axons completes the restoration of the damage.

In the CNS, simultaneous swelling, fragmentation, and eventual disintegration of axons and myelin sheaths occur in focal lesions of diverse etiologies in addition to mechanical transection of the tissue. The secondary distal degenerative change in the original sense of Wallerian degeneration is considerably slower than that in the peripheral nervous system. Attempts at regrowth of severed axons are negligible in practical terms.

2. Simple neuronal atrophy

Atrophic processes involving the nerve cell body result in slow, progressive atrophy, beaded appearance, and eventual disintegration, starting at its most distal portion and progressing toward the cell body (the "dying back" phenomenon).

3. Neuroaxonal dystrophy

This change is characterized by a series of pronounced focal enlargements and eventual fragmentation of the axon into eosinophilic homogeneous rounded bodies, beginning at the distal portion and proceeding proximally.

Changes are seen in the nucleus gracilis and cuneatus of the lower medulla in old age and vitamin E deficiency and in more widespread areas in a rare condition called "infantile neuroaxonal dystrophy." In another rare condition, Hallervorden-Spatz disease, dystrophic axons are found in basal ganglia and midbrain regions in association with iron-rich pigment granules.

4. Special form: Torpedo formation

This is a fusiform swelling in the proximal portion—of the axon before the origin of the collateral branches—of the Purkinje cell of the cerebellum in some chronic degenerative diseases.

C. **Alterations of the myelin sheath (Fig. 0–8)**

The breakdown of the myelin sheath is a prominent and

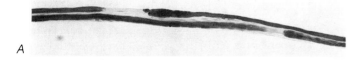

Figure 0–8. *A,* Segmental demyelination in teased peripheral nerve fibers (osmium tetroxide). *B,* Onion-bulb hypertrophy of Schwann cells in peripheral nerve. (*A* and *B, Plastic-embedded section with phase-contrast microscopy, courtesy of Dr. Peter Dyck.*)

easily recognized pathologic change in a wide range of disease processes.

1. Myelin breakdown secondary to other factors
    a. Destructive lesions resulting in death of both neuronal and glial elements, in which myelin sheaths simply share in the process of dissolution of the destroyed tissue (e.g., infarcts)
    b. Conditions that result in loss of axons, leading to loss of corresponding myelin sheaths (e.g., Wallerian degeneration)
2. Primary demyelination with little or no primary neuronal or axonal change and no loss of tissue continuity
    a. Primary involvement of myelin sheaths (presumably of the oligodendroglia or Schwann cells), with segmental demyelination. This change is more readily and more extensively studied in the peripheral nervous system. Breakdown of myelin sheaths (demyelination) occurs in one or more internodal segments in a variable, irregular fashion (best demonstrated in "teased fiber preparations"). After removal of the debris by macrophages, remyelination takes place. Multiplication of the Schwann cells at the involved internodal segment results in short internodal segments replacing it. Peripheral nerve lesions in diabetes mellitus, uremia, diphtheria, and Guillain-Barré syndrome are representative examples. In the CNS, chronic cerebral edema and carbon monoxide poisoning are thought to be characterized by this type of lesion.
    b. Primary demyelinative disease of unknown or known cause. Probably one or more components of the myelin sheath are selectively and specifically destroyed (e.g., in multiple sclerosis, acute disseminated leukoencephalopathy).
    c. A group of inherited diseases known or suspected to be due to inborn errors of metabolism—that is, defective myelin formation and, in some cases, breakdown of previously formed myelin.

In all categories, one sees a similar pattern of myelin breakdown in both the CNS and the peripheral nervous system: the sequence of change is separation and folding of the lamellae, arrangement in irregular and abnormal configuration, loss of structural integrity, coalescence of lipoprotein material to form numerous small or large globules, uptake and digestion by macrophages (CNS and peripheral nervous system) and Schwann cells (peripheral nervous system) down to neutral fat and cholesterol ester. The end results of demyelination can be summarized as follows: in the CNS, disappearance of oligodendroglia and proliferation of astrocytes (astrocytosis), with little or no remyelination; in the peripheral nervous system, Schwann cell proliferation and endoneural fibrosis.

Onion-bulb hypertrophy of the Schwann cells is a special form of end result. This represents the terminal phase of various peripheral neuropathies in which repetitive demyelination and remyelination have taken place. Multiple layers of Schwann cells are seen about nerve fibers. Previously this was regarded as specific for Dejerine-Sottas disease (familial interstitial hypertrophic neuropathy) and for certain hereditary metabolic neuropathies such as Refsum's disease, but it is now known to occur in various other chronic demyelinating neuropathies.

0.4 ALTERATIONS OF OLIGODENDROGLIA, ASTROCYTES, EPENDYMAL CELLS, AND CHOROID PLEXUS

A. Alterations of oligodendroglia (Fig. 0–9)
Most of the oligodendroglial changes noted in human pathology are of doubtful significance.

Degenerative Changes	*Reactive Changes*
1. Acute swelling (hydropic change) of the cytoplasm. This change develops so readily as an autolytic change that it is not a	1. Hypertrophy and proliferation is described in mild ischemia in animal experiments.
	2. Some believe that oli-

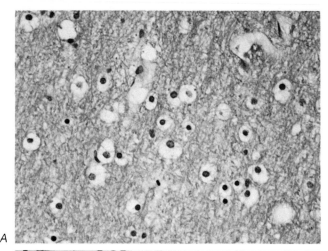

A

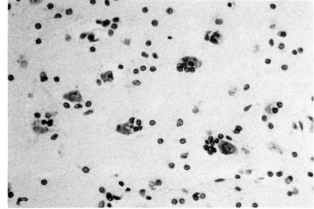

B

Figure 0–9. *A,* "Acute swelling" of oligodendroglia in cerebral white matter (H&E). *B,* Oligodendroglial satellitosis of neurons of amygdaloid nucleus (CV).

Degenerative Changes	*Reactive Changes*
useful indication of disease.	godendroglia may be converted to astrocytes and thus participate in glial scar formation under certain circumstances.
2. Viral inclusions (see Chapter 3)	
3. Cell loss. Where myelin is destroyed, oligoden-	3. Satellitosis. This repre-

droglial cells are reduced or absent. It is usually not possible, however, to determine whether the oligodendroglial cell bodies are primarily affected or the myelin sheaths are the site of primary damage.

sents an apparent increase in perineuronal oligodendroglial cells in certain chronic diseases with neuronal atrophy. It is of unknown significance.

B. Alterations of astrocytes (Fig. 0–10)

Degenerative Changes

1. Acute necrosis (as in anoxia/ischemia and other acutely destructive lesions)

The cytoplasm appears eosinophilic and ballooned. Accompanying disintegration of processes (designated as clasmatodendrosis) is more clearly demonstrable by metallic impregnation. The nucleus is shrunken and pyknotic and has irregular borders. The eventual outcome is that the cell becomes fragmented and phagocytized. The now seldom-used term ''dendrophagocytosis'' emphasizes the phagocytic activity involving the long processes of the disintegrating astrocytes.

2. Viral inclusions

See Chapter 3 for details. These are mainly eosinophilic intranuclear inclusions.

3. Chronic degenerative change

This change is characterized by increase of lipofuscin in the cytoplasm and is often seen alongside a similar change in neurons, as previously described.

4. Storage phenomena

Accumulation of specific abnormal metabolites occurs in the cytoplasm as a result of inborn errors of metabolism such as Tay-Sachs disease or mucopolysaccharidosis. See Chapter 6 for details.

5. Corpora amylacea

These are rounded basophilic structures that are found in the subpial (and subependymal) region of the spinal cord, brainstem, and elsewhere in elderly subjects. They are not considered to be expressions of any specific disease.

On electron microscopy, there is a felt-work of randomly arranged dense fibers, about 100 Å in diameter, in a

Figure 0–10. Alterations of astrocytes. *A,* Acute necrosis (H&E). *B,* Corpora amylaceae (H&E). *C,* Alzheimer type II astrocytes (H&E). *D,* Alzheimer type I astrocyte *(arrow)* (CV). *E,* Simple hypertrophy (H&E). *F,* Gemistocytic astrocytes (H&E). *G,* Fibrous astrocytosis (Cajal). *H,* Isomorphic astrocytosis (H&E). *I,* Rosenthal's fibers *(arrows)* (H&E).

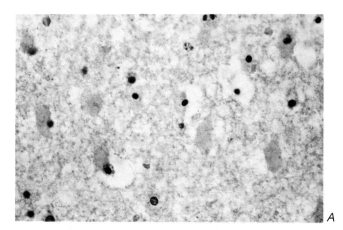

A

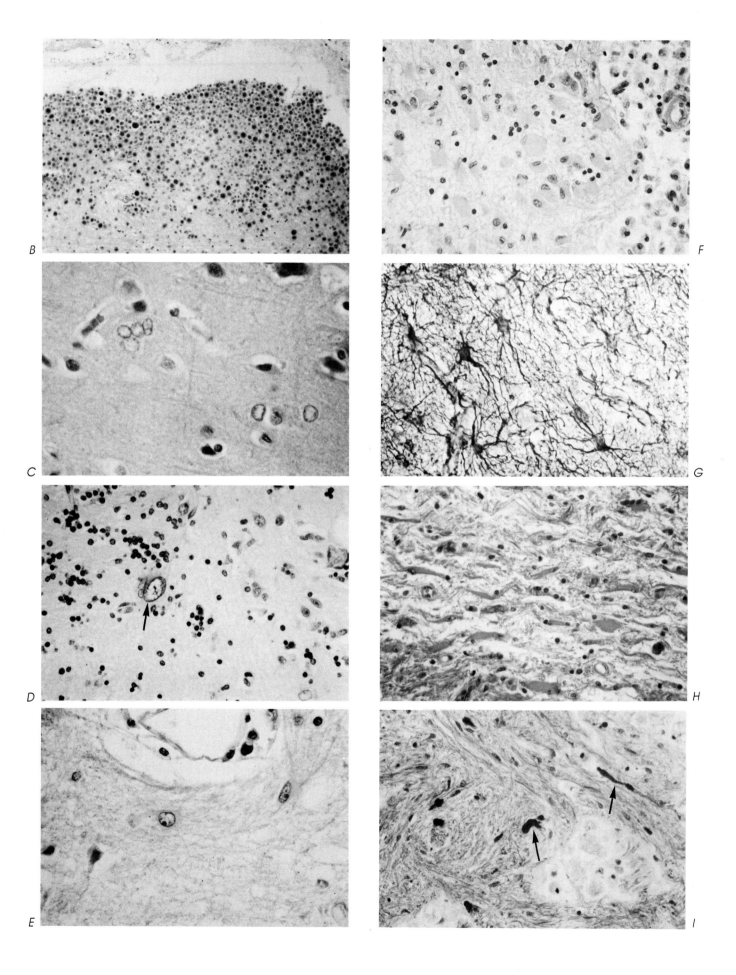

B

C

D

E

F

G

H

I

medium-dense matrix in astrocytic processes, apparently by in situ evolution. Chemically, these fibers are consistent with glucose polymers ("polyglucosan").

Progressive Changes

1. Astrocytosis (astrogliosis, or simply gliosis)

Hypertrophic changes in astrocytes are usually (but not always) associated with proliferation (numerical increase). The following distinction is made by some authors, but the two terms "astrocytosis" and "astrogliosis" are usually employed interchangeably:

• astrocytosis—increase in the number and size of astrocytes
• astrogliosis—enlargement and excessive production of astrocytic fibers = fibrous gliosis.

In most situations, astrocytosis is accompanied by subtle or clear-cut evidence of damage to other tissue components. In rare instances, astrocytosis appears to be "spontaneous," without morphologic evidence of tissue damage that the astrocytes are responding to. The astrocytosis in these situations may be referred to as secondary and primary, respectively.

Primary astrocytosis is exemplified by Alzheimer's type II astrocytes. They are characterized by large nuclei with marginated chromatin and little or no visible cytoplasm (hence, "naked" astrocytes); they can be seen in hepatic failure of diverse causes. In animal models, evidence for augmented metabolic activity devoted to ammonia detoxication is demonstrated.

Note: Alzheimer's type I astrocytes are those seen in Wilson's disease (hepatolenticular degeneration). They have large visible cytoplasm containing copper pigment granules in addition to a vesicular nucleus. Evidence of nervous tissue damage is present in this disorder, along with the appearance of those astrocytes.

Secondary (replacement) astrocytosis is a reaction on the part of (surviving) astrocytes to adjacent tissue damage, which may be obvious or more subtle. Depending on the acuteness or chronicity of the primary pathologic process, astrocytes show different morphologic features.

In acute and usually more destructive processes, the astrocytic reaction includes:

a. Simple hypertrophy (without increase in number), usually seen in early and mild lesions
b. Cell division. Virtual absence of identifiable mitoses in routine preparation leads to the notion that the astrocytes have proliferated by amitotic division. However, it is now known that mitoses can be readily demonstrable by rapid perfusion fixation.
c. Cellular hypertrophy may be pronounced (with or without multinucleation) and result in "plump (gemistocytic)" astrocytes, which are often seen in clusters or pairs with mirror-images and shapes resembling two daughter cells. When astrocytes are thought to be (arbitrarily) excessive in size and configuration, they are called "monster" (or giant) astrocytes. This term also applies to neoplastic or congenitally malformed cells.
d. New glial fiber production (in both protoplasmic and

fibrous astrocytes) resulting in fibrous gliosis (astrocytosis), in which two types may be distinguished: (1) *isomorphic gliosis,* in which astrocytic cell bodies and processes are parallel to the remaining nerve fiber bundles ("piloid" astrocytes), and (2) *anisomorphic gliosis,* which shows haphazard arrangement of astrocytes.

A special form of glial fibers, known as "Rosenthal's fibers," is seen in certain situations, both reactive and neoplastic. They appear as swollen, eosinophilic masses along the glial processes. Electron microscopy shows dense collections of granular material among glial filaments. Their genesis and significance are obscure.

C. Alterations of ependymal cells (Fig. 0–11)

Degenerative Changes	*Reactive Changes*
1. Destruction of ependymal cells occurs readily in almost any severe disorder that extends to the ventricular surfaces or when they are interrupted by stretching of the wall (e.g., in hydrocephalus). No specific histologic features of degeneration are recognized. 2. Focal gaps in ependymal lining are a common finding even among "healthy" neonates. The ependyma poses only a relatively ineffective barrier to the passage of bacteria or other foreign substances in the ventricle.	1. Regeneration is rather limited. Gaps between lost ependymal cells are filled by proliferating subependymal astrocytes, which often protrude into the ventricular cavity. Collectively, they give rise to the peppered macroscopic appearance of the affected ventricular surface (granular ependymitis). 2. Nests of (presumably regenerating or simply surviving) ependymal cells that form small rosettes are often found below the original line among the astrocytes. 3. Partial closure of the ventricular angles by a similar gliotic mechanism is not uncommon. Ependymal rosettes are seen along the line of fusion of the ventricular walls (as often seen incidentally in the frontal horns). Specific etiologic factors are usually not evident.

D. Alterations of choroid plexus (Fig. 0–12)

Degenerative Changes	*Reactive Changes*
1. Of epithelial cells. Relatively little of any significance is known about: a. Aging atrophy	1. Not known

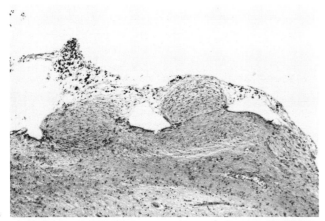

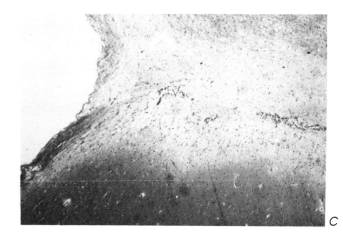

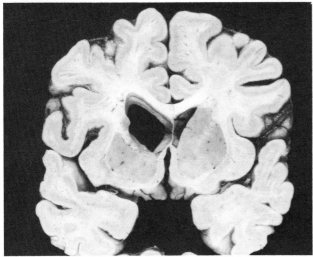

Figure 0–11. Alterations of ependymal cells. *A*, Granular ependymitis secondary to previous intraventricular hemorrhage. *B*, Partial adhesion of lateral ventricular angle. *C*, Photomicrograph of lesion similar to that shown in *B* (H&E).

b. Hematogenous pigment accumulation after intraventricular hemorrhage

2. Of the connective tissue stroma, particularly in the glomus, presumably representing a rather common "physiologic" aging phenomenon and consisting of:

a. Hyaline sclerosis of blood vessels

b. Calcification in the stroma

c. Cystic degeneration and hemorrhage, which later result in cholesteatoma or xanthoma filled with cholesterol crystals, calcific deposits, and macrophages

0.5 ALTERATIONS OF MICROGLIA, BLOOD VESSEL-CONNECTIVE TISSUE, LEPTOMENINGES, AND DURA

A. Alterations of microglia (Fig. 0–13)

Degenerative Changes

1. Death and breakdown. No specific morphologic characteristics are demonstrable.

Reactive Changes

1. Limited hypertrophy. Bipolar "rod cells" with cytoplasm containing some debris in reaction to acute but mild destructive lesions (e.g., anoxia/ischemia) or to slowly progressive lesions, particularly infectious in nature (e.g., general paresis, subacute sclerosing panencephalitis).

The following special

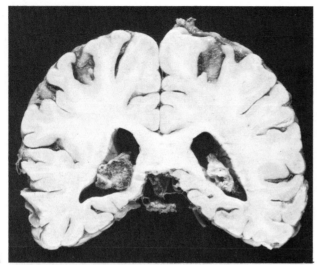

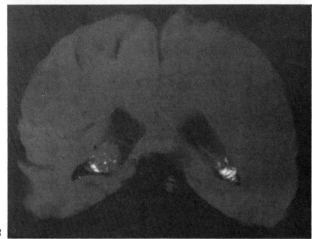

Figure 0–12. Alterations of choroid plexus. *A,* Cystic degeneration and calcification of glomi of lateral ventricles. *B,* Roentgenogram of lesion in *A.*

type of microglial collection, mainly along the dendritic arborization of a dying Purkinje cell.

2. Conversion to the usual swollen macrophage in acute massive destructive lesion. The cytoplasm becomes filled with phagocytosed and partially digested material, notably lipids. This reticulated appearance of the cytoplasm gave rise to the classic descriptions, "Gitter" (= lattice in German) cells and "compound granular corpuscles" (French).

Note: The majority of macrophages in the CNS are now believed to be derived from circulating monocytes (some from fixed histiocytes around blood vessels and in leptomeninges). As in the rest of the body, macrophages may assume the form of multinucleated giant cells, depending on the material engulfed (e.g., globoid cells of Krabbe's disease with ingested cerebrosides).

Degenerative Changes

forms have been described when they occur in clusters. *Neuronophagia:* clusters of (microglial) phagocytic cells surrounding acutely dying or dead neurons (e.g., poliomyelitis). *Microglial nodule:* collection of microglial cells and monocytes without identifiable cell structures to be phagocytosed (at least by light microscopy), as in Japanese B encephalitis. Perivascular microglial nodules are characteristic of a rickettsial disease, for the brunt of the disease is borne by small blood vessels. *Glial shrub:* more diffuse

Reactive Changes

B. Alterations of blood vessel-connective tissue

Degenerative Changes

1. Various forms of damage to blood vessels are discussed in Chapter 1 (Cerebrovascular Disease). Arteries, capillaries, and veins are involved, alone or in various combinations. Only a small amount of connective tissue is present, primarily about blood vessels and in leptomeninges and dura (see below).

Reactive Changes

1. As is the case with the other organs of the body, capillaries are primarily involved in the reparative process (granulation tissue and scar formation) of the nervous system. However, as noted above, astrocytic proliferation is the principal form of scar formation in the CNS except for special situations, for example trauma, abscess, or hemorrhage, in which connective tissue participation is very prominent.

C. Alterations of the leptomeninges (Fig. 0–14)

Degenerative Changes

1. Fibrosis. The collagen

Reactive Changes

1. Fixed histiocytes in the

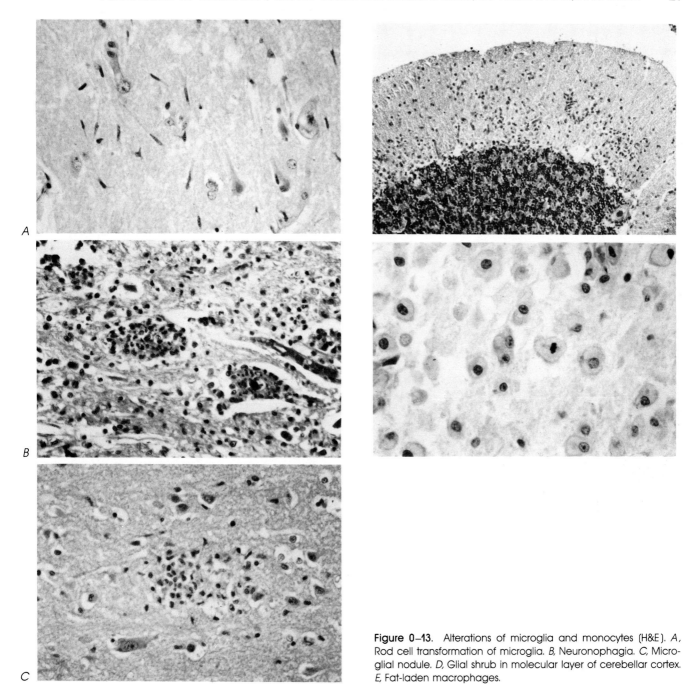

Figure 0–13. Alterations of microglia and monocytes (H&E). *A,* Rod cell transformation of microglia. *B,* Neuronophagia. *C,* Microglial nodule. *D,* Glial shrub in molecular layer of cerebellar cortex. *E,* Fat-laden macrophages.

fibers increase with advancing age and in various types of chronic cerebral disease. This change is also seen as a result of previous inflammatory or hemorrhagic conditions.

2. Focal calcification and ossification. This occurs mainly in the lower spinal cord of elderly persons. Rarely, if ever, are they any

arachnoid are thought to participate in macrophage formation in response to foreign bodies. More active inflammatory response is dependent on hematogenous elements, as in acute leptomeningitides.

2. Fibrosis may follow inflammatory or hemorrhagic diseases involving the leptomeninges. Calcifica-

more than incidental autopsy findings.

tion or ossification may also follow when the process is extensive.

3. Proliferation of the arachnoid cells occurs in advancing age in response to unknown stimuli.

4. The leptomeninges form a usually effective barrier to the processes on either side of them.

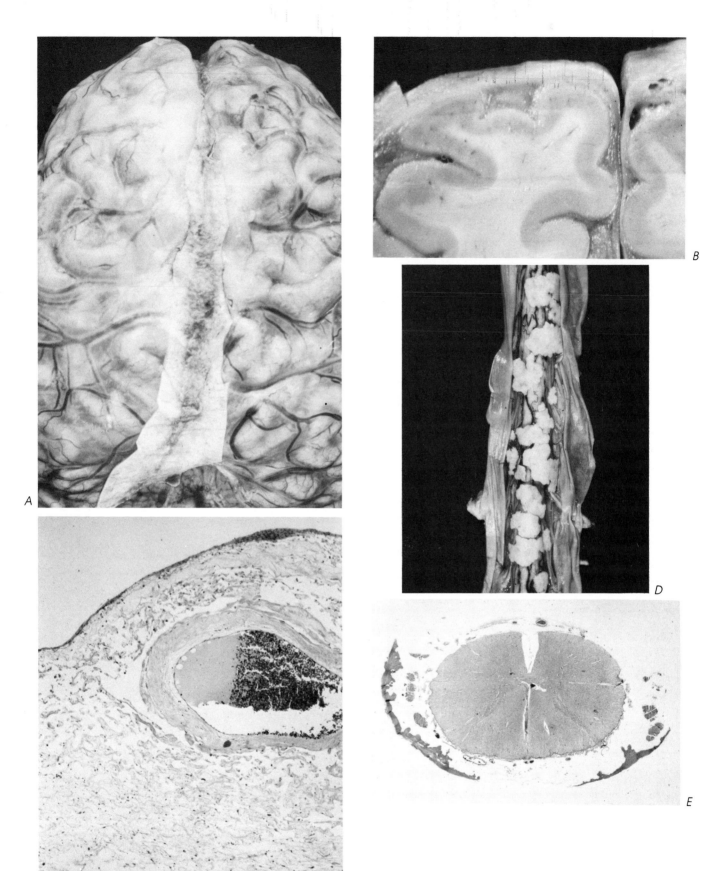

A

B

C

D

E

Figure 0–14. Alterations of leptomeninges. *A*, Mild fibrosis. *B*, Marked fibrosis. *C*, Photomicrograph of lesion in *B. D*, Focal calcification and ossification in spinal cord. *E*, Photomicrograph of lesion in *D* (decalcified, H&E).

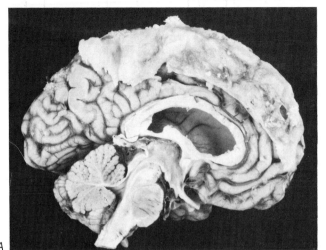

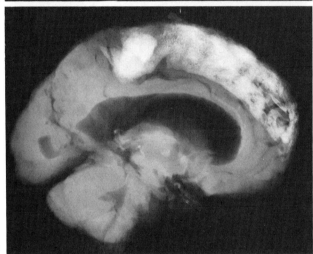

Figure 0–15. Alterations of dura. *A*, Calcification and ossification of falx. *B*, Roentgenogram of lesion in *A*.

D. Alterations of the dura (Fig. 0–15)

Degenerative Changes

1. Hyalinization of fibrous tissue, sometimes with irregular calcification or ossification. This is seen most often in the falx or along the parasagittal plane, usually as ''aging change'' rather than as a result of any known specific disease.

Reactive Changes

1. Organization of subdural foreign substance, mainly blood and inflammatory exudates. This is accomplished by activation and proliferation of the lining cells (fibroblasts) that face the subdural space.

   Calcification or even ossification may follow in severe lesions in their chronic phases.

0.6 ALTERATIONS OF THE PINEAL GLAND

Degenerative Changes

1. Calcification. This is seen in increasing frequency among persons more than 20 years old.
2. Cyst formation is similarly common.

Reactive Changes

1. Neuroglial hyperplasia (gliosis) as part of certain acute and chronic inflammatory diseases, notably general paresis (which is rarely seen nowadays).

1. *Cerebrovascular Disease*

Cerebrovascular disease, commonly referred to as "stroke," claims 500,000 victims each year in the United States, of whom 200,000 die. This makes it the third most common cause of death, after heart disease and cancer. There are 2.5 million stroke survivors in the United States; among them, 15% are totally disabled and 55% are sufficiently disabled to require special care. No other disease is as costly as this in terms of the care required.

Cerebrovascular disease is really a disease of cerebral parenchyma secondary to pathologic alterations of blood vessels that supply and drain the CNS, including those within the cranial cavity and outside of it. As such, it cannot be separated from general pathologic conditions of the heart and systemic blood vessels. The term "cerebrovascular" should not be narrowly interpreted as representing only the blood vessels of the brain. We will include in this chapter discussions of spinal cord disease of vascular etiology. The relationship between various alterations of the blood vessels serving the brain and spinal cord and types of ensuing lesions of the brain and spinal cord parenchyma are summarized in Table 1–1. Table 1–1 indicates that the effects of multitudes of vascular alterations on the CNS may be reduced to three basic patterns—(1) simple enlargement or dilatation, (2) narrowing or obstruction of the vascular lumen, and (3) disruption of the vascular wall—leading to three basic corresponding forms of parenchymal damage. The latter two, namely infarction and hemorrhage, are also capable of causing tissue displacement of the neighboring tissue. *Note:* Not included in the table are (1) extrinsic compression of arteries and veins by nonvascular conditions that may cause obstruction of blood flow and brain infarction and (2) (arterial) vasospasm.

Theoretically, any given type of vascular alteration can cause all three types of effect on the CNS parenchyma. In reality, however, one or two of these tend to predominate, as will be detailed in subsequent discussions.

Additionally, systemic factors in the absence of local blood vessel disease can cause CNS parenchymal damage, mostly in the form of infarction. These conditions are therefore discussed as part of the stroke picture.

1.0 ISCHEMIC/ANOXIC CONDITIONS OF THE CNS

The factors that cause anoxic damage to the CNS are listed in Table 1–2. There may often be concomitant involvement of various factors in a given clinical situation which make pathogenetic analysis difficult.

1.1 ARTERIAL INFARCTION

Of the above-cited factors, in the discussion of stroke we are in practice largely concerned with *ischemic anoxia* and to a lesser extent with *stagnation anoxia,* which refer to the disease processes in which adequately oxygenated blood does not circulate properly through the blood vessels. The resultant CNS tissue damage is referred to as arterial "infarct" and the pathologic process as "infarction." However, these terms are often (and sloppily) used interchangeably.

1.10 Causes of Arterial Infarction

I. General Discussion

In the clinical consideration of arterial infarction, it is convenient to reorganize the causative factors that have already been considered in the preceding section into two groups, as listed below.

A. Factors influencing *general* blood flow
1. Hemodynamic factors
   a. Reduced actual cardiac output (e.g., cardiac failure, dysrhythmia, pulmonary embolism)
   b. Maldistribution of blood into the peripheral circulation and away from the cerebral circulation (e.g., shock, carotid sinus reflex disturbance)
2. Oxygenation of the blood
   a. Reduced atmospheric oxygen
   b. Upper respiratory tract obstruction
   c. Disturbance of pulmonary gas exchange
   d. Reduced hemoglobin in blood
   - In absolute amount
   - In availability for O_2 transport
3. Altered composition of the blood (particularly increased viscosity)

B. Local vascular factors influencing *local* blood flow
1. Arterial diseases
   a. Intrinsic vascular disease leading to stenosis or ectasia

TABLE 1–1. Correlation Between Vascular and Parenchymal Lesions

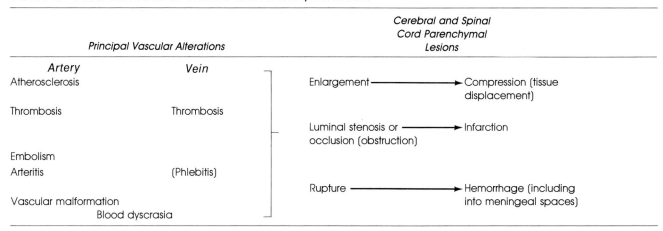

Principal Vascular Alterations		Cerebral and Spinal Cord Parenchymal Lesions
Artery	*Vein*	
Atherosclerosis		Enlargement ⟶ Compression (tissue displacement)
Thrombosis	Thrombosis	
		Luminal stenosis or ⟶ Infarction occlusion (obstruction)
Embolism		
Arteritis	(Phlebitis)	
		Rupture ⟶ Hemorrhage (including into meningeal spaces)
Vascular malformation		
Blood dyscrasia		

TABLE 1–2. Causes of CNS Anoxia (Hypoxia)

Abnormalities of:		Types of Abnormalities	
		In Relation to Blood	*In Relation to O_2 Available to Tissue*
I. Cerebral circulation "Vascular disease of CNS"	A. General: Cardiac arrest or impairment	Stagnation	Stagnation anoxia* (or hypoxia)
	B. Local: Vascular obstruction (e.g., thrombosis, embolism)	Ischemia† (or oligemia)	Ischemic anoxia (or hypoxia)
II. Circulating blood	A. Decreased O_2 saturation: 1. Atmospheric (anaeric)	Anoxic anoxemia (hypoxemia)	Anoxic anoxia (or hypoxia)
	2. Respiratory asphyxia‡ (e.g., strangulation) Paralytic (e.g., poliomyelitis, drugs) B. Decreased amount of available hemoglobin: 1. Quantity of hemoglobin (e.g., anemia, hemorrhage)	Anemic anoxemia (hypoxemia)	Anemic anoxia (or hypoxia)
	2. Availability of hemoglobin (e.g., ↑ carboxyhemoglobin)		
III. Histotoxic agents	Causing: 1. Poisoning of the brain respiratory enzyme system 2. Resulting in failure of the tissue to utilize O_2 (e.g., hydrocyanic acid)		Histotoxic anoxia (= hypoxidosis)

* "Anoxia" means a total absence of oxygen, whereas "hypoxia" represents a reduced oxygen tension. These terms are often used arbitrarily in clinical practice.

† "Ischemia" means an arrest of blood flow within the whole or some part of the circulation, whereas "oligemia" refers to some reduction in blood flow. The latter term is seldom used in practice. Ischemia implies not only an overall oxygen lack but also a reduced oxygen perfusion associated with a local accumulation of metabolites and of certain electrolytes. Concomitantly, delivery of glucose, the major metabolic substrate of the brain, to the tissue becomes reduced or is absent.

‡ "Asphyxia" literally means a pulseless state but is seldom used in that sense; it is usually taken to mean suffocation.

b. Intraluminal obstruction
  • Thrombosis
  • Embolism
2. Extrinsic compression of arteries

Actual infarction results when the cerebral (and spinal) blood flow is reduced below the critical level. In further simplification of the conditions listed above, the determining factors in most clinical situations may be reduced to the following general and local factors.

A. General factors
1. Cardiac output
2. Systemic blood pressure

B. Local factors
1. Patency of the blood vessels
2. Rate of occlusion (which in turn reflects the type of occlusion)
3. Efficacy of the collateral circulation

The relative incidence of various pathogenetic situations in the development of arterial infarcts is not completely agreed upon among the writers on the subject. Some emphasize the importance of the local stenotic/occlusive factor, and others stress the significance of the general circulatory failure.

II. Specific Vascular Lesions

Some of the major vascular lesions leading to arterial infarction are discussed below (Figs. 1–1 and 1–2).

A. Atherosclerosis

The chief etiologic factor in the production of cerebral infarction is atherosclerosis; it is the basic cause of thrombosis in 90% of cases in affluent societies. Atherosclerosis of the cerebral arteries ranks third as the cause of symptoms, after that of the limb vessels and coronary system.

Although the general morphologic features of atherosclerosis in the brain are similar to those of atherosclerosis elsewhere in the body, the following observations are pertinent.

1. Sites of predilection
  a. Extracranially, the changes occur most often and are more severe at the carotid sinus in the neck and at the base of the skull within the cavernous sinus.
  b. Intracranially, the large arteries are chiefly affected, predominantly at sites of bifurcation, at the site of curvature of the arteries, and at sites where the arteries are fixed. Only exceptionally does a plaque appear in isolation. The smaller arteries of the convexity are less often and less severely affected except when hypertension, diabetes mellitus, hypercholesterolemia, or familial xanthomatosis coexists.

Certain differences exist in the behavior of atheromatous plaques between the extracranial arteries serving the brain and the intracranial arteries as described below. The spinal arteries are rarely affected by atherosclerosis.

2. Stenosis
Stenosis of more than 75% of the lumen is considered

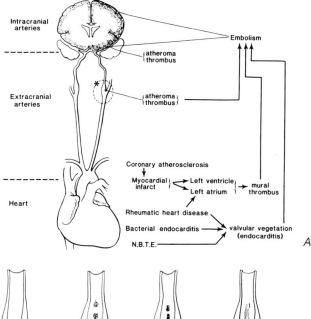

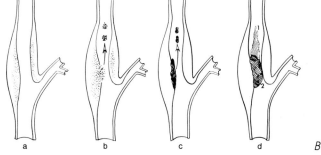

Figure 1–1. *A,* Summary of major stenotic and occlusive lesions of arteries supplying the brain. N.B.T.E. = Nonbacterial thrombotic endocarditis. *B,* Diagrammatic representation of possible consequences of atherosclerotic lesions of carotid bifurcation. *a,* Simple stenosis, at times leading to complete occlusion. *b,* Ulcerated plaque with release of atheromatous debris into bloodstream. *c,* Superimposed thrombosis with partial release of thrombus. *d,* Thrombotic occlusion: (1) laminated, older thrombus; (2) propagating red thrombus formed from stagnated blood. (*A* and *B* modified from Okazaki H: Pathology of apoplexy. 2. Vascular changes as the major cause of cerebral infarct. *Kangogaku Zasshi* 43 no. 11:1213–1216, 1979. By permission of Igaku-Shoin.)

necessary to cause a significant decrease in cerebral blood flow in the presence of normal arterial pressure. However, a drastic decrease in cerebral blood flow may occur even with mild stenosis if blood pressure falls.

3. Natural history of stenosed artery
The following changes may occur after stenosis has taken place. No distinctive clinical or radiologic features have been identified which permit prediction of the outcome of an atherosclerotically stenosed artery, hence the difficulty in clinical therapeutic decisions.
  a. Plaques may simply *increase their size* and degree of protrusion into the vascular lumen to the point of complete occlusion. A sudden occlusion by *hemorrhage* into the plaque of an intracranial artery is rarely observed as a cause of cerebral infarction, in contrast to such an event in the coronary artery. Cervical arteries, particu-

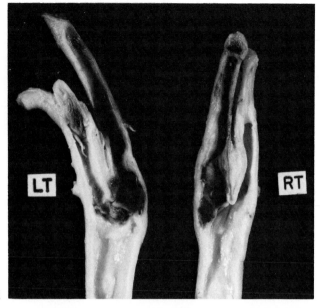

A

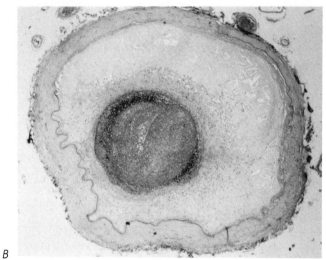

B

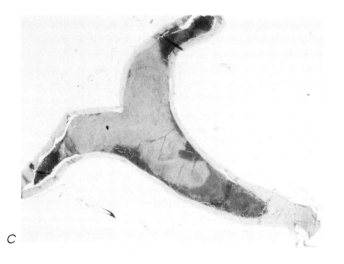

C

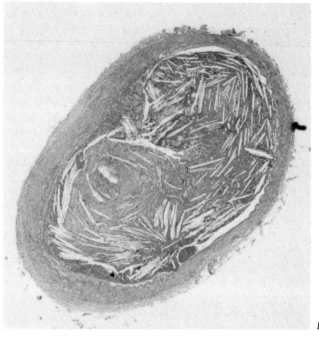

D

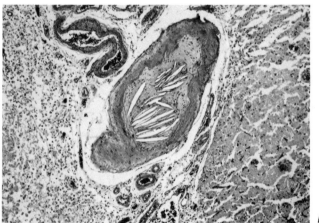

E

Figure 1–2. Various occlusive lesions of arteries leading to the brain. *A*, Longitudinal sections of cervical carotid bifurcations with atherosclerotic stenosis and superimposed thrombosis. *B*, Thrombotic occlusion of stenotic middle cerebral artery in cross section (H&E). *C*, Longitudinal section of recent bland "saddle embolus" from heart in middle cerebral artery "trifurcation" (H&E). *D*, Recent atheromatous embolus in middle cerebral artery (H&E). *E*, Organized atheromatous embolus (H&E).

larly the proximal internal carotid arteries, often show evidence of recent and old hemorrhages, but again a sudden occlusion is not a usual feature.

b. Plaques may become *ulcerated* and give rise to arterial emboli (either atheroma debris or superimposed bland thrombus). This is particularly true with the aortic arch and the carotid artery (common and internal), but is rarely, if ever, seen in the intracranial arteries.

c. Occluding *arterial thrombosis* may occur, apparently precipitated by some focal mural changes. The precise mechanism is still unclear, but in some cases an ulcerated plaque constitutes the nidus of thrombus formation. This is again more commonly observed in the cervical arteries than in intracranial arteries. A recent report suggests that intramural hemorrhage (into plaques) may play a role in initiating thrombosis of cerebral arteries more often than was previously thought. This is particularly significant among hypertensive patients. Naturally, systemic factors that favor thrombosis are also important.

d. Stagnation thrombus, which represents antegrade extension of the thrombus, may develop, usually up to the first sizable collateral branch.

e. Organization of the thrombus and plaques may occur, leading eventually to recanalization of the lumen.

f. Incorporation of the thrombus into the vessel wall is thought to be the cause in certain instances of arterial stenosis. The significance of this process in human disease is disputed by some.

g. Ectasia (dilatation) of the weakened arteries (see section 1.4) may develop and occasionally result in compression of the surrounding tissue. This develop-ment is naturally more significant in intracranial arteries. Atherosclerotic dilatation, instead of stenosis, of the cervical arteries in the vicinity of the carotid bifurcation is a relatively common occurrence in the elderly and has little clinical significance by itself.

h. Calcification of the affected arterial wall is not uncommon in the cervical arteries. Calcification per se, however, rarely contributes to significant stenosis. Some atherosclerotic arteries are ectatic (dilated) yet heavily calcified. Unlike similar-sized coronary arteries, intracranial arteries infrequently become calcified, although the internal carotid artery in the cavernous sinus and just distal to it may be more readily calcified.

B. Arteriolar sclerosis (see section 1.3)

A pathologic process that involves mainly the small intracerebral arterioles—less than 150 μm in diameter—arteriolar sclerosis affects mainly the media and culminates in progressive fibrosis of the arterial wall, with narrowing of the lumen. It appears to be physiologically related to age but is notably accelerated in hypertension and diabetes. It accounts, in the majority of cases, for the presence of small focal infarcts.

C. Embolism

Major sources and types of embolic material are listed in Table 1–3.

Note: 1. Bland or infected thrombi, atheromatous material, and neoplastic tissue, when embolized, occlude cerebral arteries of varying caliber. They tend to become lodged at arterial bifurcations. Large cervical arteries in the neck are infrequently occluded by emboli because of their relatively large lumens. Multiplicity (and different time intervals) is the

TABLE 1–3. Major Sources and Types of Emboli

Heart*	Aorta† and Neck Vessels	Peripheral Vessels

Bland thrombus in:
    Auricular appendage
    (with fibrillation)
    Ventricular wall
    (postmyocardial infarction)
    Valvulitis:
        Rheumatic heart disease
        ("verrucous")
        Systemic lupus erythematosus
        ("atypical verrucous")
        Nonbacterial thrombotic
        endocarditis
	Atheroma (ulcerated plaque and thrombus)	Fat
		
		Neoplasm (with or without pulmonary metastasis)

Infected thrombus in bacterial and fungal endocarditis (see section 3.1)		
Calcific material in rheumatic valvulitis or old calcific aortic stenosis		
Myxoma of heart (rare)		

* Left side; right-sided lesions are significant only in the presence of a right-to-left shunt

† Ascending aorta and arch

rule, but an occlusion of a major artery may dominate the ensuing clinical picture. Smaller fragments tend to be distributed in the arterial border zone, representing the most distal portions of an arterial supply. This, however, is disputed by some.

2. The histologic appearance of all bland thrombi is essentially identical. Therefore, the prediction of their source by examination of affected extracranial arteries alone is often impossible.

3. Thrombotic material found in cerebral arteries in cases of nonbacterial thrombotic endocarditis may or may not be embolic from the heart. It could represent widespread thrombotic phenomena as part of disseminated intravascular coagulation. Proof of the embolic origin of bland thrombotic material in the cerebral vessels is sometimes difficult to obtain if stringent criteria are applied, and bland emboli cannot always be differentiated from locally formed thrombi. The presence of histologically similar thrombus elsewhere, such as in the heart, is an important clue, but this may be totally dislodged. Lack of attachment of emboli to the cerebral arterial wall speaks for embolism, but the embolic material will be organized and become adherent to the wall. Emboli, particularly those of the bland thrombus type, may undergo lysis or may fragment and migrate to smaller distal branches and disappear altogether, often within 2 or 3 days of occlusion. This reestablishment of the circulation to the previously ischemic area is sometimes referred to as "recanalization." It must be remembered that to pathologists the term "recanalization" generally means the establishment of often multiple small vascular channels by way of organization of the occluding material and not a simple distal migration or lysis. As such, this type of recanalization would take a much longer time.

In any event, this reestablishment of blood flow is usually too late to salvage the ischemic (and infarcted) tissue. In fact, it carries the risk of converting an initially nonhemorrhagic infarct to a hemorrhagic one. However, it is still possible that this restoration of circulation, when rapid enough, may account for some of the clinically observed neurologic deficits that are only temporary (see section 1.14). Reported incidences of distal migration of presumed emboli vary from 40 to 75%, and this variation probably reflects differences in pathologic substrate, criteria, and time interval of angiographic observations. Previously, when infarcts were found in the absence of demonstrable arterial occlusion, hemodynamic factors were thought to have been responsible. Now it is possible that many of these, if not the majority, are examples of distal migration of emboli.

4. Calcific material is rarely released spontaneously from the affected valves. Surgical intervention upon these valves is usually responsible for distal embolization.

5. In fat embolism, fat droplets usually occlude capillaries throughout the brain. However, major parenchymal damage (small infarcts and perivascular hemorrhages) is largely confined to the white matter and is most likely due to the paucity of collateral branching here. Whether fat droplets are liberated from bone marrow and pass through the lungs or they are locally "precipitated" from the plasma has not been con-

clusively determined. These events are not necessarily mutually exclusive. (See Chapter 2.)

D. Other vascular lesions to be discussed separately later include:
1. Noninfectious inflammatory arteritides (section 1.5)
2. Arterial lesions due to traumatic agents (section 2.5)
3. Arterial lesions due to physical agents (section 6.6)
4. Primary cerebral amyloid angiopathy (section 5.1)

1.11 Pathomorphology of Cerebral Infarction (Softening, Encephalomalacia)

I. Classification

A. According to type (Fig. 1–3)
1. Anemic (ischemic, white) infarction
   This process is a coagulative necrosis of tissue with little or no hemorrhage into it (microscopic extravasations, however, are frequent), presumably because of complete cessation of blood circulation in the infarcted area. (Note: The term "anemic" here does not imply that the infarct is caused by anemia; rather, it simply suggests the gross appearance. Similarly, the term "ischemic" denotes morphologic and not etiologic significance.)
2. Hemorrhagic (red) infarction
   This is infarction complicated by frankly hemorrhagic features ranging from petechiae to confluent zones, mainly in the cortex. In venous infarction (to be discussed later), which is nearly always hemorrhagic, hemorrhage is confined largely to the white matter (see section 1.6). Mechanisms proposed to explain the production of hemorrhagic infarction include the following:
   a. Vascular endothelial damage by sudden severe reduction of cerebral blood flow, allowing extravasation of erythrocytes.
   b. Reperfusion of the infarcted area by breaking up of the occluding embolus, by resumption of effective systemic hemodynamics (hemorrhages being in the central portion of the infarct), or by perfusion through collateral circulation (hemorrhages in the periphery of the infarct, i.e., in the arterial border zone). Again, hemorrhages occur from already damaged capillary blood vessels.

Note: These explanations are not always compatible with the observed pattern of hemorrhage in a given infarct. Generally speaking, thrombosis and severe systemic hypotension tend to result in anemic infarcts and embolism in hemorrhagic ones. However, exceptions occur. No completely satisfactory explanation is offered for hemorrhagic infarction due to compression of the posterior cerebral artery by an expanding supratentorial mass.

B. According to intensity
1. In complete infarction, all cellular elements die.

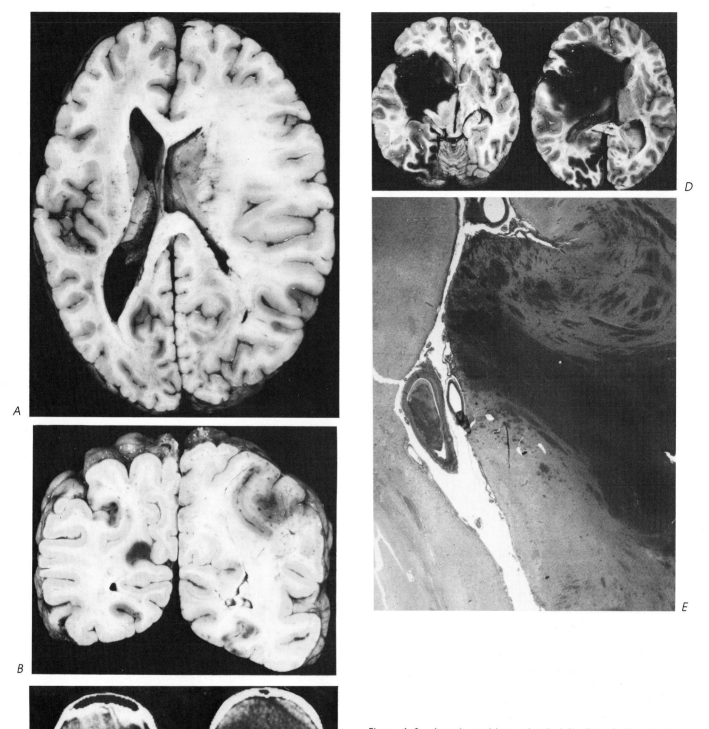

Figure 1–3. Anemic and hemorrhagic infarction. *A,* Anemic (or white) infarct of right cerebral hemisphere in its early phase. *B,* Multiple recent hemorrhagic infarcts due to multiple emboli from nonbacterial thrombotic endocarditis. *C,* Computed tomography scans of embolic infarct in left middle cerebral artery territory, apparently nonhemorrhagic at this early stage, caused by embolization to proximal left middle cerebral artery. *D,* Same infarct in horizontal section post mortem. Note extensive hemorrhagic nature of its proximal portion. *E,* Demonstration of distally migrated embolus to left middle cerebral artery branch in sylvian fissure.

2. In incomplete infarction, some of the elements, notably blood vessels and to a lesser extent astrocytes, survive.

3. In the "cellular lesion," damage is solely or largely confined to neurons.

C. According to extent

Several patterns of infarction involving the cerebral cortex or white matter are recognized. These are schematically represented in Figure 1–4 and can be described as follows (the same scheme can be applied to the cerebellum):

1. Complete cortical and subcortical pattern

On cross section, the central portion is usually continuous, whereas the periphery tends to show patchy discontinuous patterns, particularly in the white matter. Overall configuration is wedge-shaped on cross section (or cone-shaped in three dimensions), with a tapering tip toward the depth of the white matter. The tissue necrosis tends to be complete in the center but incomplete or partial at the periphery.

2.a. Largely cortical *continuous* (laminar) pattern

The necrosis may be nearly complete when extensive, but generally the damage tends to concentrate on neurons. The depth of infarcts varies from the entire thickness of the cortex and the immediately subcortical white matter to a relatively narrow band encompassing a few cortical layers. Although this is usually referred to as a "laminar necrosis," it is often irregular, being rarely limited strictly to a lamina or laminae, and purists would prefer to call it "pseudolaminar."

b. *Focal* cortical pattern, often in multiplicity and following the course of penetrator arteries. The resulting irregular pitting of the cortical surface gives rise to the term "granular atrophy."

3.a. Large white matter pattern composed of an infarct confined to extensive areas of the white matter (rare). Poorly defined, more diffuse rarefaction (incomplete ischemic necrosis) may be included under this pattern.

b. Focal white matter pattern consisting of frequently multiple small necrotic zones limited to the fields of a few penetrator arteries. The damage often varies in intensity, sometimes leading to cavitation and at other times only to rarefaction. Secondary degeneration of the tract tends to blur the margins of these lesions and simulate a more diffuse pattern of involvement.

1.12 Morphologic Evolution (Table 1–4)

The sequence of events after an infarction of a major arterial distribution (e.g., middle cerebral artery) may be best explained in terms of three different phases. Naturally, these are not three discontinuous phases; one runs into the other in a continuous evolution (Table 1–4).

A. Coagulative necrosis (Fig. 1–5)

The infarcted area appears pale and somewhat swollen, with a blurred corticomedullary junction. At first, consistency is only slightly reduced, but formalin fixation exaggerates the alteration in that the normal tissue hardens but the infarcted tissue remains soft.

In the central portion of the infarct, tissue necrosis tends to involve all elements. Neurons (with H & E stain) show eosinophilic ("ischemic") degeneration and eventual dissolution. The earliest change may be discernible after 6 hours. Astrocytes, oligodendroglial cells, and microglial cells, along

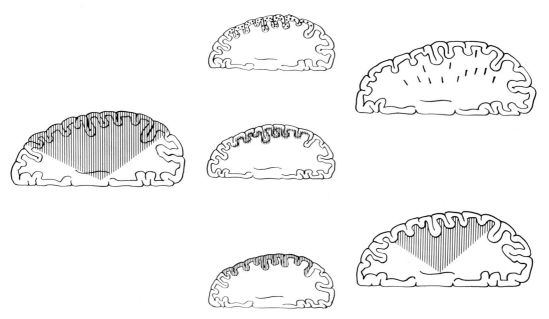

Figure 1–4. Patterns of cerebral infarction by extent. See text for explanation.

TABLE 1–4. Summary of the Evolutionary Sequence of a Complete Cerebral Infarction

Time	Macroscopic	Microscopic		
		Tissue Necrosis (of neuronal components)	Phagocytosis and Removal of Debris	Repair

Microscopic — Tissue Necrosis: *Neuron*, *Myelin*, *Axon*

Phagocytosis and Removal of Debris: *Hematogenous elements*

Repair: (By surviving elements at edge)

1 day — Macroscopic: Swelling, pallor, blurred gray-white junction; *Coagulative necrosis*

Axon: Swelling

Myelin: Swelling; poor staining

Phagocytosis: 24 hours: Polymorphonuclear cells

2 days — Tissue Necrosis: Eosin. degen.

Monocytes

Phagocytosis: Disintegration (48 hours)

Blood vessels

Lipid-laden macrophages

Capillary prominence

Macroscopic: Mushy and friable, maximum swelling

Increasingly more pronounced (5 days on)

Astrocytes

(7 days) Capillary thickening; mesenchymal fibrils

Hypertrophy and hyperplasia

Tissue Necrosis: Disintegration

2 weeks — Macroscopic: *Liquefaction begins = Disappearance of semiliquid necrotic debris*

Removal

Meshwork of richly cellular connective tissue

3 weeks — Macroscopic: *Cavitation becomes evident*

Tissue Necrosis: Limited persistence

Dense glial scar at edge of lesion

A few months — Macroscopic: Fluid-filled cavity

Few vessels remain in cavity

Fibril production completed; decrease in size and number of astrocytes

33

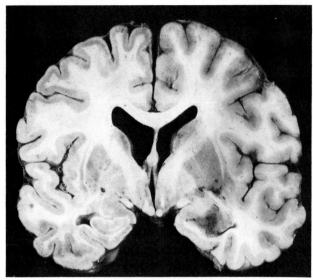

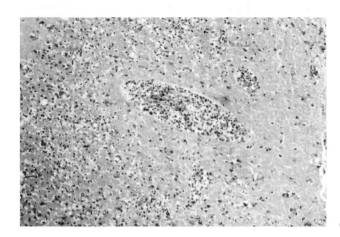

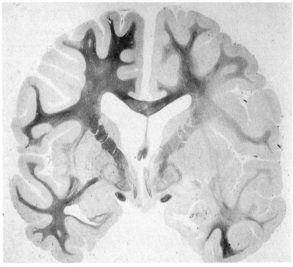

Figure 1–5. Coagulative necrosis stage of cerebral infarction. *A*, Recent (1 day) nonhemorrhagic infarct in right internal carotid artery. *B*, Myelin (LFB) stain of same hemisphere in which infarcted areas appear paler than uninvolved areas. *C*, Low-power view of an early infarcted cortex (H&E). All cellular elements are necrotic, including polymorphonuclear cell exudates.

with myelinated axons, similarly disintegrate and give rise to a somewhat granular appearance of the "background" (the neuropil). Capillaries may undergo necrosis, but polymorphonuclear cells are often seen surrounding them after 24 hours. Red cell extravasation is common to some degree even in a grossly "anemic" infarct. Edematous swelling of the infarcted tissue (see section 1.8) reaches its maximum in 3 to 4 days, and its mass effects on the uninfarcted areas and the intracranial pressure in general are of great clinical significance (see sections 1.14 and 1.9).

B. Liquefaction (or absorption) (Fig. 1–6)

Liquefaction represents removal of debris by macrophages. After the brief appearance of polymorphonuclear leukocyte infiltration (disintegration begins in 48 hours), mononuclear phagocytic cells appear on the scene in increasing numbers. The majority of these are now believed to be hematogenous in origin, rather than arising from activation of resident microglial cells, as was previously held. As

such, their activities are most prominent at the edge of the infarct where capillaries survive. These lipid-laden macrophages are referred to as "gitter cells," or "compound granular cells" in the older neuropathologic literature, as if they were different from other macrophages elsewhere. Their activities are reflected in a sharpened demarcation between the normal and infarcted tissues, which may appear as a crack in a gross specimen. The infarcted tissue becomes increasingly mushy and friable but less swollen as the tissue disintegration and clean-up by macrophages proceed. This is also the time for hypertrophy and hyperplasia of surviving capillaries and astrocytes at the edge. Characteristically, the molecular layer of the cortex usually but not always survives, even in otherwise complete infarction.

C. Cavitation (Fig. 1–7)

Continued removal of necrotic tissue by macrophages into the circulation leads to cavitation of the affected area. This cavitary process becomes evident by 3 weeks. The

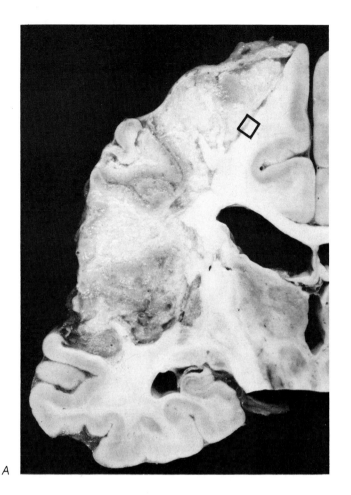

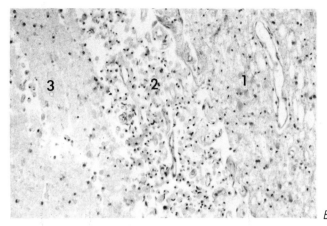

Figure 1–6. Liquefactive necrosis stage of cerebral infarction. *A*, Four-month-old infarction in left middle cerebral artery distribution, exhibiting signs of tissue breakdown and absorption. *B*, Photomicrograph of border zone in white matter (boxed area in *A*), showing three zones of tissue reaction. From right to left (1) peripheral zone of partial tissue destruction and gliosis containing hypertrophied astrocytes, (2) zone of advanced macrophage activity and residual vascular proliferation, and (3) zone of largely unabsorbed debris where only a few macrophages have entered (H&E).

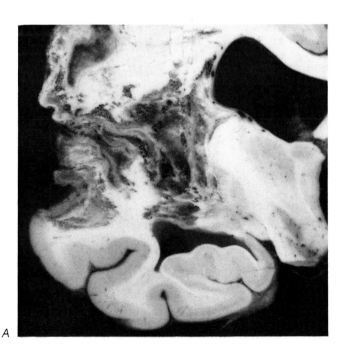

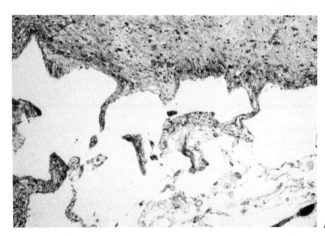

Figure 1–7. Cavitation stage of cerebral infarction. *A*, Largely empty cavity traversed by glial-vascular trabeculae that replace affected tissue. *B*, Edge of cavity with marginal gliosis and trabeculae extending toward center.

heavy network of cellular capillaries seen during the previous phase tends to decrease in prominence. Eventually, by 3 months or more, the entire lesion is replaced by a clear CSF-like fluid-filled cavity traversed by a varying number of blood vessels and gliotic trabeculae.

Unlike the situation in other somatic tissues, collagen-forming granulation tissue does not participate to any significant degree. The surrounding surviving areas are rarefied but contain many astrocytes, which are by now more stout and fibrous and have less plump cytoplasm. Double nucleation is not uncommon among them. The entire lesion is in a state of contraction and collapse, quite different from the early swollen phase.

In less complete infarction, neurons and oligodendroglial cells will die and disintegrate, but capillaries and astrocytes will survive; the result is a rarefied gliotic (astrocytic) area devoid of neurons but not a frank cavity. Individual component foci of granular atrophy described earlier are often composed of glial scars of this type. The peripheral zones of the above-described complete infarct are essentially similar to this, with certain degrees of patchiness in severity and distribution of tissue damage.

The evolution of a hemorrhagic infarct takes an essentially similar course, except for the presence of hemosiderin and hematoidin in the tissue (in macrophages, astrocytes, vascular coats, and even neurons), which gives a brown to yellowish color to the cavitating lesion.

The above descriptions must be regarded as only a rough timetable. Although liquefaction necrosis is the characteristic fate of infarcted brain tissue, it must be remembered that it first passes through the stage of coagulation necrosis. Sometimes removal of debris is markedly delayed for some reason, and a large part of the infarcted tissue may remain in a state of coagulation necrosis. This seems to hold true particularly in the elderly and debilitated. The high lipid content (myelin) and virtual absence of fibroblastic and collagenous activities in the brain infarct lead to the cavitary end stage, which is different from the densely collagenous scar tissue of infarcted somatic tissues such as the heart, kidneys, spleen, and so on.

1.13 Topographic Features

I. Discussion of Specific Factors

The factors that influence the size and extent of cerebral infarcts are (A) the presence or absence of anastomosis, (B) the site of occlusion, and (C) the type of occlusion

Note: The last two factors are largely significant because of their influence on the first factor.

A. The presence and efficacy of *anastomosis* serving as a substitution pathway ("*collateral circulation*")

Note: Strictly speaking, these terms are not synonymous (Zülch, 1971). "Anastomoses" denotes network-like intercommunications of two or more functionally separate vascular systems; the direction of the flow and the calibers of these communicating vessels are not defined. In general use, anastomosis is simply a natural or created communication between two vessels—end to end, side to side, or end to side. "Collaterals" are morphologic pathways (in this instance, arteries) in which double or triple parallel systems supply one organ and can substitute for one another in an emergency. It is, however—deplorable as this may be to purists—common practice today to use these terms interchangeably.

There are three major systems of anastomosis that may significantly influence the size and extent of a cerebral infarct resulting from an occlusion of a cranial or extracranial artery (Fig. 1–8): (1) ophthalmic artery, (2) circle of Willis, and (3) leptomeningeal vessels.

1. Anastomoses via the ophthalmic artery

These bridge the external carotid and internal carotid systems (Fig. 1–8 *B*).

2. Anastomoses of the circle of Willis

This system provides not only the alternate passage of blood between two hemispheres but also connects the anterior (internal carotid) and posterior (vertebral-basilar) systems. It is the most important system, but there are considerable individual variations in the caliber of the component arteries. It is reported that perhaps only about 20% are of the "standard" pattern (Riggs and Rupp, 1963). This accounts for the unpredictability of the site and size of infarction resulting from stenosis or occlusion of one or more of these arteries. Major variants include the following:

a. The anterior or posterior communicating artery (or both) may be hypoplastic and restrict effective circulation across the circle or between its anterior and posterior component.

b. Hypoplasia of the proximal stem of one anterior cerebral artery usually results in a takeover of its distal field of irrigation by the opposite internal carotid artery (via the anterior cerebral artery and the anterior communicating artery).

c. Hypoplasia of the proximal segment of one or both posterior cerebral arteries makes the distal segment of these arteries dependent on the anterior circulation (via the posterior communicating arteries).

d. Any number of combinations of the above is possible. Sometimes one or more of these segments are totally lacking. Selective stenosis or occlusion, most commonly by atherosclerosis of these arteries, will create situations comparable to those related to hypoplasia or aplasia.

3. Leptomeningeal anastomoses

These are connections within the arachnoid space over the surface of the brain among the major branches of the internal carotid artery, i.e., the anterior, middle, and posterior cerebral arteries. This system is significant only when the circle of Willis system is adequate.

B. Site of occlusion (Fig. 1–9)

This is closely related to the question of effective anastomoses and has already been partially discussed. Again, the

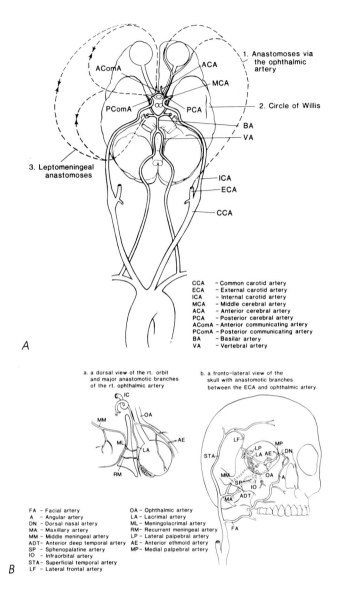

A

1. Anastomoses via the ophthalmic artery

2. Circle of Willis

3. Leptomeningeal anastomoses

CCA - Common carotid artery
ECA - External carotid artery
ICA - Internal carotid artery
MCA - Middle cerebral artery
ACA - Anterior cerebral artery
PCA - Posterior cerebral artery
AComA - Anterior communicating artery
PComA - Posterior communicating artery
BA - Basilar artery
VA - Vertebral artery

a. a dorsal view of the rt. orbit and major anastomotic branches of the rt. ophthalmic artery

b. a fronto-lateral view of the skull with anastomotic branches between the ECA and ophthalmic artery.

FA - Facial artery
A - Angular artery
DN - Dorsal nasal artery
MA - Maxillary artery
MM - Middle meningeal artery
ADT- Anterior deep temporal artery
SP - Sphenopalatine artery
IO - Infraorbital artery
STA- Superficial temporal artery
LF - Lateral frontal artery

OA - Ophthalmic artery
LA - Lacrimal artery
ML - Meningolacrimal artery
RM - Recurrent meningeal artery
LP - Lateral palpebral artery
AE - Anterior ethmoid artery
MP - Medial palpebral artery

B

Figure 1–8. *A,* Diagrammatic overview of the three major sites of collateral arterial blood flow to the brain. *B,* Representative branches connecting external (*ECA*) and internal carotid (*IC*) artery systems. *C,* Diagrammatic representation of leptomeningeal anastomoses between three major cerebral arteries. (*A* modified from Okazaki H: Pathology of apoplexy. 3. Morphology of cerebral infarct. *Kangogaku Zasshi* 43 no. 12:1325–1328, 1979. By permission of Igaku-Shoin; *B,* modified from Burnbaum MD, Selhorst JB, Harbison JW, et al: Amaurosis fugax from disease of the external carotid artery. Arch Neurol 34:532–535, 1977. By permission of the American Medical Association.)

general principle will be illustrated by various occlusions in an internal carotid artery system.

1. Proximal occlusion of the internal carotid artery may produce a limited infarct or no infarct in the territory of the middle cerebral artery.

a. When the internal carotid artery alone is occluded, the origins of the anterior and posterior cerebral arteries are not obstructed. In the presence of a good collateral circulation from the opposite side via the anterior and posterior communicating arteries, no infarct may result in this situation.

b. When an occlusion of the internal carotid artery is more distal to include these origins, a large infarct results, either in the territory of the middle cerebral artery only or in other territories, depending on the adequacy of the anterior communicating artery or posterior communicating artery leptomeningeal anastomoses with the middle cerebral artery.

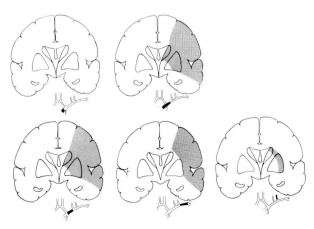

Figure 1–9. Relationship between site of occlusion in middle cerebral artery system and extent of resulting infarction.

2. Distal arterial occlusion involving a functional end artery (with no or limited leptomeningeal anastomoses) will result in an extensive infarction of the supply area.

　　a. Occlusion of the proximal part of the middle cerebral artery often results in total middle cerebral infarction, since usually the superficial collateral circulation is able to assume only a slight margin of arterial compensation.

　　b. Isolated superficial middle cerebral infarction results from occlusion distal to the origin of the perforating branches.

　　c. Occlusion of the origin of one of the perforators results in an isolated deep middle cerebral infarct in the basal ganglia. Because the anastomotic intercapillary network within the brain substance is ineffective, occlusion of an arteriole is almost always accompanied by death of the tissues that it supplies.

C. Types of occlusion

The rapidity with which an arterial occlusion occurs will influence the size and extent of the resultant infarct.

1. A *gradual* atherosclerotic stenosis of the middle cerebral artery, for example, will encourage collateral circulation from the anterior or posterior cerebral artery to take over the peripheral territory of the middle cerebral artery. When thrombotic occlusion develops later at the stenosed site, the resultant infarct will be smaller in size than that expected from the prestenotic ("normal") stage. It is also suggested that a slowly developing thrombosis itself may be sufficient to allow the development of a better collateral flow. However, severely atherosclerotic arteries are not expected to respond with compensatory dilatation.

2. In contrast, when *rapid* occlusion by an embolus takes place, the resultant infarct tends to be "total" in extent.

II. Discussion of Resultant Topographic Features of Cerebral Infarcts

Because of the natural variation of these factors, vascular occlusions at the identical position may result in infarcts of different size and extent in different patients.

The general principle involved is best explained by the example of an occlusion or stenosis of a major artery in the carotid system on one side. The variable extent of resulting infarcts is diagrammatically illustrated in Figure 1–10.

A. Total infarction

A proximal occlusion of the middle cerebral artery will result in an infarct in the entire area of its distribution in the face of inadequate or absent collateral blood flow to its territory from the anterior and posterior cerebral arteries.

B. Reduced infarction resulting from a partially adequate collateral circulation

1. Proximal zone of supply type

This represents a reduction or contraction in the size of an infarct to the proximal portion of the middle cerebral artery with occlusion of that vessel. The most distal field is maintained by blood flow from the meningeal anastomoses of other (i.e., anterior and posterior cerebral arteries)

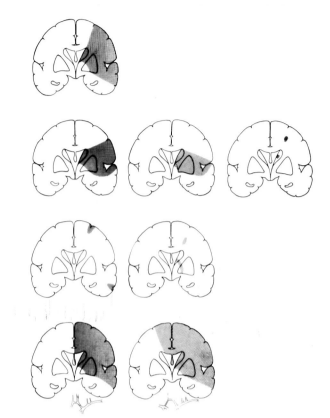

Figure 1–10. Variable extents of infarction in distribution of middle cerebral artery (see text for explanation).

neighboring territories. Because of individual variation in the extent of anastomosis, the external border of the resultant infarct is variable.

2. Center of supply area type

This results from stenosis of the middle cerebral artery, leading to sufficient irrigation of the proximal area but a reduced blood supply to the distal area. With adequate leptomeningeal anastomotic supply from the anterior and posterior cerebral arteries, the endangered area is concentrically reduced in size to the center of the middle cerebral artery distribution zone, with sparing of the most distal and proximal areas. An infarct of this type is characteristically localized in the frontal operculum and the upper insular cortex, and it may be barely visible from the outside.

3. Terminal zone of supply type

This is typically found in the form of circumscribed cysts deep in the centrum semiovale, often in association with small infarcts in the terminal area of the striolenticular arteries (perforators of the middle cerebral artery). Similarly, small infarcts in the posterior white matter in or close to the optic radiation are in the terminal supply zone of the anterior choroidal artery. Naturally, these lesions could be a result of occlusion of a local arterial branch (see section 1.3).

C. Arterial border (or boundary) zone infarction

1. Single medium or large infarcts or, more frequently, multiple small cortical (or immediately subcortical) infarcts

are found between the areas served by the middle cerebral artery and the anterior cerebral artery and less frequently by the middle cerebral artery and the posterior cerebral artery, when there is concomitant reduction in the blood supply of all territories due either to stenosis of the cervical internal carotid artery or to proximal stenosis of the three major cerebral arteries. Systemic hypotension will aggravate focal ischemia and in fact may be sufficient, when severe enough, to cause this type of infarction in the absence of significant intrinsic vascular lesions. The previously popular term ''watershed zone infarct'' is conceptually incorrect, for the direction of the flow implicit in this term is away from the watershed and not to the area in question. The real situation is analogous to irrigation of fields or sprinkling of the lawn with two or more sources of water supply connected to a main source.

2. In the deep cerebral tissue, an infarct may be found passing through the head of the caudate nucleus and putamen, representing an arterial border zone between Hubner's artery (anterior cerebral artery), the lenticulostriate (middle cerebral artery), and the anterior choroidal artery and leptomeningeal branches of the middle cerebral artery.

D. The extension of an infarct beyond the anatomic borders of the vascular supply area

1. A long-standing severe stenosis of the anterior cerebral artery may cause a shift of the border and an increase in size of the supply territory of the middle cerebral artery.

2. As one of the anatomic variations, one or both anterior cerebral arteries may be nearly completely dependent on the internal carotid artery (of the same side). Occlusion of the internal carotid artery will then result in an infarct, including one or both anterior cerebral artery territories in addition to the area of the middle cerebral artery.

III. Individual Arterial Systems

The internal carotid system is thought to supply 90% of blood flow to the brain. The distribution of cerebral infarcts appears to reflect this roughly. Of 220 consecutive Mayo Clinic patients with infarctive stroke admitted within 36 hours of onset, infarcts were in the internal carotid artery distribution in 179 patients (81%) and in the vertebral-basilar artery territory in 38 patients (17%) (Jones and Millikan, 1976).

A. Internal carotid system

Many aspects of infarction of the internal carotid artery system have been discussed above.

1. Internal carotid artery (Fig. 1–11)

Disease of the internal carotid artery is most likely to give rise to complications in relation to the middle cerebral arteries.

In humans, a sudden natural occlusion of a common or internal carotid artery in the neck is rarely observed. These arteries, particularly at the carotid sinus region, are most often affected by atherosclerosis, which causes first stenosis and eventually complete occlusion (see section 1.4). Because of a naturally endowed adequacy of collateral circulation or

thanks to ample time given for the collateral channels to increase their caliber, infarction may not develop. These patients generally show a good cross-filling of the ipsilateral middle cerebral artery at the time of angiography of the contralateral carotid or vertebral-basilar system.

When the collateral circulation is less adequate, the cerebral hemisphere becomes infarcted along a band of tissue that represents the border zone between the irrigation territories of the anterior cerebral artery and middle cerebral artery. Arterial border zone infarcts, being nonfatal, are usually seen at autopsy as a series of minute to small cortical and immediately subcortical scars; these give rise to the external appearance of granular atrophy. The width of this zone and the number and density of these component scars vary from case to case. In some instances, an arterial border zone infarct may be relatively narrow but deep, its tip reaching down toward the ventricular wall.

The infarcts may also involve the border zone between the middle cerebral artery and the posterior cerebral artery (1) when the posterior cerebral artery receives most of its blood supply from the internal carotid artery, as seen in cases in which the posterior communicating artery and posterior cerebral artery were direct extensions of the internal carotid artery system; (2) when there is a concomitant reduction in the territory of the posterior cerebral artery, due to compromise of the proximal posterior cerebral artery itself; or (3) when the posterior cerebral artery is a direct extension of a vertebral-basilar system that has been compromised by stenosis or occlusion.

It must be remembered, however, that small, multiple embolic occlusions of small leptomeningeal branches from the affected but nonoccluded cervical arteries can result in similar pathologic changes, perhaps infarcts rarely being as multiple as those due to the hemodynamic factor.

It is also not unusual to find loosely organized occlusive changes in multiple segments of these arteries overlying the zone of granular atrophy. These are regarded as evidence of previous platelet thrombi due to circulatory stagnation rather than of embolism. It appears that some of the previously reported examples of cerebral endarteritis obliterans (Buerger's disease) are in fact cases involving occlusive changes.

If the collateral flow from the contralateral internal carotid artery (via the anterior communicating artery) is grossly inadequate, a various extent of the middle cerebral artery territory and, in some cases, the anterior cerebral artery territory as well, may become infarcted, as discussed previously. Characteristically, before the patient experiences sudden permanent hemiplegia from this massive infarct, he has experienced multiple attacks of transient motor or sensory impairment with pronounced or complete recovery (so-called transient ischemic attacks). The question of the relative significance of hemodynamic factors and embolic occlusions in the explanation of these episodes has not been completely settled.

Whether it is segmental or total, thrombosis (or severe stenosis) of the internal carotid artery between its origin and the origin of the ophthalmic artery may result in a similar

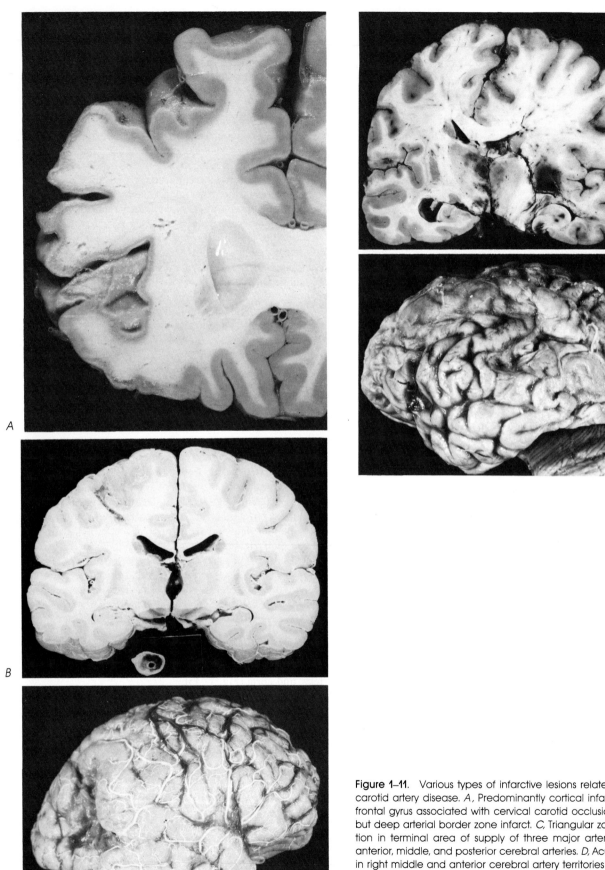

Figure 1–11. Various types of infarctive lesions related to internal carotid artery disease. *A,* Predominantly cortical infarct of inferior frontal gyrus associated with cervical carotid occlusion. *B,* Narrow but deep arterial border zone infarct. *C,* Triangular zone of infarction in terminal area of supply of three major arteries—namely, anterior, middle, and posterior cerebral arteries. *D,* Acute infarction in right middle and anterior cerebral artery territories with marked edema resulting in distortion of various tissue components (see details in section 1.9). *E,* External sectional view of more irregular areas of infarction encompassing anterior and middle cerebral artery territories in patient with occluded cervical internal carotid artery.

cerebral lesion or lack of it, because there is no alternate passage between these two points. If the occlusion extends beyond the origin of an ophthalmic artery that has been significant in collateral circulation, the arterial border zone cerebral infarct will be larger. If the thrombus extends beyond the bifurcation of the internal carotid artery and occludes the origins of both the middle and the anterior cerebral artery, it is more likely to result in infarction of the entire territories of these vessels unless, again, the collateral flows via the anterior and posterior communicating arteries are adequate to salvage portions or possibly all of them. An occlusion of the intracranial portion of the internal carotid artery (with or without further distal extension) also occurs in the absence of cervical occlusion.

2. Middle cerebral artery (Fig. 1–12)

Stenotic and occlusive involvement of the middle cerebral artery and its ischemic consequences have already been discussed. Either directly or indirectly (by occlusion of the internal carotid artery), this territory is infarcted in some 50% of all stroke accidents. This makes the middle cerebral artery the most often-affected single artery of the brain. Our own analysis of 100 consecutive infarcts of the middle cerebral artery (of less than 2 weeks' duration) in relation to the site of arterial occlusion is presented below (Fig. 1–13).

From these data, it is clear that clinical signs and symptoms resulting from ischemic focal cerebral tissue destruction are not reliable for determination of the sites of arterial occlusion. An adequate arteriographic study is essential not only for this determination but also for determination of the extent of occlusion and evaluation of collateral circulation, which are important factors in making an accurate prognosis and in determining the proper type of therapy.

3. Anterior choroidal artery

Isolated infarction of this territory is seldom seen. The posterior part of the internal capsule, pallidum, optic tract, and amygdaloid nucleus may be infarcted. Involvement of these areas in cases of internal carotid-middle cerebral artery thrombosis is not uncommon because of blockage of the origin of this artery by the thrombosis.

4. Anterior cerebral artery (Fig. 1–14)

A large isolated infarct in the territory of the anterior cerebral artery is relatively rare, largely because of the presence of adequate anastomotic flow through the anterior communicating artery, even if the proximal anterior cerebral artery (A-1 segment) is totally occluded. An occlusion distal to the anterior communicating artery may result in total distal infarction. More often, small, old infarcts involving only portions of its territory are found incidentally at autopsy, usually involving the anterior corpus callosum and adjacent white matter or cingulate gyrus.

Note: 1. The functional competence of individual arteries is difficult to assess from the autopsy material, even with the aid of postmortem angiography. In practice, the distribution of an infarcted tissue allows speculation as to the functional competence of the arteries along the line of reasoning described above. It must, however, be remembered that embolic material may fragment and dislodge from the occlusive sites.

2. Concomitant stenosis of two (e.g., middle and anterior) or three (middle, anterior, and posterior) major cerebral arteries will result in infarction of the arterial border zone between them, as is apparent from the discussion of the internal carotid artery involvement. These infarcts are often discontinuous and consist of series of small cortical infarcts, creating a condition known as granular atrophy when they are old. Fresh lesions of this type are rarely seen at autopsy because these are not fatal conditions by themselves. Multiple embolization from the neck arteries (see section 1.0) can produce a similar type of lesion. Whether stenotic or embolic in origin, the area of granular atrophy may become swallowed up by a new, larger area of infarction in the distribution of one of the component arteries (most commonly the middle cerebral artery) as the stenosis progresses to a complete occlusion.

B. Vertebral-basilar system

Several important anatomic considerations should be made before discussion of infarction in this territory.

1. The vertebral arteries are often unequal in size and contribute unequally to the flow in the basilar circulation. The smaller one is often totally occluded by atherosclerosis without creating lesions in the brain tissue.

2. Branches from the vertebral arteries and the basilar artery are quite variable in origin, and so are the size and area of their irrigation, from individual to individual. Isolated obstruction of one or more of these vessels will result in greatly variable patterns of infarction.

3. The source of blood supply to the posterior cerebral arteries also varies, depending on the configuration of the circle of Willis (which is often asymmetric). When the posterior communicating artery is large and the proximal posterior cerebral artery is small, the distal posterior cerebral artery becomes the direct extension of the internal carotid artery, whereas if the proximal posterior cerebral artery is large and the posterior communicating artery is small, the basilar artery contributes mainly to the blood flow of the posterior cerebral artery.

4. The vertebral arteries have several anastomoses between their own branches and also extensive communications with branches of the external carotid artery, subclavian artery, and aorta (Fig. 1–15).

Prediction, based on occlusion of individual arteries, as to the location and extent of resultant infarction in the vertebral-basilar system is often impossible. Also, the clinical signs and symptoms may indicate areas of involvement, but they do not necessarily indicate which artery is occluded.

1. Vertebral artery (Fig. 1–16)

When severe stenosis or occlusion of a vertebral artery occurs in the neck, the location of infarction is difficult to predict, partly because of the variability of the branching pattern as indicated above and partly, and more importantly, because of the possibility of preferential atheromatous stenosis of the origin of any of the penetrating arteries of the brainstem which makes its distribution more vulnerable to otherwise marginal vascular insufficiency.

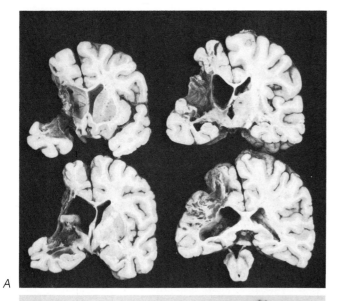

A

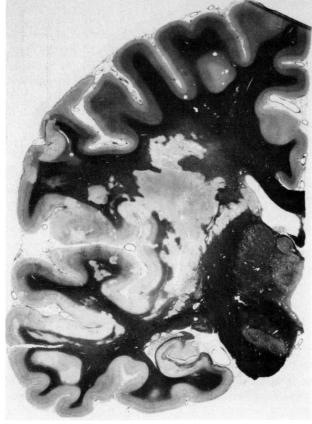

B

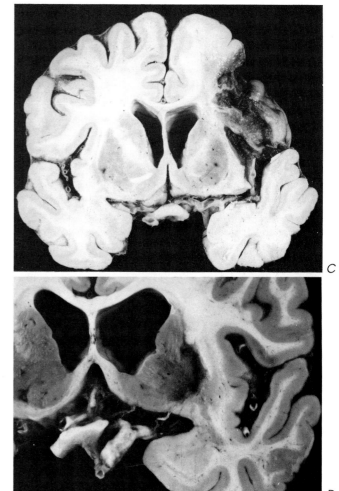

C

D

Figure 1–12. Infarctive lesions related to middle cerebral artery. A, Old infarct of "entire" left middle cerebral artery territory. Note that in more proximal portion of involvement, tissue breakdown is complete, but peripheral portions show irregular mixture of destroyed and surviving tissues and do not exactly follow an "anatomy textbook pattern." B, More irregular and patchy infarction of the left middle cerebral artery territory, due to occlusion of proximal portion of middle cerebral artery (LFB/CV). C, Old infarct limited to "cortical" portion of right middle cerebral artery territory (also exclusive of right temporal lobe), due to occlusion distal to perforators and anterior temporal branch. D, Infarct in territory of middle cerebral perforator, due to atheromatous occlusion at its origin.

With minimal stenosis of the basilar artery but with inadequate collateral circulation from the internal carotid arteries (via the posterior communicating arteries), the arterial border zone of the cerebellar arteries may be infarcted. An additional arterial border zone (of the three penetrating branches) that may become infarcted lies at the junction of the base and tegmentum of the pons.

When the subclavian artery is occluded, with obliteration of the origin of the vertebral, thyrocervical, and costocervical arteries, there is greater impairment of the flow in the posterior circulation because of the compromise of the collateral pathways described above.

If the subclavian artery is occluded proximal to the origin of the vertebral artery, the blood supply to the arm may

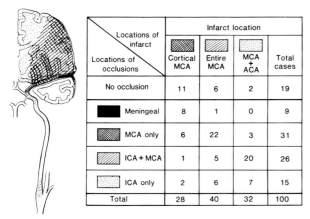

Locations of occlusions	Infarct location			
	Cortical MCA	Entire MCA	MCA + ACA	Total cases
No occlusion	11	6	2	19
■ Meningeal	8	1	0	9
▦ MCA only	6	22	3	31
▨ ICA + MCA	1	5	20	26
▒ ICA only	2	6	7	15
Total	28	40	32	100

Figure 1–13. Correlation of middle cerebral artery (MCA) and anterior cerebral artery (ACA) distribution infarcts and sites of arterial occlusion (when present) based on recent autopsy studies of 100 patients who had died within 35 days of the clinical onset of stroke. ICA = internal carotid artery.

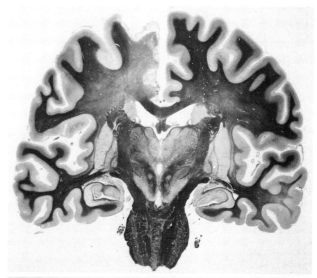

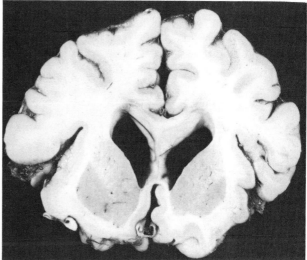

Figure 1–14. Infarcts in territory of anterior cerebral artery. *A,* Predominantly cortical old infarct in distribution of left anterior cerebral artery, with pallor of underlying white matter, due to secondary fiber degeneration (LFB/CV). *B,* Old infarct on both sides of anterior corpus callosum associated with atheromatous stenosis of anterior cerebral arteries.

be largely dependent upon retrograde flow from the basilar artery (and the anterior circulation via the circle of Willis) or the opposite vertebral artery. A greatly increased demand for blood during exercise of the arm could precipitate clinical evidence of cerebral ischemia. This is known as "subclavian steal syndrome."

When the intracranial portion of the vertebral artery is occluded, the collateral connection in the neck is no longer helpful, and the chance of infarction increases.

The occlusion of the origin of the posterior inferior cerebellar artery or of the small medullary branches will further increase the possibility of infarction, particularly in the lateral sulcal region of the medulla. The resulting clinical syndrome is referred to as Wallenberg's syndrome or the lateral medullary syndrome. Variation in size of this infarct depends on the difference in the efficacies of the leptomeningeal anastomoses. The distal territory of the posterior inferior cerebellar artery (the inferior medial surface of the cerebellar hemisphere) may additionally or independently become infarcted in the absence of adequate collateral flow from the superior cerebellar artery or anterior inferior cerebellar artery.

The simultaneous occlusion of both vertebral arteries results in a similar pattern of infarction as that of basilar artery thrombosis. More commonly, one vertebral artery is rudimentary or severely or totally compromised before the other, which has been acting as virtually the single source of blood supply to the basilar artery, becomes occluded. Unilateral occlusion of the smaller of the two vertebral arteries (as is usually the case) may not cause any infarction.

2. Basilar artery (Fig. 1–17)

Occlusion of the basilar artery may result in total infarction of its entire anatomic territories, including both the thalami and occipital lobes in addition to the brainstem and cerebellar structures. However, in more than half of the cases of complete thrombosis of the basilar artery, scattered patchy infarction in various combinations of involved anatomic areas of the brainstem, cerebellum, and pons occurs in an utterly unpredictable manner. This is naturally affected by variable extents of anastomoses between the terminal portions of the branch arteries of the basilar artery and also by the efficacy of collateral flow from the anterior circulation.

Penetrating brainstem branches of the basilar artery are often occluded by a segmental clot in the main artery, and this accounts for the ready occurrence of infarction of their territory, even when other areas are spared. This differs from the effect of bilateral occlusion of the vertebral arteries.

Some of the small infarcts in the brainstem are likely to be the result of arteriolar sclerosis of the penetrating arterial branches (see section 1.3).

Isolated occlusion of vertebral and basilar artery

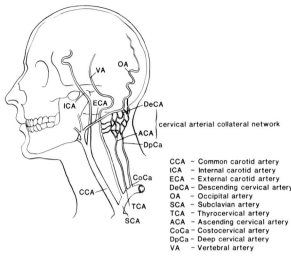

CCA – Common carotid artery
ICA – Internal carotid artery
ECA – External carotid artery
DeCA – Descending cervical artery
OA – Occipital artery
SCA – Subclavian artery
TCA – Thyrocervical artery
ACA – Ascending cervical artery
CoCa – Costocervical artery
DpCa – Deep cervical artery
VA – Vertebral artery

cervical arterial collateral network

Figure 1–15. Collateral pathways between the vertebral artery and the extracranial arteries. (Modified from Bosniak MA: Cervical arterial pathways associated with brachiocephalic occlusive disease. Am J Roentgenol 91:1232–1244, 1964. By permission of the American Roentgen Ray Society.)

branches is relatively infrequent. Of these, the posterior inferior cerebellar artery is most often affected, either at its origin or in its proximal segment and mostly by atherosclerosis or thrombosis (or both). Resulting infarction is in the inferior aspect of the ipsilateral cerebellar hemisphere. Many of these infarcts are apparently clinically silent or are dismissed as minor events unless accompanied by Wallenberg's syndrome, for old, scarred infarcts in this territory are not rare at autopsy without corresponding anamnesis.

The superior aspects of the cerebellar hemisphere may be infarcted with or without involvement of the dorsolateral aspect of the upper brainstem, as a result, for instance, of occlusion of the superior cerebellar artery.

Occasionally, a large cerebellar infarction accompanied by significant edema compresses the brainstem, particularly the medulla, and results in a fatal outcome. Clinical localization of such an infarct is often difficult without the aid of a computed tomography scan or arteriography.

Infarcts in the posterior circulatory region, without associated thrombotic occlusion (but with stenosis), are seen in

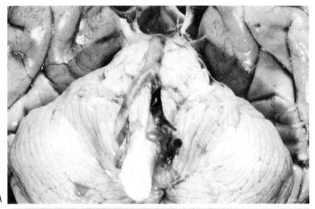

A

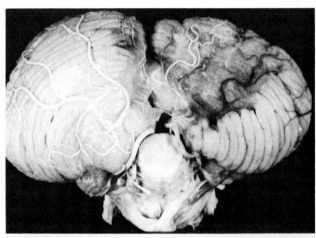

C

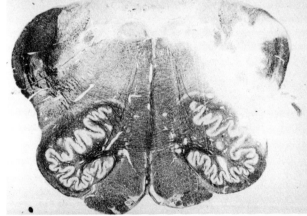

B

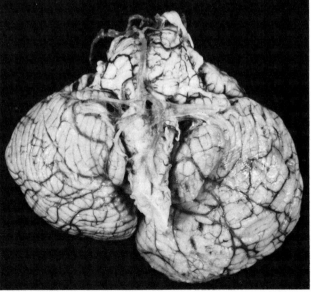

D

Figure 1–16. Infarctive lesions of vertebral artery. A and B, Left vertebral artery thrombosis resulting in infarction of lateral medullary area (Wallenberg syndrome). (B, LFB/CV.) C, Old infarct associated with occlusion of distal inferior cerebellar artery. Arteries are injected with white contrast medium. Nonfilling arteries appear black. D, Extensive left cerebellar infarction due to thrombosis of ipsilateral vertebral and posterior inferior cerebellar arteries. Note pronounced swelling with tonsillar herniation of involved side.

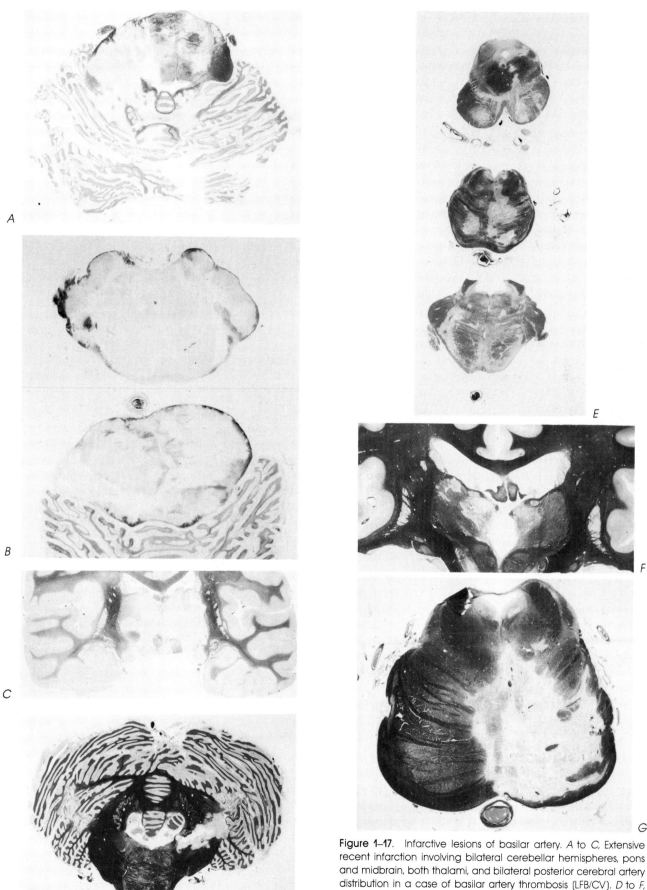

A

B

C

D

E

F

G

Figure 1–17. Infarctive lesions of basilar artery. *A* to *C,* Extensive recent infarction involving bilateral cerebellar hemispheres, pons and midbrain, both thalami, and bilateral posterior cerebral artery distribution in a case of basilar artery thrombosis (LFB/CV). *D* to *F,* More patchy but similarly widespread pattern of infarction due to basilar artery thrombosis. *G,* More one-sided infarction of pons in basilar artery thrombosis.

10 to 20% of angiographically studied cases. These are due either to hemodynamic factors or to breaking up of an embolus.

Sometimes the effects of severe compromise of the vertebral-basilar system may be felt, not in the area directly supplied by it but in the anterior circulation, often in an arterial border zone distribution. This is expected when the anterior circulation has already been restricted but has been receiving an adequate collateral flow from the vertebral artery and basilar artery before they have been compromised.

3. Posterior cerebral artery (Fig. 1–18)

In most instances, the posterior cerebral artery is a direct extension of the basilar artery, and as such its territory becomes infarcted, often bilaterally, when there is insufficiency in the posterior circulation. In other instances, this artery is an extension, via the posterior communicating artery, of the anterior circulation, either unilaterally or bilaterally, and shares the fate of that artery. Isolated occlusion of this artery, either at its proximal trunk or at its branches, by atheroma or embolism also occurs. Its compression by an expanding supratentorial mass is discussed in section 1.9.

C. Spinal arterial system (Fig. 1–19)

Involvement of identifiable individual intraspinal arteries, such as the anterior spinal artery, by atherosclerosis, thrombosis, or embolism is rare.

More commonly, the disease (usually atherosclerosis) of the aorta, particularly the thoracic and upper abdominal aorta above the renal artery, is responsible for infarction within the spinal cord.

In humans, only a few (5 to 10) significant radicular arteries supply the spinal cord. Two areas of the spinal cord are vulnerable to infarction, as follows:

1. The midthoracic (roughly at T-4) segments, which constitute a longitudinal arterial border zone, often with complete cross-sectional infarction at this level and with rostral and caudal tapering ends. The tapering ends represent a cross-sectional arterial border zone between the anterior and posterior spinal arteries. This type of infarction is thought to result from sudden total ischemia to this zone, usually as a result of systemic hypotension or lesions of the thoracic aorta such as dissecting aneurysm and surgical ligation of the aorta at this level.

2. The lumbar segment, with predominantly anterior spinal infarction involving principally the ventral horns. This area is thought to be a distal area of supply by the single large artery, the arteria radicularis magna of Adamskiewicz, without potential substitution by way of an invariably slender midthoracic arterial network.

Note: Small ischemic foci may be found in elderly patients with aortic atherosclerosis, particularly in the cervical (C-5 to C-6) and lumbar segments. These lesions are found in the anterior horns or their bases and have no clear-cut relationship to the position of the radicular arteries, and no intramedullary vascular lesions are demonstrated to explain them.

1.14 Natural History of Ischemic Cerebral Vascular Disease

It is a common clinical observation that when a cerebral infarct occurs, the development of neurologic deficit is relatively rapid—reaching its maximum usually within a few hours. If the patient survives, there is a clinical improvement in the deficit over a variable period of time, and in the end the patient is left with some or no residual deficit.

After the conclusion of this stroke episode, over a longer period of time, if not the patient's lifetime, he or she may or may not have additional stroke(s).

There are three different standpoints from which one looks at the natural history of ischemic stroke episode(s) without regard to other factors, such as etiology or pathology. These are based on the length of clinical observation: brief initial observation, the entire course of the illness, and the patient's lifetime.

I. Brief Initial Observation

The brief period of examination or clinical observation (a few minutes to hours) usually relates to the initial handling of the patient, with particular reference to the possible progression, stabilization, or improvement of clinical signs and symptoms. Three separate categories of the "temporal profile" have been described (Millikan et al., 1975): transient ischemic attacks, progressive stroke or stroke-in-evolution, and completed stroke.

It must be realized that the term "temporal profile," as applied to progressive stroke or stroke-in-evolution and completed stroke at least, does not refer to the "entire course" of a single stroke episode but rather indicates a "clinical stage" of a stroke as a segment of its totality. Transient ischemic attack is defined as *temporary* focal cerebral dysfunction of vascular origin which usually lasts only 2 or 3 minutes to 30 minutes but rarely as long as 24 hours. Naturally, if an episode as long as 24 hours in duration is to be included, a brief (hours) clinical observation may not permit a designation of transient ischemic attack for this episode.

The designation of transient ischemic attack is possible only when the entire course of the event has been run.

II. Entire Course of Illness

The entire course of a single stroke episode may be reviewed retrospectively at the "end point" (that is, when the deficit disappears completely or when it reaches the stable residual level). This standpoint fits more closely the common usage of the term "profile" than that applied to the mode of observation in cases of transient ischemic attack. Naturally, a stroke episode of very short duration can likely be observed in its totality.

Most ischemic strokes have three phases when the severity of neurologic deficits is plotted against the lapsed time, as indicated in Figure 1–20.

The first is the *developing phase* (A). This is the phase in which there is progressive worsening of deficits or the inter-

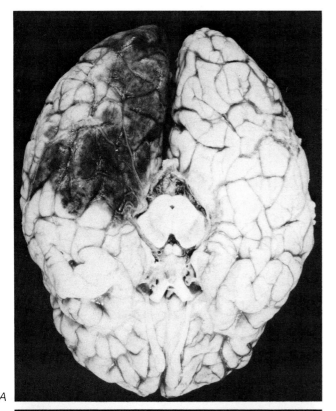

A

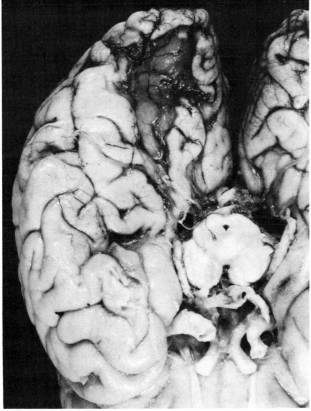

B

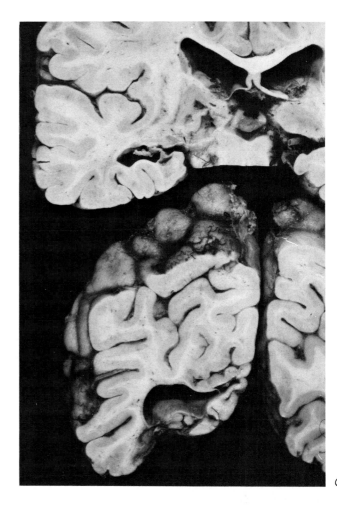

C

Figure 1–18. Infarctive lesions of posterior cerebral artery. *A*, Acute hemorrhagic infarction involving large area of left posterior cerebral artery, due to embolic occlusion in its proximal portion from postinfarctive mural thrombus in left ventricle of heart. *B*, More restricted old infarct in posterior cerebral artery distribution (clinically 20 years old, presumably embolic in origin). *C*, Old infarcts involving left posterior thalamus, hippocampus, and occipital and adjacent temporal lobes, due to atherosclerotic stenosis of proximal posterior cerebral artery.

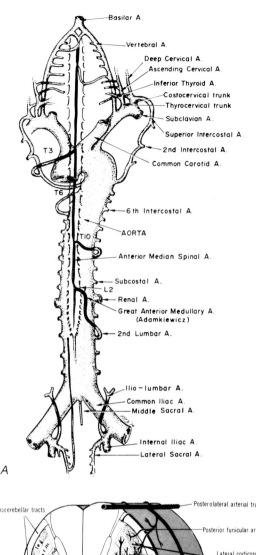

A

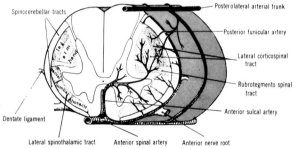

B

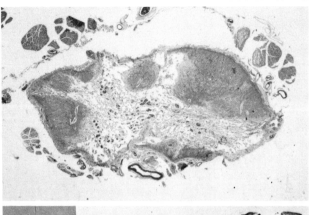

C

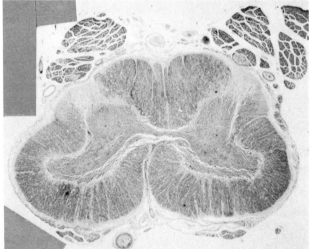

D

Figure 1–19. Infarctive lesions of spinal arterial system. *A,* Diagram of major arterial supply to spinal cord. *B,* Cross-sectional distribution pattern of intraspinal blood supply. *C,* Actual case of old lower spinal cord infarction due apparently to compromise of blood supply at some point external to spinal canal (LFB/PAS/H). (No intradural arterial occlusion was demonstrated.) Note irregular zone of ischemic necrosis. *D,* Predominantly gray matter involvement secondary to hypoxic episode resulting from thoracic aortic surgery. (*A* from Herrick MK, Mills PE Jr: Infarction of spinal cord: two cases of selective gray matter involvement secondary to asymptomatic aortic disease. *Arch Neurol* 24:228–241, 1971. By permission of the American Medical Association; *B,* from Schneider RC, Crosby EC: Vascular insufficiency of brain stem and spinal cord in spinal trauma. *Neurology* [Minneap] 9:643–656, 1959. By permission of Harcourt Brace Jovanovich.)

val between the onset and the "peak." With a sudden occlusion of a major artery, such as by embolism, this phase takes a rather sharply ascending course with an abrupt onset of symptoms, which reach their maximal intensity within a matter of minutes. With thrombosis, which is presumed to take longer to establish a complete arterial obstruction, there tends to be a stuttering onset and a stepwise development of symptoms over a period of time, sometimes extending for several hours. This corresponds to the phase of stroke-in-evolution. It is not possible to predict with certainty, at any given point of this phase, the future course of the stroke.

The patient may succumb during this phase, either from the direct effects of cerebral tissue necrosis or, more likely, particularly in cases of massive supratentorial infarction, from secondary mass effects of the swollen necrotic tissue and surrounding edema upon the brainstem, as detailed in section 1.9. This phenomenon reaches its maximum 3 to 4 days after the onset of a stroke and is usually accompanied by deteriorating state of consciousness, pupillary paralysis, and decerebrate posture.

The *peak period* (or, rarely, *point*) (*B*) is reached when all of the areas destined to be involved become ischemic or,

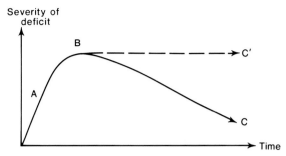

Figure 1-20. Three phases of a stroke episode. *A* = developing phase; *B* = peak; *C* = recovery phase (total or near-total recovery of deficit), and *C'* = stable permanent deficit. See text for explanation.

in fact, infarcted. The symptoms are maximal (that is, maximal for this particular episode, and not necessarily "complete") and remain so for some time—that is, the deficit becomes fixed and stable. In infarction of the territory of the internal carotid artery, 18 to 24 hours, and in infarction of the vertebral-basilar territory longer than 24 hours and perhaps up to 72 hours of this plateau period, are necessary before one can predict that further progression of deficit is unlikely. This corresponds to the phase of "completed stroke."

The plateau phase may be short and be followed by a rapid deterioration of the clinical status due to the development of the secondary changes described above.

The third stage is the *recovery phase* (C). The rate and extent of return of impaired neurologic functions vary considerably from case to case. When disturbances of function are due to actual necrosis (that is, death of neurons), recovery of that function is not likely. However, if it is due to reversible ischemia, as might be expected at the margin of the necrotic focus, or is due to tissue compression by edema of the infarcted and surrounding area, good functional recovery is expected. A relatively rapid improvement (over the next several hours) of major symptoms is often ascribed to disintegration and distal passage of an embolus with reopening of the obstruction to blood flow, assuming that the involved area has been ischemic but not irreversibly damaged (or infarcted). Naturally, the longer the duration of the deficit, the less likely is the possibility of eventual recovery of the area.

A great deal of attention has been given in recent years to a clinical type of stroke episode (presumably ischemic) that is characterized by complete resolution of any neurologic deficit—"stroke with full recovery." One may distinguish two types:

A. Transient ischemic attacks (TIA) (Fig. 1-21) (transient cerebral ischemia, transient vascular insufficiency), which are defined as episodes of temporary focal cerebral dysfunction of vascular origin. Symptoms are often minor but usually stereotypical. The duration of these episodes is variable but short, often between a few minutes to 30 minutes. Some authors allow as much as 24 hours. These episodes are often recurrent and repetitive and have varying intervals. A considerable latitude in definition is observed in numerous reports on the subject, resulting in a wide difference in the

interpretation of their data in regard to the frequency, significance, and pathogenesis.

B. Reversible ischemic neurologic deficits (RIND) (prolonged ischemic attacks). This category was created to accommodate a group of transient stroke episodes characterized by a slower development and a longer persistence of symptoms over 24 hours and up to 3 weeks (or even up to 60 days by some authors).

For both of these conditions, it is presumed that the episodes are due to temporary (i.e., reversible) ischemic dysfunction of neurons short of cell death. In some patients with transient ischemic attacks, no structural lesions in the CNS parenchyma can be demonstrated at autopsy. It is, however, quite clear that some, and perhaps many, of these episodes are in fact due to small infarcts with or without demonstrable vascular occlusion. The issue is complicated by the frequent finding at autopsy of small, often multiple infarcts for which no clinical counterparts are recorded. Naturally, it is not known whether this is due to omissions in anamnesis or actual absence of clinical symptoms. It is true that some are located in the so-called silent areas of the brain, but others are clearly in the areas, such as the motor cortex, where a functional deficit is expected.

Several partially understood mechanisms are thought to be involved in the production of TIA or RIND (or both).

1. Angiospasm

Spasm of cerebral arteries was once a popular concept, but the current consensus is that it does not occur in the cerebral arteries except in the presence of subarachnoid hemorrhage or migraine.

2. Embolism

Mural thrombus on or atheromatous material from ulcerated plaques in the extracranial arteries, particularly at the cervical internal carotid arteries, is known to embolize and obstruct small cerebral arteries at least temporarily before breaking up to disappear into the distal circulation. A similar phenomenon can actually be observed in the retina of living patients. Some authors object to this pathogenetic explanation, claiming that the repetitive nature of cerebral symptoms is not adequately explained by the unpredictability of embolic scattering in the brain. There are, however, experimental data to suggest that embolic material of the same size tends to reach the same general area of the brain. Other sources of emboli listed previously may occasionally be involved. At present, the embolic genesis of transient ischemic attacks is the most popularly held view.

3. Hemodynamic factors

Temporary disturbance of cerebral perfusion can occur as a result of fluctuation in blood pressure or cardiac output (as in cardiac arrhythmia), particularly in the presence of stenosis or occlusion of cervical or cerebral arteries. The lesions are expected to be in arterial border zones. Relatively infrequent documentation of such episodes in relation to transient ischemic attacks is cited by some authors as the reason for objecting to this pathogenetic explanation.

4. Disturbance of intracranial vascular autoregulation

Severely arteriosclerotic vessels are incapable of normal

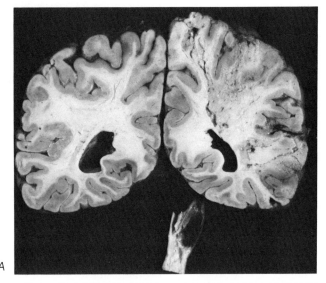

A

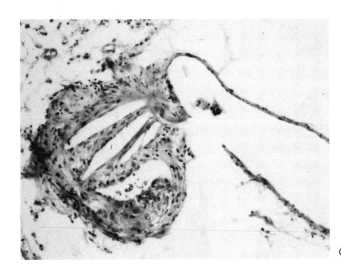

C

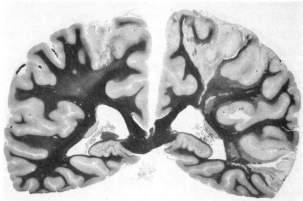

B

Figure 1–21. Transient ischemic attacks and major stroke. A, Gross photograph of posterior cerebral hemispheres and right carotid bifurcation shows atheromatous stenosis and superimposed recent thrombosis. B, Corresponding brain slice stained for myelin (LFB) shows smaller and older (paler in this preparation) arterial border zone infarcts (greater on right) and more extensive and recent infarction of right middle cerebral artery distribution. Older lesions show evidence of old atheromatous embolization as at least part of cause. C, Example of leptomeningeal arteries over older arterial border zone infarcts on right containing organized atheromatous embolus, which evidently came from ulcerated plaque at carotid bifurcation before total occlusion and accounts for repeated transient ischemic attachs (H&E).

response to changing blood pressure and may permit a temporary circulatory disturbance.

5. Arterial thrombosis

Some form of disturbance of the coagulation mechanism may be present to cause thrombotic occlusion of small cerebral arteries. A quick establishment of collateral circulation is invoked to explain the temporary nature of the attacks. The possibility exists that changes related to atherosclerosis serve as triggering factors for various hematologic changes that promote thrombosis.

The major significance of transient ischemic attacks is that one-third or more of affected patients will have a stroke within 5 years or less, which is nearly 10 times as frequent as the incidence of stroke among the general population of comparable age. Another third will continue to have recurrence of transient ischemic attacks, and in the last third, transient ischemic attacks will cease. It is impossible to predict the prognosis in each individual case, and the only practical rule appears to be to investigate all cases of transient ischemic attacks expeditiously so that either a medical or a surgical treatment can be instituted when appropriate to prevent the occurrence of a major stroke.

Recent Mayo Clinic experience (Jones and Millikan, 1976) with 179 patients with recent stroke, presumably in-

volving the internal carotid artery, who were seen during the first 7-day period is tabulated in Table 1–5.

The different outcomes in relationship to these grades are displayed in Table 1–6.

It was found that if hemiplegia developed within 3 hours of the onset of symptoms and persisted for 36 hours, there was a 90% or greater chance that the patient would have a permanent incapacitating motor deficit. This group of patients has an entirely different prognosis from the group in which a grade 2 hemiparesis develops within 6 to 12 hours of onset.

For the small number of cases with relapse (4 and 5 of Table 1–5), there was no clinical clue to help identify these cases in advance of the relapse. No pathologic explanation was offered for this particular type of course.

Of 44 patients who had a −4 deficit accompanied by any alteration of consciousness, 18 (41%) died, whereas of 64 patients with a −4 deficit alone, only 1 (<2%) died. From these figures, it is obvious that alteration of consciousness carries a very poor prognosis. This is understandable since the altered (depressed) state of consciousness in patients with supratentorial infarction is almost invariably due to the secondary compression of the brainstem (see section 1.9). The overall mortality (10.6%) in these 179 patients is only slightly below the figure of 13% for the group of 144 patients

TABLE 1–5. Course in 179 Patients With Recent Internal Carotid Artery Territory Stroke

Type of Course	Number of Patients	Percent with −4 Deficit*
1. Progressive worsening of deficit associated with deterioration of consciousness	34 (19%)	13/34 = 38%
2. Essentially unchanged deficit	66 (37%)	61/66 = 92%
3. Improved deficit without exacerbation	62 (35%)	26/62 = 42%
4. Remission and early relapse	6 (3%)	5/6 = 83%
5. Late exacerbation (after stabilization within 48 hours)	8 (4%)	6/8 = 75%

* The severity of the initial neurologic deficit is graded as −1 through −4.

reported more than 20 years ago (Millikan and Moersch, 1953) from the same institution. From another series of ischemic stroke patients of the Rochester, Minnesota, population (Whisnant et al., 1971), the death rate at the end of 1 month was 27%. This corresponds to the report for a previous general hospital series of 612 patients by Carter (1964), which gives the figure of 26%. In contrast to early death by secondary brainstem compression occurring within the first few days of a stroke episode, later death is usually due to intercurrent infection, mainly pneumonia, or to cardiac failure from coronary arteriosclerotic heart disease.

The above classification is limited to observation of single stroke episodes without regard to underlying pathology or pathogenesis and is of little value in the long-term study of patients.

III. Patient's Lifetime

Another important aspect of the true and complete temporal profile, therefore, is the question of stroke recurrence in a patient's lifetime. It is well recognized that some patients

TABLE 1–6. Comparison of the Severity of Initial Deficit and Outcome in 179 Patients With Recent Internal Carotid Artery Territory Stroke

	Severity of Initial Deficit			
	−1 (N = 18)	−2 (N = 34)	−3 (N = 16)	−4 (N = 111)
Full recovery	33%	24%	12%	4%
Improved with deficit	44%	59%	69%	24%
Unchanged or worse	22%	17%	19%	55%
Death				17%

may have a major stroke with no subsequent recurrence until death by other causes, whereas others will have multiple transient ischemic attacks or prolonged strokes with residual deficit and may eventually die of a major stroke. The latter group of patients may be termed as having an "active" form of cerebral vascular disease. Hypertension is implicated as a predisposing factor for this active form in some of the clinical series. However, it is apparent that some of these patients are, in fact, suffering from small intracerebral hemorrhages or small infarcts related to arteriolar sclerosis of deep penetrating vessels (see section 1.3), both of which may present themselves clinically as episodes of transient ischemic attack or reversible ischemic neurologic deficit.

It is evident that more data are necessary before an accurate picture of the natural history of stroke can be drawn.

1.2 CENTRAL NERVOUS SYSTEM DAMAGE DUE TO SYSTEMIC CIRCULATORY FACTORS (ANOXIC OR HYPOXIC ENCEPHALOPATHY)

1.21 Types of Conditions That Lead to Hypoxic Encephalopathy

These conditions are identical to those listed in section 1.0. We are naturally more concerned here with systemic factors that tend to affect the whole brain (cerebral hypoxia or anoxia) rather than the consequence of local vascular abnormalities (cerebral infarction). These include hypoxia, stagnation, and hypoglycemia.

A. Hypoxia
Hypoxia, or reduced oxygen content of the inspired air, results in reduced oxygen tension in the blood (hypoxemia) that reaches the brain. This situation occurs clinically in asphyxiation, severe pulmonary infection, respiratory insufficiency or arrest, anesthesia, and so on.

B. Stagnation
1. *Oligemia* is local or generalized reduction in cerebral blood flow.
2. *Ischemia* is local or generalized arrest in cerebral blood flow.

Major clinical situations in which these changes occur include exsanguination, cardiac arrhythmia, cardiac arrest, and so on. Humans who are resuscitated after episodes of cardiac arrest which lasted longer than 3 to 5 minutes often either die within a short time or suffer severe brain injury. Episodes of arrest briefer than 3 minutes may leave patients with neurologic impairment.

C. Hypoglycemia
In hypoglycemia, there is nonutilization of available oxygen, due to the lack of glycogen to be "burned" for energy production. The net effects are similar to those of anoxia.

1.22 Morphologic Changes Seen in Hypoxic Encephalopathy (Figs. 1–22 to 1–24)

All conditions listed above have similar effects on the brain. Neurons are most susceptible, but other elements will also suffer as the degree of insult increases—a situation comparable to that seen in the development of an infarct (see section 1.1). If death occurs within several hours (3 to 6 hours), morphologic evidence of cellular necrosis may be entirely lacking. Eosinophilic (''ischemic'') degeneration of neurons becomes more evident as time passes. Not all neurons are equally affected, and there appear to be patterns of ''selective vulnerability.''

These characteristic patterns of tissue necrosis become more apparent as the survival time extends after the anoxia/hypoglycemia episode. The histologic evolution of tissue damage and of the reparative process is the same as described for cerebral infarcts of various degrees of severity. A clearer understanding of various patterns of tissue damage in relation to varied types and degrees of stagnation anoxia (or hypoxia) has been gained in recent years both from clinical observations and from experimental data (Brierley, 1972).

A. The belief was held that brain damage can result from a simple reduction in the oxygen tension of arterial blood (hypoxemia) for a sufficient time. The reported pattern of brain damage was indistinguishable from that following profound arterial hypotension with normal arterial oxygenation. It is now recognized that primary *hypoxia* can bring about brain damage only through the medium of a secondary reduction in cerebral perfusion, due to a reduced cardiac output. The reduced cardiac output results from the vulnerability of the heart to hypoxia.

B. The brain damage due to *overall oligemia* (as opposed to ischemia, i.e., total cessation of flow) is determined by the rate at which the blood pressure falls, the lowest pressure attained, its duration, and the rate at which it returns to normal. A moderate decrease in brain perfusion pressure does not result in a reduction in cerebral blood flow, because of autoregulatory vasodilatation and the consequent reduction in cerebral vascular resistance. When this autoregulatory process fails after a maximal vasodilatation, cerebral blood flow will then decrease in parallel with the perfusion pressure. Three patterns of brain damage are described as the result of cerebral oligemia due to systemic arterial hypotension (Adams et al., 1966), as follows:

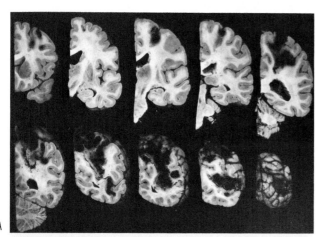

A

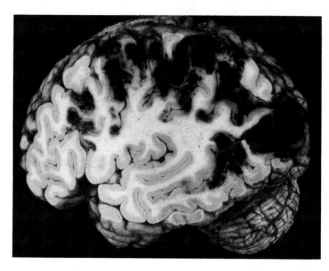

C

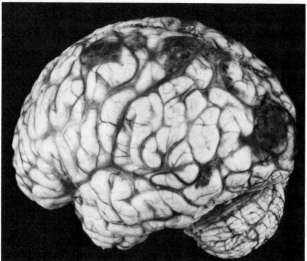

B

Figure 1–22. Hypoxic encephalopathy with arterial border zone-type damage (hemorrhagic infarction). *A,* Frontal sections of right cerebral hemisphere. *B,* External view of left cerebral hemisphere. *C,* Left cerebral hemisphere sectioned along plane of arterial border zone.

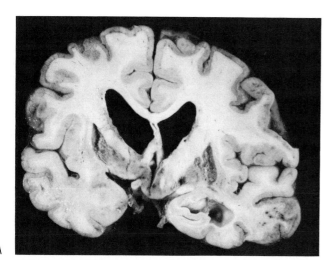

A

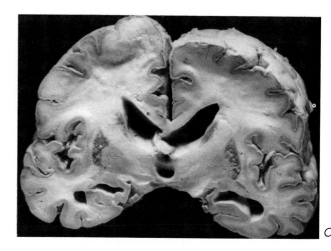

C

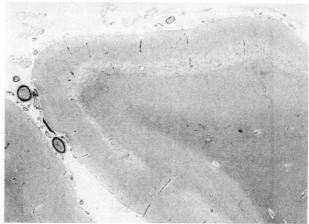

B

Figure 1–23. Laminar necrosis pattern of hypoxic encephalopathy. *A,* Deeper layers of cerebral cortex show more or less continuous pattern of necrosis accentuated in arterial border zones, coupled with necrosis of basal ganglia, particularly of putamen and caudate. *B,* Lower-power view of midcortical layer of ischemic damage (LFB/PAS/H). *C,* More extensive cortical involvement with pronounced atrophy (reduction in thickness) of entire cortical layers yet still showing laminar accentuation of damage.

1. Arterial border zone pattern

Ischemic changes are concentrated along the arterial border zones between the territories of the major cerebral and cerebellar arteries; they are minimal or absent in the hippocampus. The most frequently and severely affected is the parieto-occipital region, which constitutes the junction of the three cerebral arteries. This pattern is a consequence of a major and abrupt fall in systemic blood pressure. Since reperfusion of the damaged area usually occurs after the insult, infarction, when present, is often hemorrhagic as a result of leakage through damaged capillaries.

2. Generalized and cortical (laminar necrosis) pattern

Both the cerebral and cerebellar cortices are affected. The depth of sulci and the third, fifth, and sixth cerebral cortical laminae are more vulnerable. In the cerebellum, the Purkinje cells are most vulnerable.

In the hippocampus, Sommer's sector (h-1) is most vulnerable, and h-2 is the most resistant portion ("the dorsal resistant zone"). (See note below.) The caudate nucleus and putamen are not invariably involved, and their involvement varies in degree and extent. Ischemic damage is less frequent in the globus pallidus.

In the neonate, foci of tissue necrosis are usually symmetrically located in the inferior colliculi and other

brainstem nuclei rather than in the cerebral cortex. Adult cases may show this pattern of brainstem damage in addition to the usual supratentorial lesions.

It appears that this generalized pattern is associated with hypotension of relatively slow onset but of long duration. Early vasodilatation combined with a slowly falling perfusion pressure is thought to ensure that a critical level of blood flow is not restricted but affects all arterial territories more or less equally.

Note: The pyramidal layer of the hippocampus, particularly Sommer's sector, is often preferentially affected in anoxia and hypoglycemia (see below). The chronic damage to this area may be the only evidence of anoxia, as in persons with repeated episodes of generalized convulsive seizure with attendant sublethal episodes of apnea. A scarred state (gliosis) is known as "hippocampal sclerosis," or "mesial temporal lobe sclerosis" when the damage extends beyond to include the neighboring structures.

3. Combined pattern

This type shows the combination of generalized ischemic alterations in the cerebral and cerebellar cortices, with a pronounced accentuation along the arterial border zones. This combination is quite frequent and suggests sudden

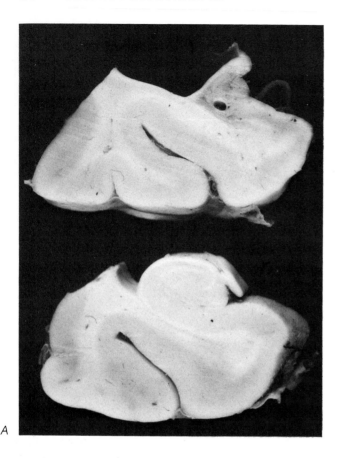

A

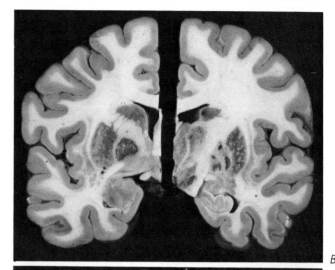

B

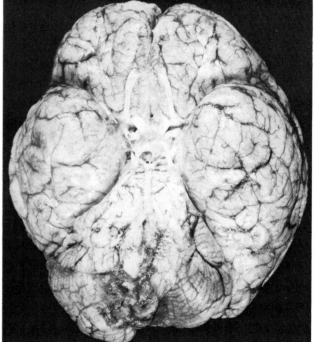

C

Figure 1–24. Other lesions of hypoxic encephalopathy. *A,* Unilateral hippocampal sclerosis (*Top*). Compare with uninvolved hippocampus (*Bottom*). *B,* Predominantly basal ganglionic pattern in patient with respiratory distress. Note asymmetry. *C,* Markedly swollen appearance with tonsillar necrosis in "respirator brain."

hypotension (for the arterial border zone lesions) and then a more sustained period of hypotension with reduced cerebral blood flow (for the generalized alterations).

4. Arterial supply territory pattern

Although not strictly considered as hypoxic encephalopathy, this pattern may be seen in association with systemic circulatory failure. When focally severe stenosis exists in one of the major cerebral arteries or thin branches, infarction may result in its territory only, the degree of generalized oligemia being insufficient to cause more widespread damage. This has already been discussed in section 1.1.

Overall ischemia is most commonly the result of cardiac arrest. If the arrest is of abrupt onset and termination, brain damage will be generalized in at least the neocortex and cerebellum.

Appreciable periods of reduced blood flow before or after a short period of cardiac arrest will lead to a concentration of ischemic alterations along the arterial border zones. Similarly, hitherto unrecognized and untreated hypotension occurring after arrest appears to account for the development of hemispheric brain injury among patients sustaining relatively short (4 to 5 minutes) episodes of circulatory arrest.

C. Hypoglycemia

The changes in the brain are essentially similar to those of hypoxia. The hippocampus is reported to be more preferentially affected, whereas the Purkinje cells are less involved. Hypoglycemia is often complicated by hypoxia, and this feature makes difficult a clear and separate delineation of the effects of pure hypoglycemia.

1.23 The "Respirator Brain"

The subject of the "respirator brain" is still plagued with conceptual difficulties. Many pathologists (Adams, 1976; Walker, 1976) believe that it represents what happens when a brain, after having sustained irreversible anoxic-ischemic damage, is supported by artificial means that are not sufficient to resuscitate or maintain neuronal activities. Autolytic changes of the brain proceed ("intravitam autolysis"), but with little or no reactive changes on the part of the supportive elements. Some suggest the term "brain death and autolysis" in lieu of the more colloquial "respirator brain." Others, however, believe that the "respirator brain" is due at least in part to premortem phenomena and the changes seen are not like those observed in the brain when autopsy is delayed for some days. For example, the brain changes appear to them to be a combination of severe hypoxic changes and severe edema, the edema itself being a hypoxic change possibly related to the acidosis that occurs in patients with deficient respiration and requiring a respirator. As the edema increases the intracranial pressure beyond arterial pressure, cerebral blood flow to the brain ceases and a vicious cycle ensues. In fact, a severe deficit of cerebral blood flow, as determined by failure of radioisotopic bolus injection clinically, has been shown to correlate with the characteristic neuropathologic features (Pearson et al., 1977). Regardless of the lack of total unanimity concerning the pathogenesis of this condition, the following morphologic features are generally agreed on.

A. Characteristic gross changes
1. Necrosis occurs, manifested by extreme softness and swelling (edema) and associated with evidence of circulatory stagnation, i.e., vascular congestion with or without petechial hemorrhage or venous (or arterial) thrombosis.
2. Herniation and necrosis of cerebellar tonsils develop, and these often fragment and descend into the spinal canal.
3. Even the spinal cord, particularly the gray matter, may be similarly affected. The upper cervical segments are more consistently affected, but necrosis may extend into the lumbar region.

B. Histologic changes (aside from those of a primary intracranial lesion)
1. There is eosinophilic ("ischemic") degeneration of some neurons, which appears to have occurred during the time when the brain was functioning metabolically.
2. Absence of vascular filling with fresh blood, lack of endothelial swelling, and absence of macrophage response or gliosis are noted.

1.3 HYPERTENSIVE VASCULAR DISEASE OF THE CNS

1.31 Hypertensive Lesions of the Arteries

It is convenient to consider various hypertensive CNS lesions schematically in relation to two major types of vascular changes—namely, those affecting large and those affecting small arteries (arterioles)—for both are age-dependent processes that are accelerated by arterial hypertension. Naturally, the transition between large and small arteries is gradual, and consequently both pathologic changes may be seen in intermediate-sized arteries (Table 1–7).

A. Atherosclerosis and its consequences
These have already been discussed. In hypertensive patients, atherosclerosis tends to be more severe in larger vessels and appears in smaller arteries that are not affected in normotensive individuals, such as superficial branches of the middle, anterior, and posterior cerebral arteries and major branches of the vertebral arteries and basilar artery. Proximal portions of deep penetrating arteries of the basal gray matter also become affected.

B. Hypertensive arterial changes (arteriosclerosis, arteriolar sclerosis) (Fig. 1–25)
Major types of pathologic alteration of the wall of arterioles are as follows.
1. Hyaline degeneration (synonym: hyalinosis, medial fibrosis)
The media (lamina muscularis) becomes replaced by collagenous tissue; the intima is also thickened with fibrous tissue, and this results in narrowing of the vascular lumen. Some arterioles show luminal dilatation instead.
2. Fibrinoid necrosis (synonym: plasmatic angionecrosis and others)

TABLE 1–7. Correlation of Vascular Alterations and Parenchymal Lesions in Arterial Hypertension

Types of Vessels	Pathologic Changes	Resultant CNS Lesions
A. Large arteries	Accelerated atherosclerosis (with or without thrombi)	Major infarct / Multiple small infarcts
B. Arterioles	Arteriolar sclerosis / Hyalinosis / Fibrinoid necrosis	Micro-aneurysms → Small hemorrhages / Massive hemorrhage
	Acute fibrinoid necrosis	(Hypertensive encephalopathy)

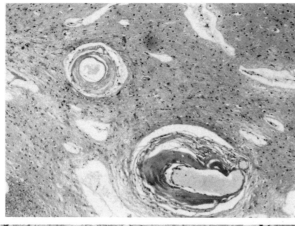

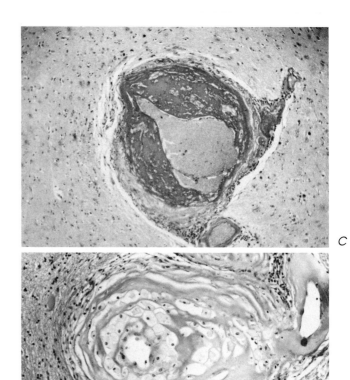

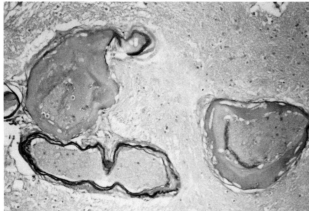

A

B

C

D

Figure 1–25. Arteriolar sclerosis in basal ganglia. *A,* Arteriole with muscular layer converted to fibrous tissue (hyalinosis) in left upper corner and arteriole whose hyalinized wall is further saturated with plasma (fibrinoid necrosis) in right lower corner (H&E). *B,* Arterioles with fibrinoid necrosis as viewed in EvG preparation. Note disruption and disappearance of internal elastic lamina. *C,* More extensive mural fibrinoid degeneration with early aneurysmal dilatation of lumen (H&E). *D,* Arteriolar sclerosis accompanied by numerous fat-laden macrophages within plasma-soaked, thickened wall (H&E).

Blood plasma permeates the vascular wall, which is already altered as above, and renders the wall an amorphous eosinophilic mass. Fibrin is demonstrable in the wall by histochemical means.

Note: C. M. Fisher (1971) introduced the term "lipohyalinosis" to separate these hypertensive arteriolar changes from the more common hyaline changes of aging arteries by adding the qualifying prefix "lipo," because the hyaline material in the wall also stains positively for fat. He also emphasized the presence of fat-laden macrophages within the altered arterial wall, and he noted that when they were present, the lesion might be related to the atherosclerosis.

3. True microaneurysm (Fig. 1–26)

One form of microaneurysm results from focal bulging of the arteriolar wall that has been weakened by the above-described changes (under pressure), with dilatation of the lumen either concentrically or eccentrically. C. M. Fisher (1972) called this form "lipohyalinotic aneurysm" or "miliary aneurysm in lipohyalinosis." In another form, the focally bulged arterial wall appears to be composed almost entirely of a layer of fibrin thrombus with evidence of red cell

extravasation outside of it. Fisher called this form "saccular miliary aneurysms" (or microaneurysms). Contrary to the previously popular view, he considered the latter form a focus of limited bleeding and not a stage in evolution of a lesion that will produce a massive hemorrhage. The true microaneurysms are most frequent in the putamen, then the cerebral cortex, thalamus, and caudate nucleus (seldom in the pallidum). The unique hemodynamics of the cerebral circulation (the relatively high arterial pressure that exists in the regional perforating blood vessels that originate directly from the main trunk of the middle cerebral artery) is considered the reason for the special frequency of microaneurysms in the basal ganglia.

Note: Fisher (1972) expressed the belief that the lesions that Charcot and Bouchard described in 1868 without detailed microscopic examination include these true microaneurysms as well as the false microaneurysms (bleeding globes of Matsuoka) to be described below in connection with gross hemorrhages (see section 1.32, B, 3).

4. Thrombotic obliteration of previously altered vessels (with a resultant infarct distally)

5. Healing of above changes

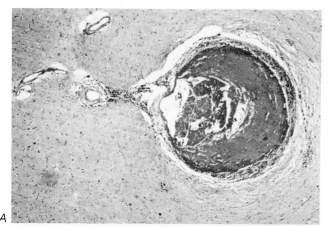

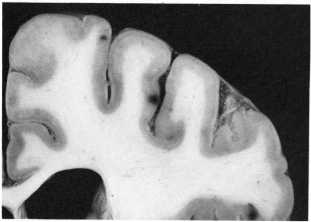

Figure 1–26. Hypertensive microaneurysm. *A,* Microaneurysm with extensive intraluminal but nonocclusive thrombosis in putamen. *B,* Multiple recent and old petechiae in cerebral cortex.

This consists of small fibrous nodes with obliterated lumens (0.4 to 1 mm in diameter) and often with evidence of previous perivascular hemorrhage.

1.32 Effects of Arteriolar (and Arterial) Sclerosis on Brain Parenchyma

A. Small infarcts (in the gray and white matter).

These tend to be multiple and therefore to create the following special forms.

1. État lacunaire (lacunar state) (Fig. 1–27).

This is a collection of multiple, small infarcts in the basal ganglia and thalamus. Small hemorrhages also result in similar small cavities. The original term "lacunes" refers to small cavities of both causes, which often coexist.

Note: Continued reference to individual small infarcts simply as "lacunes" represents a throwback to the macroscopic description of the mid-19th century. Although the term "état lacunaire," referring to a collection of such small holes, is still useful, these individual lesions should be described, when possible, by their rightful pathologic terms. It is also important to remember that a small number of these small infarcts may be due to transient (by embolism) or permanent

(by atheroma or thrombosis) occlusion of the parent arteries (middle cerebral artery, posterior communicating artery, and posterior cerebral artery) near the origin of the perforations, rather than due to intrinsic lesions of the intraparenchymal arterioles.

2. "Binswanger's disease" (subcortical arterio-(lo)-sclerotic encephalopathy) (Fig. 1–28)

This disorder consists of patchy or diffuse degeneration of white matter usually associated with multiple, more discrete focal necrosis (infarcts). Arteriolar sclerosis (mostly hyalinization) of long penetrating arterioles is usually present. It is assumed that this condition represents a particular variety of distal ischemic necrosis, but the vascular changes are disproportionately milder than the changes in the white matter in some instances. Although the diffuse component may be a result of secondary tract degeneration due to actual focal infarction, the paucity of such foci in some instances in the face of rather widespread degeneration requires explanation. An alternate theory is proposed which implicates the late effect of cerebral edema initiated by some aspects of hypertensive disease and relegates the vascular change to a secondary phenomenon resulting from the hypertensive disease itself and to the cerebral edema. This view may hold some truth, but the validity of the hypothesis in the total picture of this disease has yet to be determined.

As might be expected, the clinical picture of Binswanger's encephalopathy is that of subacute (or chronic) progressive deterioration of mental capacity without clear focal neurologic symptoms. However, there does not appear to be a close clinicopathologic correlation, for these changes, albeit mild, can be found incidentally at autopsy.

Note: Collections of the small cavitary lesions described above should be distinguished from "état criblé" (cribriform atrophy), which is not a true form of tissue damage due to hypertension and is commonly seen in elderly persons, sometimes in association with the above lesions. In the white matter, the individual component of this condition consists of a dilated perivascular space that often has, in longitudinal sections, a beads-in-a-string contour, containing varying numbers of collagenous fibers and mononuclear cells, often with pigment granules in their cytoplasm. A normal-appearing or slightly fibrotic blood vessel is found in the center. There is usually no evidence of degeneration of the surrounding tissue from this alteration alone. Therefore, the term "atrophy" is probably a misnomer. Early alteration of this type can be seen even in young adults, particularly in the anterior temporal and insular white matter. In Hurler's syndrome (see section 6.1), this change is often very prominent despite the tender age of the patient.

An identical change may be found in the basal ganglia around penetrating arteries. Additionally, there are dilatation of the perivascular space and rarefaction of the surrounding tissue about smaller, apparently normal blood vessels, including capillaries. Some believe that an essentially slow disintegration of parenchyma is responsible for this tissue rarefaction, and they use the term "encephalolysis" for this appearance.

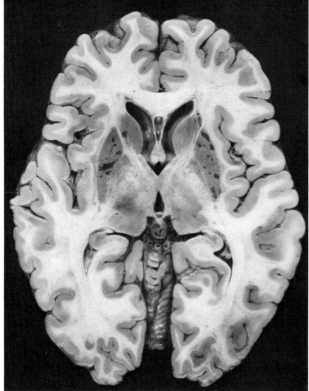

A

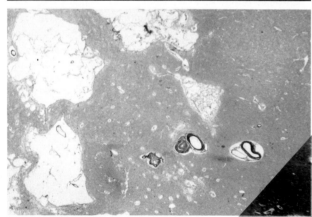

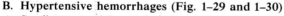

B

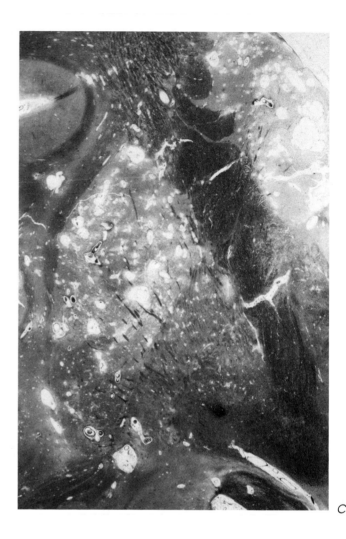

C

Figure 1–27. Small infarcts related to arteriolar sclerosis. A, Bilateral état lacunaire of basal ganglia, consisting of multiple small, old, cystic infarcts. B, Lower-power microscopic view of left putamen shown in A (LFB/PAS/H). C, État criblé of putamen and caudate, consisting of dilated perivascular spaces without tissue necrosis (Weil's).

B. Hypertensive hemorrhages (Fig. 1–29 and 1–30)

1. Small (punctate) hemorrhages

There are good grounds for believing that intracerebral aneurysms leak to give rise to small hemorrhages (up to 2 to 3 cm) at almost any site within the brain, but with predilection for the gray matter or the junction of the cortex and the white matter, and also the basal gray matter.

When fresh, they appear as round or oval, well-circumscribed dark-red spots. When old, they appear as tiny areas of softening, brown to golden yellow in color (due to blood pigment-laden macrophages). The immediately subcortical lesions usually result in "slit hemorrhage" described below. Many of these are apparently asymptomatic.

2. "Slit hemorrhages"

These are slitlike blood pigment-stained areas of soft-

ening extending along the plane of U fibers and created by previous small hemorrhages situated at the corticomedullary junctional zone. In the depth of a sulcus, these tend to take on a crescent shape.

3. Gross hemorrhages

These may be small (up to 1 to 2 cm in diameter) or massive (up to several centimeters in diameter) hemorrhages and are less frequent than small hemorrhages but are clinically more significant and often prove fatal.

The precise nature of the underlying vascular lesion(s) and the mechanism of arterial rupture have long been discussed and have not been completely settled. C. M. Fisher (1972) disputed the previously popular view that true microaneurysms are necessary precursors of massive hemorrhages and that the diseased arterial segments that are

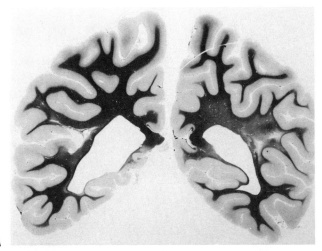

A

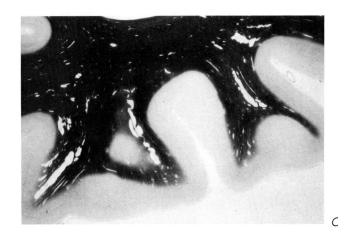

C

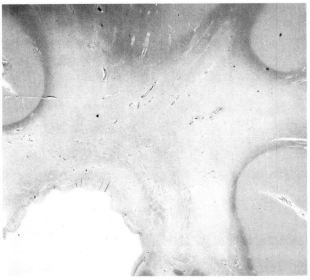

B

Figure 1–28. *A* and *B*, Binswanger's encephalopathy. Multiple focal white matter infarcts and more diffuse fiber degeneration in parietotemporal regions bilaterally (*A*) (hematoxylin myelin, Loyez modification). Low-power microscopic view of diffuse periventricular white matter degeneration with thickened arterioles (LFB/PAS/H) (*B*). *C*, État criblé of cerebral white matter, not to be confused with Binswanger's encephalopathy (Loyez).

responsible would be totally destroyed by the massive hemorrhages. Instead, he held responsible multiple, small "bleeding globes" found at the edge of such large hemorrhages. These globes (also known as pseudoaneurysms, hemostatic globes, or fibrin globes) consist of a mass of platelets at the end of an arterial stump which are surrounded by concentric layers of fibrin containing extravasated red cells. Characteristically, these small arteries may show hyalinization of the media but no "lipohyalinosis," arterial dilatation, or fibrin thrombosis. He further expressed the belief that a primary hemorrhage occurs from one or more of these arterioles and that the majority of the bleeding globes represent secondary disruption, which in turn results in further bleeding, in avalanche style. Others believe that simultaneous rupture of multiple, small arterioles is responsible for large hemorrhages, and still others implicate rupture of a single larger artery to account for the extent of bleeding. Fisher conceded the possibility that actual rupture points may have contained more severely damaged arterial segments and stated that the weight of evidence suggests that some element of the lipohyalinotic process underlies massive hypertensive hemorrhages.

The predilection sites of these gross hemorrhages are areas supplied by the penetrating type of branches from such arteries as the middle cerebral and basilar which include the putamen (mainly the external portion), thalamus, and pons. However, the cerebellar hemispheres (usually in the central portion) and the cerebral white matter are also occasionally affected. Almost any region may be involved, but the midbrain and medulla or spinal cord are rarely, if ever, involved by hypertensive hemorrhages of any size.

Roughly speaking, the relative frequencies of the various sites are the cerebrum 10 to 13, the pons 2, and the cerebellum 1. This appears to reflect the relative volume of the tissues involved. However, in the cerebral tissue, the basal ganglia and thalamus are affected much more often than other areas, as stated above, roughly representing 60% and 10 to 20% of the overall incidence, respectively.

The extension of the lesion follows the path of least resistance, often along the white matter tracts, in a manner similar to that seen in "slit hemorrhages." Rupture into the ventricular cavity is common with the large hemorrhages that are located in the medial aspect of the basal ganglia and thalamus. On the other hand, rupture through the cortex into

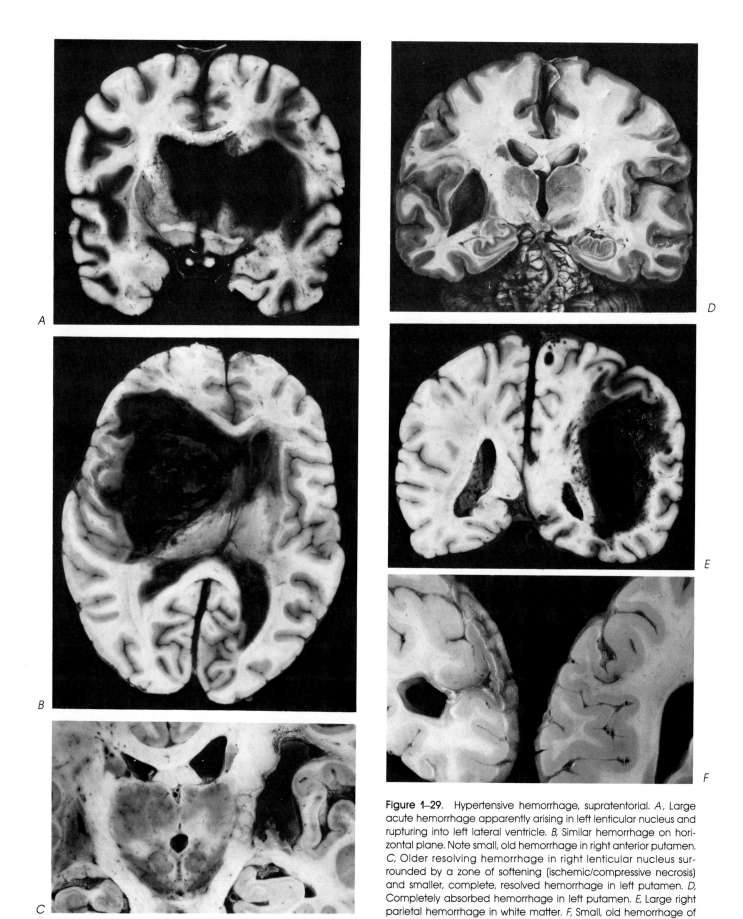

Figure 1–29. Hypertensive hemorrhage, supratentorial. *A*, Large acute hemorrhage apparently arising in left lenticular nucleus and rupturing into left lateral ventricle. *B*, Similar hemorrhage on horizontal plane. Note small, old hemorrhage in right anterior putamen. *C*, Older resolving hemorrhage in right lenticular nucleus surrounded by a zone of softening (ischemic/compressive necrosis) and smaller, complete, resolved hemorrhage in left putamen. *D*, Completely absorbed hemorrhage in left putamen. *E*, Large right parietal hemorrhage in white matter. *F*, Small, old hemorrhage of right posterior temporal white matter (left side) and small old "crescent" hemorrhage in subcortical white matter (right side).

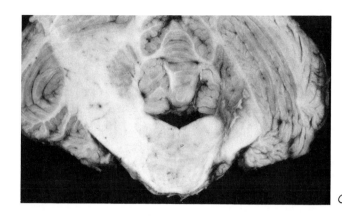

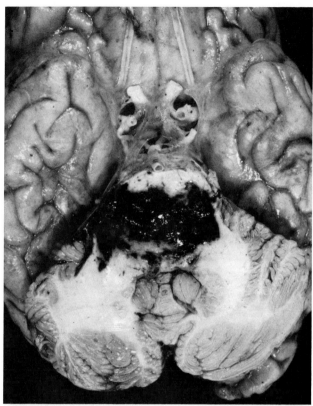

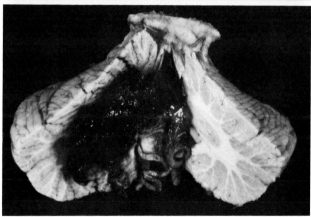

Figure 1–30. Hypertensive hemorrhage, infratentorial. A, Acute, extensive pontine hemorrhage. B, Acute, extensive left cerebellar hemorrhage with rupture into fourth ventricle. C, Old, small right cerebellar hemorrhage extending into middle cerebellar peduncle.

the subarachnoid space is rare. Although blood in the CSF is a good indication of cerebral hemorrhage, less extensive, strictly intraparenchymal hemorrhages are associated with clear CSF. Undoubtedly, some of these lesions were clinically diagnosed as infarcts before computed tomography became available.

Naturally, the size and location of the hemorrhages will determine the clinical symptoms and the outcome. Generally speaking, because of the speed with which hypertensive (and therefore arterial) hematoma accumulates, its effects, direct or indirect, on the neighboring tissue, particularly the rostral brainstem, become manifest quite rapidly. When the lesion is large, its temporal profile is characterized by a sudden onset of "stroke" symptoms (often with headache and vomiting),

which steadily reach their maximum within a few minutes to hours. Disturbance of consciousness occurs early. This is in contrast to the situation involving a massive cerebral infarct (see sections 1.14 and 1.9).

The massive hemorrhage consists of masses of blood with no recognizable tissue left in the center because the extravasating blood displaces, compresses, and to some extent disrupts the adjacent brain tissue; its edges are irregular, and small petechial hemorrhages and pseudoaneurysms are usually present along its borders. The surrounding white matter is edematous and soft.

Unlike infarction, much of the effect of a hematoma appears to be secondary to its compressive force on the neighboring tissue rather than to the actual destruction of the central tissue. The longer the hematoma remains, however, at least in the acute phase, the more permanent will be the damage to the surrounding tissue. This provides a rationale for early evacuation of intracerebral hematomas, if their exact locations can be clinically determined. This task has been made considerably easier by the advent of computed tomography.

The morphologic evolution of hemorrhage is similar to that of hemorrhagic infarct. When the hemorrhage is circumscribed and nonfatal, red cells and necrotic debris at the edge will be digested by macrophages; this process eventually leaves a cystic cavity with orange-yellow borders and marginal gliosis. Mesenchymal reaction is often intense within the central portion of small to medium-sized hemorrhages. Resultant fibrotic plaques, which appear white on gross inspection, may partially fill the site of hemorrhage instead of leaving a cavity. Limited intraventricular extensions often heal with a gliotic band(s) across the ventricular cavity.

C. Hypertensive encephalopathy (Fig. 1–31)

The clinical syndrome of hypertensive encephalopathy consists of a rapid increase in blood pressure accompanied by severe headache, nausea, vomiting, alterations of consciousness (apathy through coma), and convulsions. Cases due to cerebral infarct or hemorrhage must be excluded. Therapeutic lowering of the high blood pressure often results in a dramatic resolution of the syndrome. Earlier, the pathogenesis was thought to be vasospasm (constriction). More recent studies suggest that a failure of cerebrovascular autoregulation is the basic mechanism. This pressure-forced arterial dilatation leads to damage to the blood-brain barrier with focal leakage of plasma fluid and the formation of cerebral edema.

The characteristic arteriolar lesion is necrosis of medial muscle fibers and insudation of fibrin in the vascular wall and beyond. This, however, is not demonstrable in all autopsied cases.

1.4 MALFORMATIVE VASCULAR LESIONS

The major lesions are focal saccular aneurysms and collections of multiple dilated vessels, which are usually referred to as vascular malformations. Other lesions that are commonly referred to as aneurysms will be discussed here as well.

A. Saccular ("congenital") aneurysm (Fig. 1–32 to 1–35)

This is a true aneurysm—that is, a lesion with dilatation of the vascular lumen due to weakness and yielding of all components of the wall. A false aneurysm does not exhibit enlargement of the lumen, even though the external diameter of the affected vascular segment may enlarge.

Although the exact pathogenesis has not been fully elucidated, saccular aneurysms are believed to arise on the basis of a congenital defect. This primary defect is thought to be focal absence of the media, leading to a subsequent

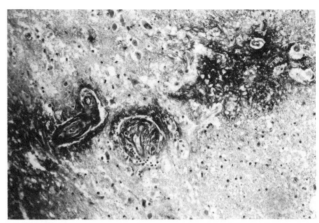

Figure 1–31. Acute "fibroid" necrosis of arterioles and exudation of fibrin material into surrounding tissue in a case of hypertensive encephalopathy (H&E).

gradual ballooning out because of the arterial pressure effect over the years. This defect is usually present at the arterial bifurcation.

These aneurysms are first seen at about the time of puberty; they occur with relatively the same frequency in all subsequent decades. The size varies from 1 mm to 3 to 4 cm, the average being 9 to 10 mm. The gross configuration of a saccular aneurysm may be divided into two types: (1) rounded—this type may be broad-based on, or connected by a narrow stalk to, the parent vessels; and (2) narrow and cylindric—this type is seen much less frequently and is believed by some to represent a blind-ended rudiment of embryonal arterial channels whereas others have involuted during embryogenesis. It is most commonly seen at or near the anterior communicating artery.

The sac of the aneurysm is basically composed of the thickened intima and adventitia. The media ends abruptly at the mouth of the sac, whereas the internal elastica often extends for a short distance into the sac from the parent artery. Atherosclerosis often develops prematurely in the wall, and thrombosis may partially obliterate the lumen.

These aneurysms occur in the major arteries at the base of the brain, especially in the anterior half of the circle of Willis. Most of them occur at the distal angle of an arterial branching or bifurcation. They usually lie in the subarachnoid space, but may, to a greater or lesser extent, lie embedded within the cerebral tissue. Approximately 90% of aneurysms are situated in the internal carotid artery system and 10% in the vertebral-basilar system. In about 10 to 20% of these persons the aneurysms are multiple. In 75% there are two aneurysms.

What is the natural history of saccular aneurysms?

1. Asymptomatic

Saccular aneurysms are often incidental findings at autopsy. Asymptomatic aneurysms occur five to six times more often than those that rupture.

2. Rupture

Rupture of the sac occurs primarily from the dome or at the edge of the atheromatous plaque. Six percent of the pa-

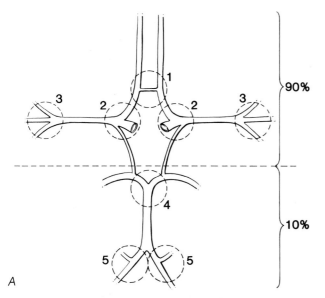

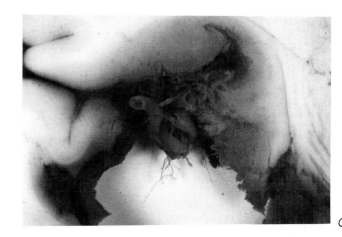

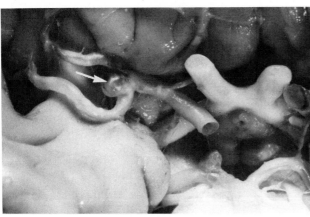

Figure 1–32. Saccular aneurysm. *A*, Distribution pattern at base of brain. In anterior circulation: 1, vicinity of anterior communicating artery (approx 30%); 2, internal carotid artery and its branching (approx 30%); 3, middle cerebral artery "trifurcation" (approx 30%). In posterior circulation: 4, basilar artery bifurcation; 5, vertebral artery. *B*, Unruptured, small, thin-walled aneurysm (*arrow*) at middle cerebral bifurcation (so-called trifurcation). *C*, Ruptured small saccular aneurysm of middle cerebral artery trifurcation (fresh dissection with blood washed away and photographed under water). (*A* from Okazaki H: Pathology of apoplexy. 7. Cerebral arterial aneurysm. *Kangogaku Zasshi* 44 no. 4:429–432, 1980. By permission of Igaku-Shoin.)

tients are less than 30 years old at the first rupture, and 90% are between 30 and 70 years of age. Rupture or even the presence of an aneurysm of this type is rare below the age of 15.

The exact events leading to rupture of the aneurysmal sac are not understood. Hypertension is common among many of the patients, but many of them are also absolutely normotensive. Intracranial hemorrhage resulting from a rupture of the aneurysm may be considered in the following forms.

a. Subarachnoid hemorrhage

This is the main form of bleeding. Although the blood spreads diffusely through the subarachnoid space, a heavy local accumulation is not uncommon. It occasionally ruptures into the subdural space. The blood may also dissect into the brain substance (see below). Acute hydrocephalus may result from a sudden blockage of the subarachnoid space. Hydrocephalus may also develop as a consequence of leptomeningeal fibrosis after healing (organization) has taken place.

b. Significant intracerebral hemorrhage

Intracerebral hemorrhage of significant extent occurs in 60 to 70% of fatal cases in addition to subarachnoid hemorrhage. The site of intraparenchymal hemorrhage depends on the location of the aneurysm and the direction in which the dome projects. In some instances, intracerebral hemorrhage is massive whereas subarachnoid hemorrhage is minimal. Further extension of hemorrhage into the ventricular system may follow. Aneurysms of the anterior communicating artery are notorious for their tendency to rupture almost directly into the frontal horns.

The first hemorrhages prove to be fatal in 30% of cases. As many as 20 to 30% of the survivors of the first episode are expected to have a fatal recurrence within 6 weeks.

3. Cerebral infarction

Cerebral infarction may occur, and one or more of the following factors may be responsible.

a. Arterial spasm (vasospasm or angiospasm), as demonstrated by angiography, particularly after subarachnoid hemorrhage

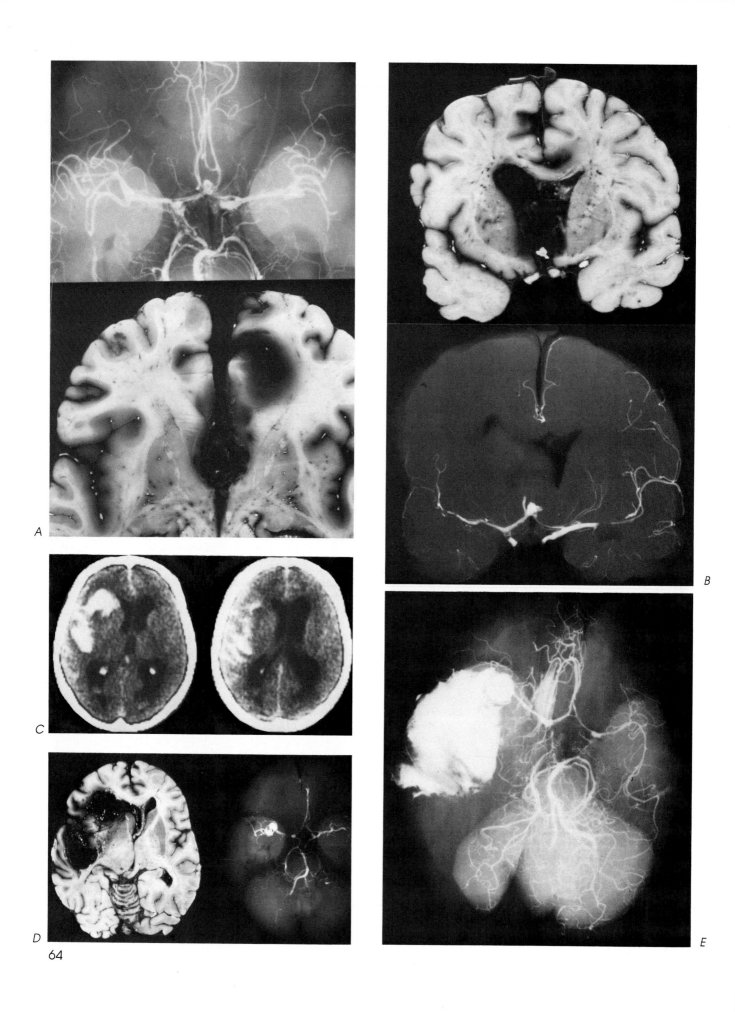

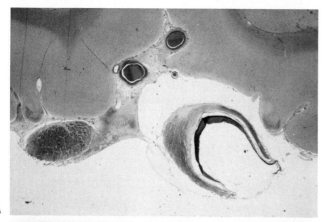

A

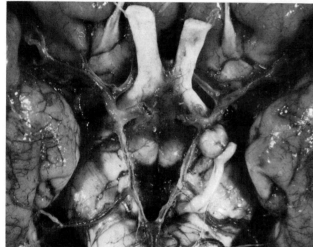

B

Figure 1–34. Saccular aneurysm. *A,* Saccular aneurysm of right internal carotid artery (supraclinoid portion) partially embedded in right optic nerve (LFB/PAS/H). *B,* Small saccular aneurysm at left internal carotid artery and posterior communicating artery, compressing left third cranial nerve.

b. Embolus breaking off from a thrombus in the sac and obstructing a distal arterial branch

c. Compression of adjacent arteries by the sac and by extravasated blood

d. Cerebral atherosclerosis with or without hypotensive episodes

4. Compression of cranial nerves

Compression of some of the cranial nerves, especially the third and the second, by the enlarged sac may occur. The brain parenchyma may be compressed by the aneurysm, especially in the hypothalamic and pituitary regions.

5. Closed aneurysmal sac

The aneurysmal sac may be spontaneously closed by thrombosis. This often affords a protecting mechanism against rupture.

The therapeutic ligation of the cervical internal carotid artery may cause sufficient stagnation within the sac to allow thrombosis.

6. "Giant aneurysm" variants

These are large aneurysms measuring up to 5 cm in diameter and usually occurring at or near the circle of Willis. Three-fourths of them are seen in patients who are 50 years of age or older. Although little actual documentation of their natural history is found in the literature, some are thought to have grown within a few months. Others are said to have been present for more than 20 years. Previously confirmed subarachnoid hemorrhage is reported in fewer than 1% of cases. In some of the fast-developing lesions, incorporation of a hematoma into the aneurysmal wall is thought to explain the rapid increase in size. Some of the other features of the giant aneurysm include the following

a. Normal roentgenographic findings in 60% of cases

b. Calcification, often curvilinear in contour, in 18% of cases

c. Large mural thrombus in 50% of cases

d. Persistent capability of bleeding despite layers of thrombosis

B. So-called vascular malformations

There are numerous, often confusing arrays of terminologies and classifications for these lesions. This subject may be relatively simplified if one determines where the abnormalities lie in reference to the artery-capillary-vein continuum. There are certain relationships between the type of lesion and its natural history and clinical behavior. As is true with saccular "congenital" aneurysms, the lesions under discussion are probably based on congenital abnormalities but appear to attain their clinically significant sizes during the growth of the patient.

Three major types of vascular malformation are represented diagrammatically in Figure 1–36 to indicate the sites of abnormalities in reference to the artery-capillary-vein continuum.

1. Capillary telangiectasia (Fig. 1–37)

The lesion consists of congeries of dilated capillary blood vessels separated by neural parenchyma and often accompanied by a tortuous, enlarged draining vein or veins. Most of these are small and clinically silent and are found only incidentally at autopsy in middle-aged and elderly persons. Some degrees of extravasation may have occurred, as

Figure 1–33. Ruptured saccular aneurysm with intracranial hemorrhage. *A,* Postmortem angiogram with horizontal section of brain, showing small saccular aneurysm of anterior communicating artery with rupture leading to subarachnoid hemorrhage. *B,* Brain slice and postmortem angiogram showing much intraventricular but little subarachnoid hemorrhage from ruptured aneurysm of anterior communicating artery. *C* and *D,* Computed tomography scans (*C*) and brain slice and postmortem angiogram (*D*) in a case of ruptured aneurysm of left middle cerebral trifurcation which resulted in extensive frontal and temporal lobe hematoma near base and subarachnoid hemorrhage at higher level. *E,* Medium-sized aneurysm of right middle cerebral artery trifurcation with rupture into right temporal lobe as seen in basal view of postmortem angiogram. (*E* from Okazaki H, Campbell RJ: Nervous system. *In Current Methods of Autopsy Practice.* Second edition. Edited by J Ludwig. Philadelphia, WB Saunders Company, 1979. By permission.)

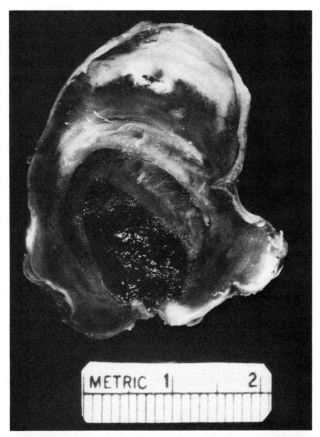

A

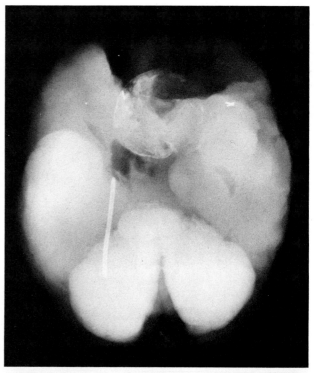

C

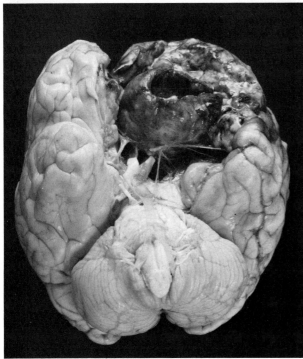

B

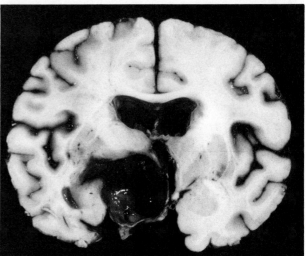

D

Figure 1–35. Saccular aneurysm. *A*, Large (3.5 by 3.0 by 2.5 cm) saccular aneurysm at left internal carotid artery bifurcation with markedly reduced lumen as a result of extensive thrombosis. *B* and *C*, Giant aneurysm of left internal carotid artery bifurcation which had been explored and packed recently through left frontal craniotomy (*B*), and corresponding roentgenogram (*C*). *D*, Giant aneurysm of right internal carotid artery proximal to bifurcation, with limited pericapsular intracerebral hemorrhage.

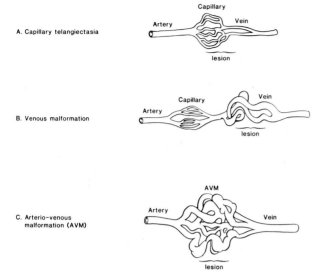

A. Capillary telangiectasia

Capillary
Artery   Vein

lesion

B. Venous malformation

Capillary   Vein
Artery

lesion

C. Arterio-venous
malformation (AVM)

AVM
Artery   Vein

lesion

Figure 1–36. Three basic types of vascular malformation in the central nervous system. Certain morphologic overlaps among these three simplified models are discussed in the text. (Modified from Okazaki H: Pathology of apoplexy. 8. Cerebral aneurysm and cerebral arteriovenous malformation. *Kangogaku Zasshi* 44 no. 5:541–544, 1980. By permission of Igaku-Shoin.)

evidenced by the presence of old blood pigment and some gliosis at autopsy. Sites of predilection include the pons (the base near the midline), cerebral cortex, and white matter. They rarely reach the surface of the brain. A rare, multiple, familial form is known as hereditary hemorrhagic telangiectasia (Rendu-Osler-Weber disease).

2. Venous malformation (Fig. 1–37)

This lesion consists of many large vascular spaces of varying size which are packed closely toward the center (''cavernous hemangioma''). The vascular wells resemble normal venous channels and often have secondary changes (e.g., fibrous thickening and calcification). The older literature distinguished between (1) cavernous types (when no neural element is present between vascular channels), and (2) racemose types (when channels are separated by neural tissue). Both can be seen in a single lesion, the latter type being found predominantly in the periphery. The distinction, therefore, does not constitute a fundamental difference. Some of these, as will be discussed below, may in fact be arteriovenous malformations.

They are usually found incidentally in middle-aged and elderly patients, but small amounts of old hemorrhage into the surrounding tissue or calcification may be present at autopsy. Multiplicity (up to four or five) is not uncommon; it is found in one-third of incidental cases.

Note: 1. Distinction between the above two types (1 and 2) is not always clear, and what should be considered transitional forms occur not infrequently. These may be called capillary-venous malformations.

2. *Varix* is a single dilated vein that takes a tortuous course. It is rarely, if ever, of clinical significance.

3. Arteriovenous malformation (Fig. 1–38 to 1–41)

An arteriovenous malformation is formed by a network of abnormal, thick-walled vascular channels that are neither purely arterial nor entirely venous in type. They are sometimes referred to as arterialized veins. The channels are fed directly by one or more arteries and are drained by many abnormally dilated veins; thus they constitute an arteriovenous shunt.

The arteriovenous malformation itself constitutes a relatively closed system, and the arteries and veins of the normal brain tissue surrounding it remain relatively uninfluenced and establish no collateral channels with the malformation. Arteriovenous aneurysm or fistula is a synonym occasionally seen in the literature.

Some of the ''venous malformations'' described above may, in fact, demonstrate a direct arteriovenous shunt by angiography, which qualifies them to be true arteriovenous malformations. However, because of their usually asymptomatic nature, angiography is rarely performed during life for these lesions.

This is the most important subtype of vascular malformation, being found clinically among young adults and middle-aged persons. Sixty-four percent of these lesions are diagnosed before the age of 40. This is in sharp contrast to the relatively low (26%) incidence of symptomatic saccular aneurysms occurring during the same period.

The majority (90%) of arteriovenous malformations are found in the cerebral hemispheres; more than half of these are found in the middle third and the rest in the posterior and anterior thirds, in that order of frequency; 10% are found in the brainstem or cerebellum. They rarely involve the dural sinuses, particularly the lateral or sigmoid sinuses.

In its typical configuration, the lesion lies in the subarachnoid space and extends through the gray matter in the shape of a cone. The base of the cone rests on the cortex, and the apex points toward the ventricle. The amount of the parenchymal tissue varies, but the abnormal vessels tend to be more dispersed at the periphery.

Secondary changes, e.g. thrombosis and calcification of the abnormal blood vessels, are common.

Important pathologic consequences of these lesions include *atrophy* of the parenchyma by chronic ischemia or compression leading to neurologic deficits and seizures and *hemorrhage,* which may be limited or massive and fatal. The frequency of intracranial hemorrhage is inversely proportional to the size of the lesions. In a Mayo Clinic series the incidence of hemorrhage in relation to the angiographic size of the arteriovenous malformations was small arteriovenous malformation 77%, medium 67%, and large 50%. The large lesions are characterized by progressive neurologic deficits and seizures, whereas small ones tend to cause a massive hemorrhage, which often proves fatal the first time.

There are two important variants of arteriovenous malformation.

a. Arteriovenous malformation of the vein of Galen (Fig. 1–40)

The term refers to a vascular lesion with huge aneurysmal dilatation of the vein of Galen or internal

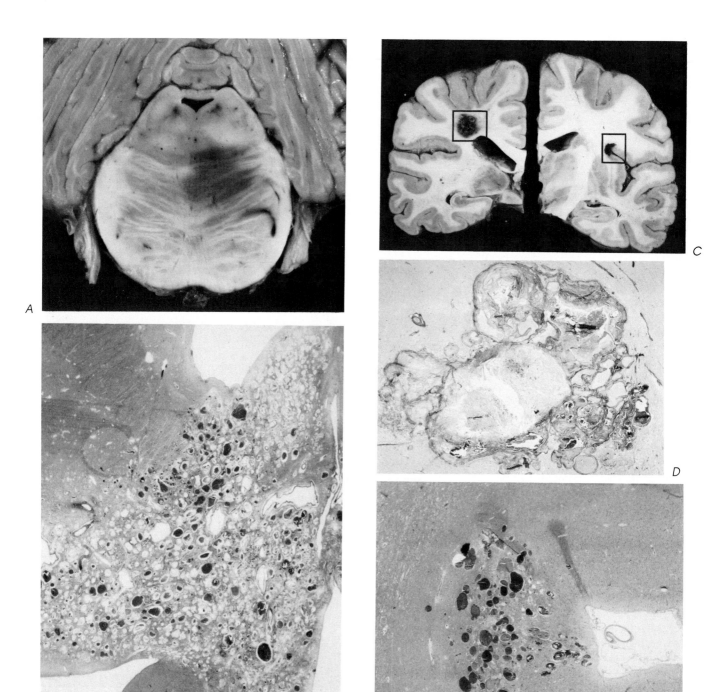

Figure 1–37. Capillary and venous malformations. *A,* Incidental small vascular malformation, consisting largely of dilated capillaries (capillary telangiectasia) in base of pons. *B,* Small vascular malformation of hypothalamus with more thick-walled venous channels than thin-walled capillaries (trichrome). *C,* Incidental capillary te-

langiectasia on right (at upper corner of insula) and predominantly venous malformation on left (in centrum semiovale). *D* and *E,* Histologic appearance of right-sided lesion (*D*) from area shown in left box in *C* (H&E) and left-sided lesion (*E*) from area shown in right box in *C* (EvG).

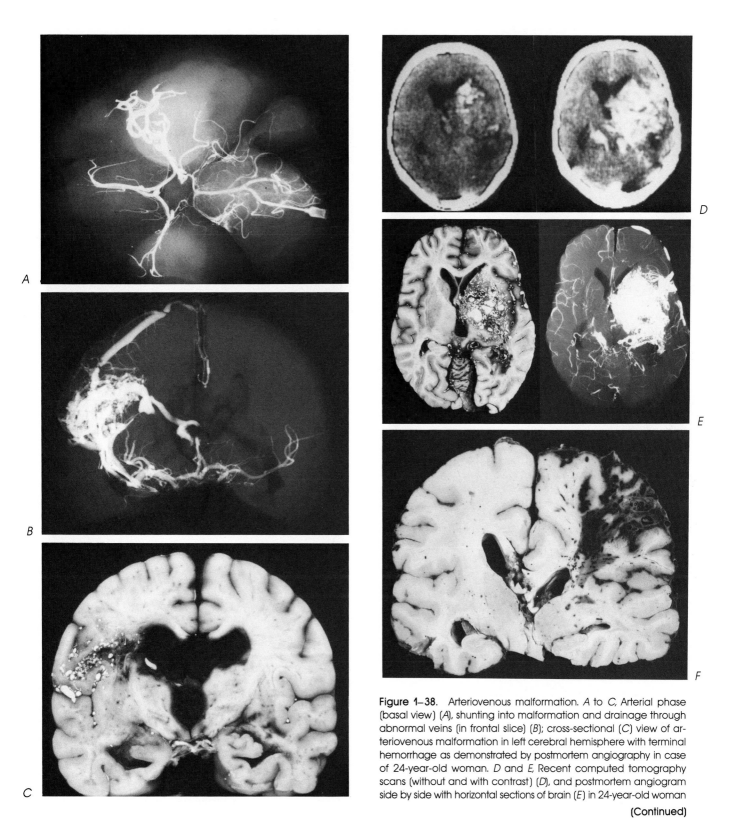

Figure 1–38. Arteriovenous malformation. *A* to *C*, Arterial phase (basal view) (*A*), shunting into malformation and drainage through abnormal veins (in frontal slice) (*B*); cross-sectional (*C*) view of arteriovenous malformation in left cerebral hemisphere with terminal hemorrhage as demonstrated by postmortem angiography in case of 24-year-old woman. *D* and *E,* Recent computed tomography scans (without and with contrast) (*D*), and postmortem angiogram side by side with horizontal sections of brain (*E*) in 24-year-old woman

(Continued)

69

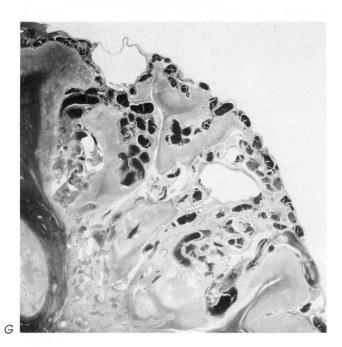

G

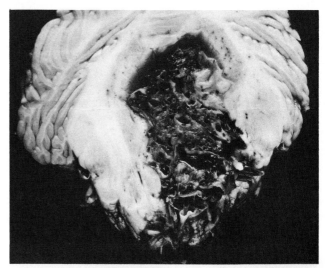

H

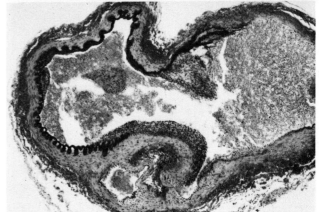

I

with terminal bleeding from deep-seated arteriovenous malformation. *F* and *G*, More superficially located cerebral hemispheric arteriovenous malformation (*F*), and its low-power histologic features (*G*) (EvG). *H* and *I*, Brainstem arteriovenous malformation in 20-year-old woman (*H*), in which direct transition between artery and vein was demonstrable in one of the sections (*I*) (EvG).

cerebral veins (strictly speaking, a varix) associated with arteriovenous malformation in their tributary areas.

Three clinical syndromes, related to the age at clinical onset, are recognized.

• Neonatal. This type is characterized by congestive failure secondary to the massive arteriovenous shunt.

• Infancy. This is marked mainly by hydrocephalus (at times acute) and convulsions.

• Childhood and adolescence. This type is characteristically manifested by headache, mental retardation, subarachnoid hemorrhage, or focal neurologic deficits (loss of vision, hemiparesis, ataxia, and so on).

b. Spinal cord arteriovenous malformation (Fig. 1–41)

The spinal cord lesion consists of one or more longitudinal anomalous large vessels, which often take a very tortuous course on the surface of the cord and roots. Some of them penetrate into the parenchyma. More often, however, only diffusely scattered, small vessels with thick fibrous walls are seen in the parenchyma, and the intervening tissue shows ischemic atrophy. Often

erroneously, the large external vessels are referred to as veins and the entire lesion as a "venous malformation." However, these vessels are a direct extension of the feeding radicular artery(ies) without interposed capillaries. Thus, the lesion is basically the same as the cerebral arteriovenous malformation. Thrombosis, calcification, or hemorrhage from these vessels may occur and add to the parenchymal tissue damage.

"Subacute necrotic myelitis" of Foix-Alajouanine is now generally recognized to be due to the presence of spinal arteriovenous malformation of the lower cord.

C. **Other vascular lesions that are often referred to as aneurysm include the following.**

1. Atherosclerotic aneurysm (Fig. 1–42)

This lesion is also known as a "fusiform" aneurysm. It is an exaggerated form of arterial ectasia due to atherosclerosis, as discussed already in section 1.10. The stretching of the arterial wall results from a more or less circumferential weakening of the arterial wall over some length. The most common vessels involved are the vertebral and basilar arteries, and the internal carotid arteries in the cavernous sinus and immediately distal to it.

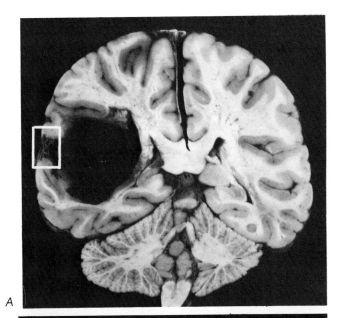

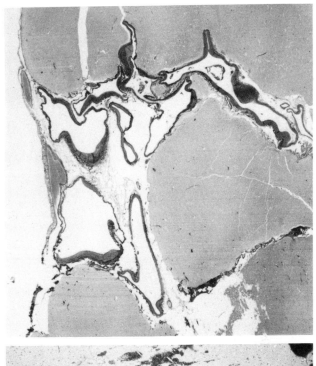

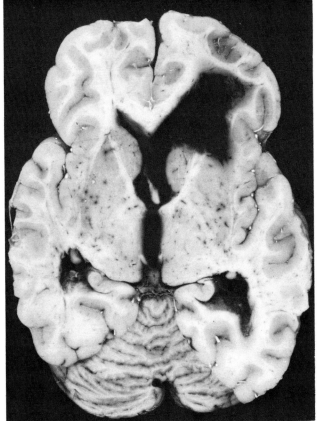

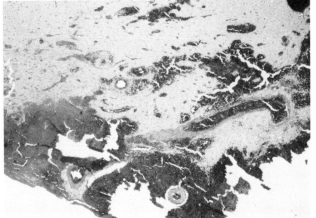

Figure 1–39. So-called cryptic arteriovenous malformation. *A* and *B,* Large acute hemorrhage from small surface arteriovenous malformation (*A*) and, from area boxed in *A*, magnified view (*B*) in 14-year-old previously healthy boy (EvG). *C,* Sudden intracerebral hemorrhage in 19-year-old woman as demonstrated at autopsy. *D,* Small group of scattered abnormal vessels found at anterior margin of hemorrhage in the same case.

The clinical signs and symptoms are caused by compression of the brain parenchyma, particularly the pons and medulla, and by thrombosis of the involved segment with resultant brainstem infarction. Rarely, these result in subarachnoid hemorrhage by rupture.

2. Dissecting aneurysm (Fig. 1–43)

This is a false aneurysm in which blood accumulates within the thickness of the wall. The cervical arteries, particularly the common carotid arteries, may become involved by extension of the disease process from the arch of the aorta. Because of its stenotic effect on the lumen of the affected arteries, cerebral infarction may result. Rarely, isolated intracranial arteries are involved, usually independently of the systemic disease.

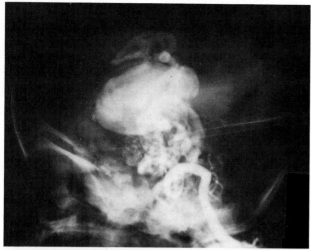

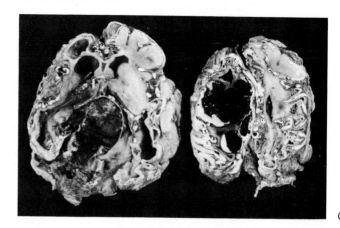

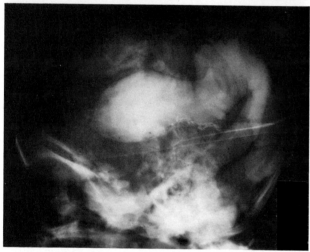

Figure 1–40. So-called aneurysm of vein of Galen. *A* to *C,* Early (*A*) and later (*B*) phases of cerebral angiography. Horizontal slices of neonatal brain (*C*) show bilateral extensive arteriovenous malformation, including hugely dilated vein of Galen.

3. Carotid-cavernous sinus aneurysm

In this condition, there is fistula formation between the internal carotid artery and the cavernous sinus that surrounds it. The commonest etiologic factor is a traumatic tear of the artery.

4. Infectious or "mycotic" aneurysm

This lesion is discussed in section 3.1.

1.5 NONINFECTIOUS VASCULITIDES OR INFLAMMATORY ANGIITIS ("CONNECTIVE TISSUE DISEASE")

A. Systemic lupus erythematosus (Fig. 1–44)

This disease involves the CNS frequently (about 75%) and the peripheral nervous system rarely (about 8%).

Cerebral microinfarcts (cortex and brainstem) are the most prevalent findings, associated with changes involving the arterioles and capillaries of the brain. Necrotizing arteritis with "fibrinoid degeneration" of the wall leading to thrombosis is described in the literature as one of the essen-

tial features of the disease. However, complicating factors of arterial hypertension via renal involvement and embolization from the cardiac lesion (e.g., Libman-Sacks endocarditis) must be taken into account in the interpretation of these lesions. In noncomplicated cases, cerebral vascular alterations may be strikingly meager despite the presence of small infarcts. Certainly onion-skin arterial change that is seen elsewhere is not found in or near cerebral microinfarcts. It is conceded that disturbances of mental function which are frequently noted (one-third of cases) may not be fully accounted for by the anatomic alterations alone.

Mononeuropathy multiplex, which may be present, presumably results from vascular lesions within nerves. Distal sensorimotor neuropathy and Guillain-Barré syndrome are occasionally seen. They probably have different (yet unknown) bases.

B. Panarteritis (periarteritis) nodosa (Fig. 1–45)

The disease shows predominant involvement of the skeletal muscle and the peripheral nervous system; the CNS is uncommonly involved (10%). Vascular pathology consists of segmental necrotizing panarteritis attended by polymorphonuclear leukocytes, eosinophils, and lymphocytes. The

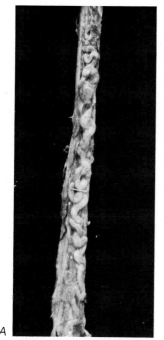

A

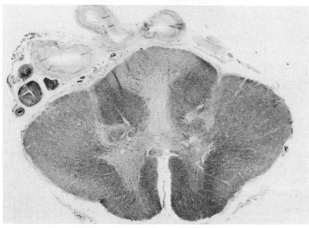

B

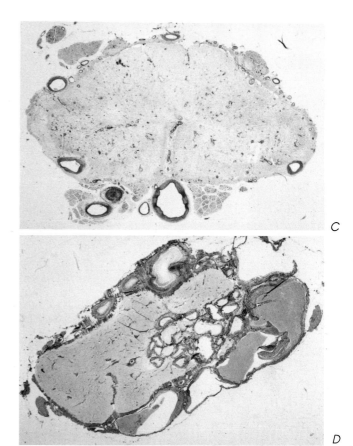

C

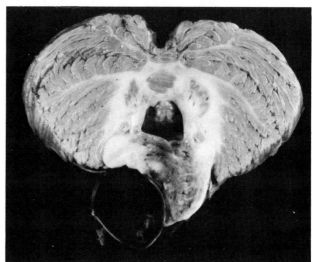

D

Figure 1–41. Spinal arteriovenous malformation. *A* and *B,* Posterior view of lower thoracic and lumbar cord (*A*) and cross section of lower thoracic cord (*B*), with abnormal vessels primarily outside of cord parenchyma (EvG). *C,* Cross section of upper lumbar segment, with a few large abnormal vessels outside of cord parenchyma and numerous small abnormal vessels within cord substance associated with extensive tissue degeneration (LFB/PAS/H). *D,* Cross section of spinal cord with arteriovenous malformation consisting of large abnormal vessels both inside and outside of cord parenchyma (EvG).

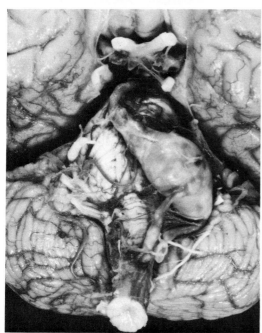

A

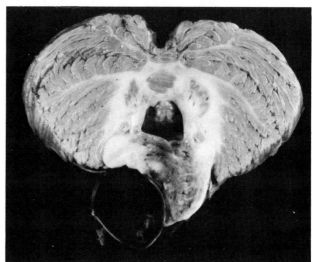

B

Figure 1–42. Atherosclerotic aneurysm. *A,* Fusiform dilatation involving distal left vertebral and proximal basilar arteries. *B,* Cross-sectional view of fusiform aneurysm of basilar artery with recent thrombosis causing pronounced chronic compression and recent infarction of pons.

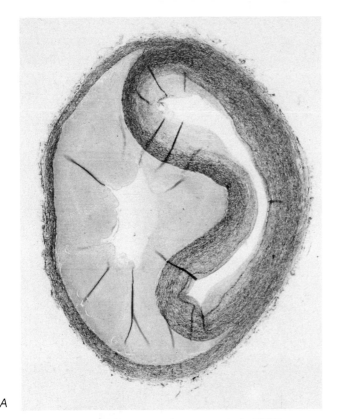

A

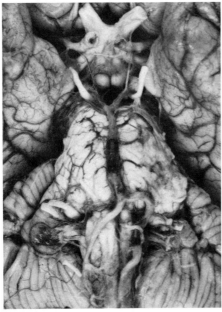

B

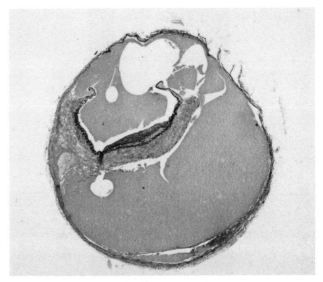

C

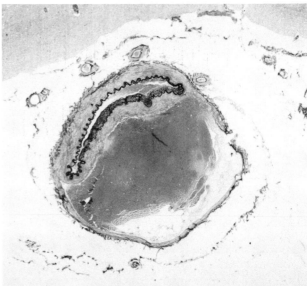

D

Figure 1–43. Dissecting aneurysm. *A*, Cross section of common carotid artery involved by cephalad extension of dissecting aneurysm of aortic arch (EvG). *B* to *D*, Focal dissecting aneurysm of basilar artery (*B*). Cross section of affected segments shows point of rupture (*C*) and longitudinal dissection within wall (*D*), luminal compromise of which resulted in pontine infarction (not shown).

lesion often leads to thrombosis. Fibrotic healing will follow. Vascular lesions of different ages in a given area (as in biopsy) are a frequent and important finding. Results are tiny foci of ischemic necrosis at any level of the neuraxis; hemorrhage may rarely occur (both peripherally and centrally). Renal involvement with hypertension (which is common) may lead to intracranial hemorrhage or hypertensive encephalopathy.

C. Scleroderma (progressive systemic sclerosis)

The rarity of CNS involvement with scleroderma is attributed to the lack of collagen in the brain and the histologic

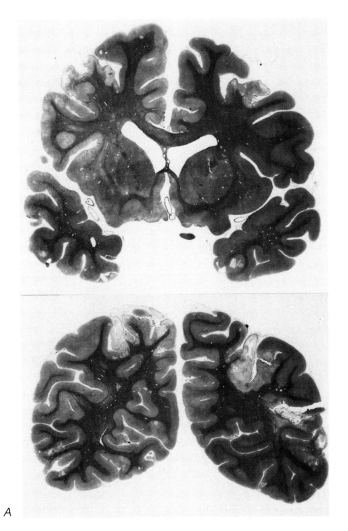

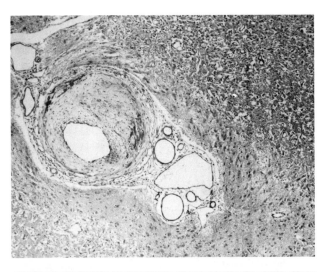

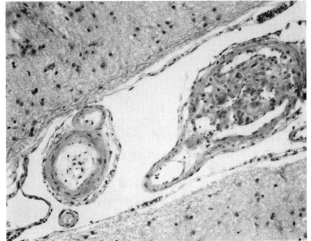

Figure 1–44. Systemic lupus erythematosus. *A* to *C*, Typical distribution (*A*) of multiple small infarcts (mostly old in this case) in bilateral arterial border zones (LFB/CV). Underlying vascular lesions responsible include what appears to be intrinsic focal necrotizing and proliferative lesion (*B*) or multiple embolic occlusions from Libman-Sachs endocarditis (*C*) (H&E).

difference between cerebral and other arteries. The rarity of recorded peripheral nervous system involvement is thought by some to be due to incomplete examination. The muscle is somewhat more commonly involved. However, the pathogenesis and nature of scleroderma are incompletely understood.

D. Rheumatoid arthritis

This disease may produce necrotizing arteritis similar to that of panarteritis nodosa. It usually affects the peripheral nerves more than the CNS.

E. Giant cell arteritis (temporal arteritis) (Fig. 1–46)

Giant cell arteritis is known primarily as the disease of the external carotid arteries, particularly the temporal arteries, among elderly (over 60) persons. Ischemic neuropathy of the optic nerves and of the oculomotor nerves is the principal neurologic complication.

This form of granulomatous panarteritis may involve arteries at the base of the brain in addition to the ophthalmic arteries. The lesion is characterized by subintimal cellular proliferation, a chronic inflammatory reaction with giant cells, concentrated in the vicinity of the elastic lamina, which becomes largely destroyed. More acute necrotizing changes can be seen in the media. Parenchymal damages are ischemic in nature and result from stenosis or obliteration of the lumen.

F. Granulomatous angiitis of the CNS (Fig. 1–47)

Initially, this rare condition was reported as a diffuse but focally accentuated granulomatous vasculitis involving, often exclusively, arteries and, to a lesser extent, veins of the CNS and as being characterized by the prominence of giant-cell (both Langhan's and foreign-body types) reaction among proliferating mesenchymal cells in the intima, adven-

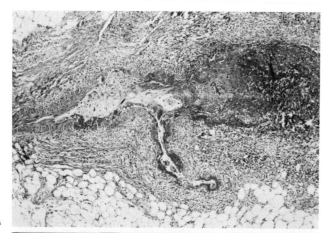

A

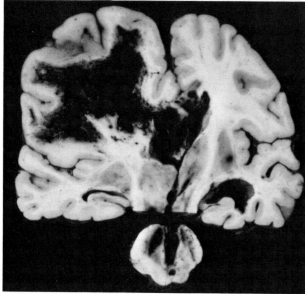

B

Figure 1-45. Panarteritis nodosa. *A*, Acute, segmental, necrotizing arteritis characteristic of acute phase of this disease, involving medium-sized artery in soft tissue of limb (H&E). *B*, Deep cortical and subcortical hemorrhages seen in case of panarteritis nodosa with cerebral vascular involvement.

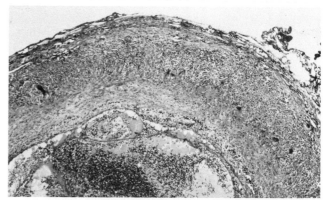

A

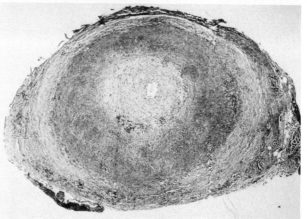

B

Figure 1-46. Giant cell (temporal) arteritis. *A*, Portion of arterial wall of temporal artery in acute phase, with necrotizing changes in media, multinucleated giant cells in close proximity to internal elastic lamina, and thrombus formation in lumen (H&E). *B*, Less active phase with more proliferative changes in intima, leading to severe stenosis of lumen (H&E).

titia, or all layers and lymphocytic infiltrates. Some of the subsequently reported cases have shown additional features of fibrinoid necrosis. Some cases are reported in association with Hodgkin's disease and herpes zoster. As such, histologic features overlap with other vasculitides. It is probable that the reported cases constitute a heterogeneous group. The clear establishment of a nosologic entity awaits discovery of the cause or a pathogenetic mechanism.

G. Thrombotic thrombocytopenic purpura (Moschcowitz disease) or thrombotic microangiopathy (Fig. 1-48)

Arterioles and capillaries of the cerebral gray matter are obstructed by granular, hyaline masses, which may appear to infiltrate the wall, leading to multiple small perivascular hemorrhages and microinfarcts. Occasionally, large hemorrhages also occur. These often result in death of the patient

(particularly in adults). These changes are identical to those seen in other organs.

1.6 VENOUS DISEASES: VEIN AND DURAL SINUS THROMBOSIS (FIG. 1-49)

These disorders were much more common in the past when severe infantile malnutrition and dehydration and uncontrolled suppurative lesions in the head and neck at any age were common. Intracranial venous thrombosis is classified according to underlying etiologic factors.

A. Secondary (or septic) thrombosis

This type is secondary to cranial or intracranial pyogenic infection. Local infections include osteomyelitis of cranial bones, often secondary to paranasal sinus or otitic infections.

Remote suppurative infections in the rest of the body may also lead to intracranial venous thrombosis via retrograde septic embolization. Resulting venous thromboses under these conditions may be either bland or infected (sep-

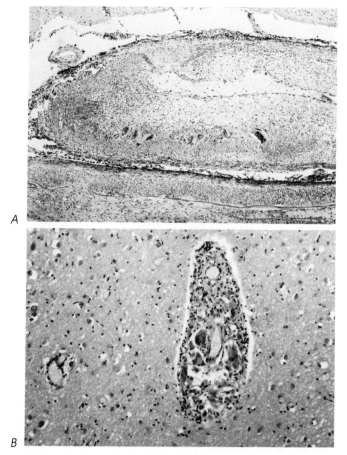

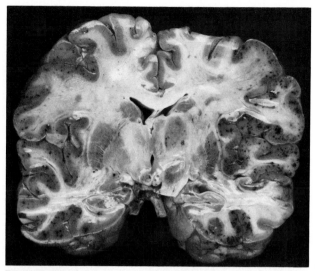

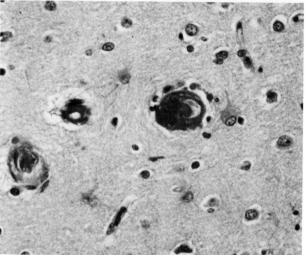

Figure 1–47. Granulomatous angiitis. *A,* Medium-sized leptomeningeal artery with chronic intimal proliferative change containing giant cells (H&E). *B,* Chronic inflammatory cell reaction with giant cells about small vessel within brain parenchyma (H&E).

Figure 1–48. Thrombotic thrombocytopenic purpura. *A,* Multiple petechiae, mostly confined to cortical gray matter. *B,* Granular-hyaline mass in walls and lumens of cerebral cortical arterioles which will eventually lead to petechiae or microinfarcts (H&E).

tic). The sites of thrombosis are generally in close proximity to the focus of infection, e.g., the cavernous sinus in facial infections and the lateral sinus in otitic infections.

B. Primary idiopathic or "marantic" type

No concrete etiologic factors are known in this type, aside from the presence of general debility, malnutrition, dehydration, or febrile diseases. Children are predominantly affected; among adults, females are more susceptible. The puerperal state was (and is still to a lesser extent now) one of the underlying conditions. The superior sagittal sinus and its tributaries are predominantly involved.

C. Mechanical type

This type is caused by venous compression during surgery or at the edge of a craniectomy defect through which edematous brain herniates.

Because of the richness of anastomosing venous networks, isolated nonseptic thrombosis of one of the intracranial sinuses rarely results in parenchymal tissue damage. However, when thrombosis extends into tributary veins for some distance, there may be cerebral infarction in their fields of drainage. The resultant infarcts are characteristically

hemorrhagic in type, the hemorrhages being more prominently distributed in the white matter.

Principal anatomic types are considered separately below.

Sites of Thrombosis	*Tissue Damage*
1. Superior sagittal sinus, lateral sinus, cavernous sinus	Infarction of the brain practically never results unless the clot extends into the tributary veins.
2. Cortical veins (mostly by extension from venous sinuses)	Infarction of the underlying brain (cortical and subcortical) usually occurs, and its extent varies according to the extensiveness of tributary involvement.

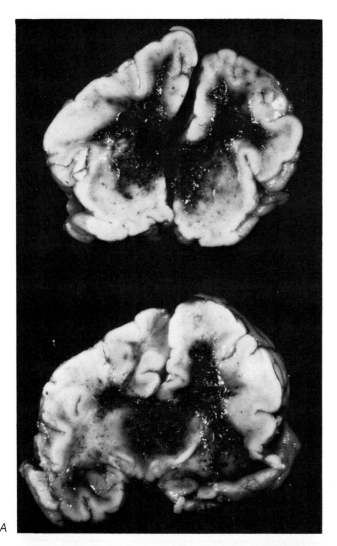

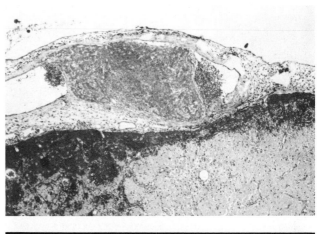

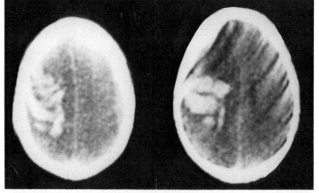

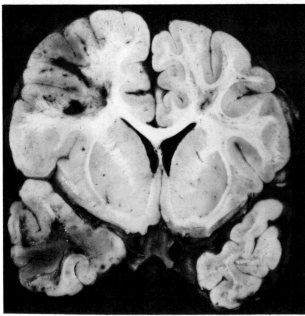

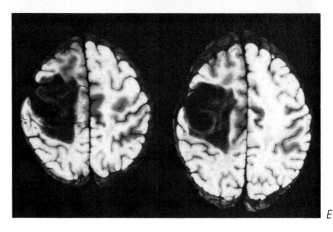

Figure 1–49. Intracranial venous thrombosis. *A*, Extensive hemorrhagic infarction of cerebral white matter, caudate nucleus, and thalamus bilaterally due to thrombosis of internal cerebral vein system in neonate. Veins of cerebral white matter are markedly distended with thrombi and show perivascular hemorrhages. *B* and *C*, Multifocal hemorrhagic infarcts with hemorrhages primarily occurring in white matter in 1-year-old boy (*B*), associated with multifocal organizing leptomeningeal venous thrombosis (*C*) (H&E). *D* and *E*, Typical pattern of hemorrhagic infarction (with hemorrhages mainly in gyral white matter) secondary to superior sagittal sinus thrombosis with extension into tributaries, particularly on left, as seen on computed tomography scans (*D*) and horizontal sections of brain (*E*) in 41-year-old man.

Sites of Thrombosis	*Tissue Damage*
3. Internal cerebral veins or vein of Galen (most often in infants and usually of primary type)	Hemorrhagic infarction of the entire field of drainage of the deep venous system results.
4. Spinal (rarely)	Tissue damage in this type is rare. The "phlebitis" described in subacute necrotic myelitis of Foix-Alajouanine is now considered an example of arteriovenous malformation (see section 1.4).

1.7 BLOOD DYSCRASIA

Any systemic disease that causes a bleeding tendency will also produce hemorrhagic phenomena within the intracranial cavity. *Leukemia* is the most frequent example of this type of pathologic change, and therefore this section will concentrate primarily on this disorder (Fig. 1–50). Cellular infiltration and tumefaction associated with leukemia will be discussed in conjunction with neoplastic disorders (see section 7.5).

In leukemia (particularly in the acute myelomonocytic and lymphocytic varieties), bleeding into the neural tissue occurs as part of a generalized hemorrhagic diathesis (thrombocytopenia is the essential underlying factor). Another factor that appears to be of importance is the rapidly increasing number of abnormal leukocytes ("blastic crisis"). When the white blood cell count is more than 300,000/mm^3 (even with higher platelet counts), 70% of persons will have fatal hemorrhages.

A. Precise mechanisms for the hemorrhages have not been clearly established, but the following factors are considered significant.

1. Occlusion of vessels with white blood cells leads to infarcts, which in turn weaken the vessels.

2. Leukostasis leads to local nutritional impairment, which means excessive vascular permeability.

3. Intravascular growth of leukemic cells causes damage to blood vessels.

B. Hemorrhagic lesions take various forms in terms of their localization.

1. Parenchymal hemorrhage

This is a common cause of death in acute leukemia. It takes (not mutually exclusive) two forms.

   a. A solitary or multiple large collection of blood in the centrum semiovale or elsewhere. Characteristically, patches of gray areas are seen within hemorrhages, representing collections of white blood cells. These hemorrhages appear to be of an oozing type rather than an explosive example seen in hypertension. Secondary rupture into the ventricular cavities and into the subarachnoid space may occur.

   b. Multiple petechial hemorrhages associated with minute infarctions. Patients may survive minor episodes of this type.

2. Leptomeningeal and subdural hemorrhages

These are seldom extensive, although cerebral compression may result from the subdural type.

3. Hemorrhage in the cranial and spinal roots

Hemorrhage in the substance of the cranial and spinal nerve roots is also occasionally seen, often in association with cellular infiltration.

4. Hemorrhage in peripheral nerves

This type is infrequently seen. When present, it is often, but not always, preceded by leukemic infiltration.

1.8 CEREBRAL EDEMA (FIG. 1–51)

The term "cerebral edema" is defined as an abnormal accumulation of the fluid associated with volumetric enlargement of the brain tissue. Two major types are recognized relative to the essential underlying mechanisms and are contrasted for discussion purposes.

A. *Vasogenic Type*	B. *Cytotoxic Type*
1. This type is related to injury of the wall of the cerebral blood vessels. It leads to an escape of conventional blood-brain barrier indicators into the surrounding parenchyma.	1. In this type, a noxious factor affects the structural element of the parenchyma directly, producing intracellular swelling. Vascular permeability remains relatively undisturbed.
2. Edema fluid basically represents filtrate, including plasma proteins. This explains eosinophilic and PAS-positive reactions in histology.	2. Basically, plasma ultrafiltrate is involved. Its composition is influenced by the type of agents.

In individual cases, the situation is usually complex. Undoubtedly, extravasated plasma fluid adversely affects the structural elements of the parenchyma, and conversely, their swelling may eventually interfere with vascular permeability. In addition, it is not unusual for some injurious agent to act simultaneously on both blood vessels and parenchyma.

3. The injury to cerebral vasculature is usually of a *local* character, such as occurs in the vicinity of brain tumors, traumatic lesions, inflammatory foci, and so on. A *generalized* disturbance of vascular permeability can be envisaged resulting from some toxic agent that injures blood vessels diffusely or from severe interference with hemodynamics at a central level.	3. This type has been explored far less than the vasogenic type, and the available information is based mainly on experimental investigations of edema produced by triethyltin poisoning, water intoxication, and certain anoxic conditions. The cellular swelling (intracellular overhydration) itself is a nonspecific reaction, which can be induced by agents of varying nature that dis-

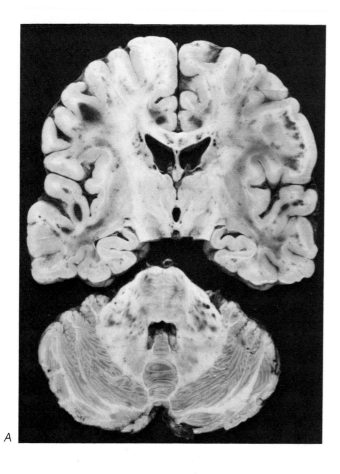

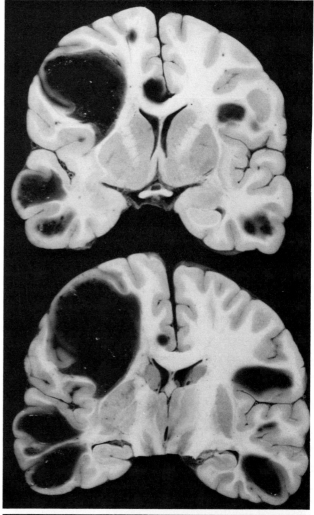

Figure 1–50. Leukemic hemorrhage. *A,* Multiple petechiae and small hemorrhages. *B,* Multiple large and small hemorrhages. *C,* Small and large foci of hemorrhagic infiltration with necrosis in brachial plexus.

A. *Vasogenic Type*

turb cell osmotic regulation.

The crucial event is suspected to be interference with the sodium pump of the glial cells. Astrocytes are thought to be especially susceptible to swelling because of their high sodium content.

4. Most examples of significant cerebral edema appear to have a major vasogenic component.

B. *Cytotoxic Type*

4. In man, the manifestations of cytotoxic edema are superimposed or even modified by a vasogenic component.

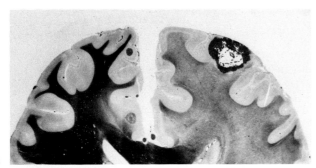

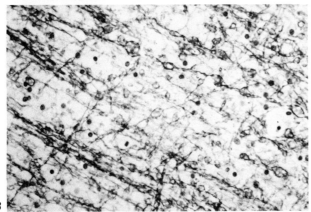

Figure 1–51. Cerebral edema. A, Extensive edema of white matter (right side) incident to superficial invasion of white matter by cortical metastatic tumor as manifested by pallor of affected area due to separation of individual myelin sheaths and their eventual breakdown caused by presence of edema fluid. Note absence of edema when metastasis is confined to cortex (LFB/CV). B, Close-up view of edematous area showing irregularly beaded appearance of myelin sheaths (LFB/CV).

5. This type of edema is predominantly localized in the white matter.

6. Ultrastructurally, there is enlargement of extracellular spaces in the white matter associated with cellular swelling. The latter predominantly affects astrocyte foot processes.

5. The gray or white matter is involved, depending on the type of cytotoxic agent that is involved.

6. Ultrastructurally, there is no enlargement of the extracellular space. The main feature is swelling of various cellular tissue components, depending on the type of agents that are used.

C. Hydrocephalus

A third type of cerebral edema exists in cases of hydrocephalus. The stretched ventricular walls cause tears in the ependymal lining, resulting in escape of fluid, which consists essentially of CSF seeping into the extracellular space of the periventricular white matter. Some swelling of astrocytes is also seen.

In commonly encountered human conditions in which edema is associated with a focal lesion, the edematous brain tissue appears swollen, somewhat softened, and semitranslucent. In long-standing edema, the affected tissue becomes yellowish and quite soft; it eventually becomes microcystic. In the presence of jaundice, as in metastatic liver disease, edematous areas will also show bile staining as an expression of a disturbed blood-brain barrier.

Histologically, the tissue elements appear separated by accumulated fluid. Myelin sheaths, followed by axons, become irregular, beaded, and vacuolated. They eventually break down. This may attract macrophage formation. In chronic edema, there is widespread astrocytic hypertrophy and hyperplasia (gliosis), which, in a small cerebral biopsy, may resemble a low-grade astrocytic tumor and may lead to a diagnostic error. Any sizable increase in the volume or mass of the brain (hematoma, neoplasm, infarct, or edema)—which is enclosed within a rigid, nonexpansible bony skull—will be reflected in a reciprocal diminution in the volume of cerebral fluid and intravascular blood. When this compensatory mechanism is exhausted, elevation of intracranial pressure ensues. Secondary effects on the brainstem occur, particularly on the cardiocirculatory and respiratory centers, and cause eventual impairment of cerebral perfusion, nutrition, and metabolism. In addition, ischemia and hypoxia contribute to edema formation, and thus a vicious cycle is established. They cause an additional increase in intracranial pressure and thus result in decompensation and death. These phenomena will be dealt with in the next section (1.9).

1.9 CEREBRAL HERNIATIONS AND THEIR SECONDARY VASCULAR EFFECTS

Any intracranial mass lesion, whether vascular, inflammatory, or neoplastic in origin, will necessitate readjustments of the tissue relationships within the confines of the skull, which is essentially a closed vessel except in early infancy. This is particularly true if the lesion is accompanied by cerebral edema, which also adds to the intracranial tissue mass.

Adjustment usually results in a projection of the swollen tissue into free space that can accommodate it. This process is referred to as "cerebral internal herniation." The primary clinical concern here is that the herniating tissue may cause pressure effects on the vital brainstem structures. It may also compress or stretch blood vessels within the swollen tissue or the compressed brainstem structures. This results in irreversible tissue damage, which may be either hemorrhage or infarction.

The major forms of cerebral internal herniation and their consequences are shown in Table 1–8 as a flow sheet. These are concerned mainly with the effects of a supratentorial mass on the rostral portion of the brainstem across the tentorium. An infratentorial mass lesion will also cause a "reverse" herniation. The former affects the vital functions of the medulla oblongata more directly and rarely gives sufficient time for this reverse herniation to be significant.

TABLE 1–8. Summary of Various Forms of Cerebral Tissue Herniation and Their Consequences*

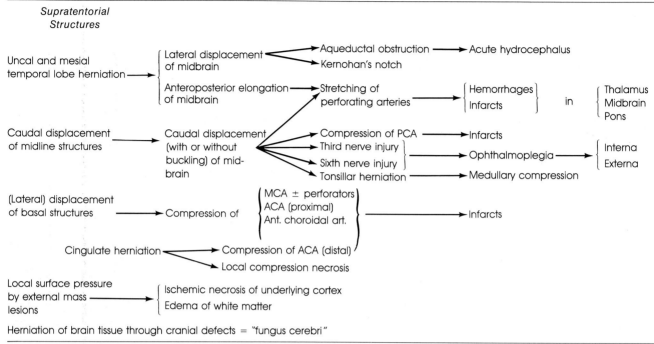

* ACA = anterior cerebral artery; AP = anteroposterior; MCA = middle cerebral artery; PCA = posterior cerebral artery.

Some of the more important features will be explained below (Fig. 1–52). A unilateral expanding supratentorial lesion is postulated here. The ipsilateral uncus and eventually the entire mesial temporal lobe go over the tentorial edge. This competes with the midbrain for space encompassed between the rigidly held tentorial edges. The contralateral cerebral peduncle is pushed against and injured by the opposing tentorial edge. This damage appears as a linear surface indentation known as "Kernohan's notch." In a frontal section of the peduncle, this appears as a sharp horizontal cut. The ipsilateral peduncle is usually not injured, because it is positioned against the soft temporal lobe tissue. A notch, at times resulting in a focal hemorrhagic necrosis, appears on the ventral aspect of the herniating mesial temporal lobe. The posterior cerebral artery is also compressed against the tentorial edge underneath this herniating tissue; the result is an infarction, almost invariably hemorrhagic, of its supply territory.

In addition to the anteroposterior elongation resulting from the lateral compression, the midbrain is usually displaced caudally. These two deforming forces result in stretching of the arterial perforators to the rostral brainstem (from the thalamus to the pons). Focal rupture of small arteries results in hemorrhages (sometimes referred to as "Duret hemorrhages") along these vessels. Typically, they are in the midline of the midbrain and in the lateral tegmentum of the pons, at least initially. Hemorrhages may occur along the perforators in the thalamus. Sometimes, hemor-

rhages extend into the base of the pons or rupture into the fourth ventricle. Infarcts may also occur in the distal region of these affected vessels.

Distortion and obstruction of the aqueduct may lead to internal hydrocephalus.

Cranial nerves, particularly the third and sixth nerves, are stretched out as the brainstem is pushed caudally. The third nerve tends to be injured by being pressed against the plica retroclinoidea medialis and the caudally descending proximal portion of the posterior cerebral artery. Focal hemorrhages may occur at these points. The descent of the uncus also presses on the third nerve.

The supratentorial pressure is also transmitted to the cerebellar tonsils, which descend into the foramen magnum and compete with the medulla for the limited space. The medulla is often compressed anteriorly and deformed (posterolateral flattening) by the tonsils.

Compression and distortion of the other arteries, such as the middle cerebral artery with its perforators, anterior cerebral artery, and anterior choroidal artery, may occasionally result in infarction in their distribution.

The cingulate gyrus also herniates underneath the free edge of the falx, which is more flexible than the tentorium. Compression of the local arteries causes hemorrhagic infarction in a manner similar to that seen with the posterior cerebral artery, in addition to a focal compressive necrosis.

When the expanding mass is over the brain tissue, as is the case with a subdural hematoma (see section 2.2), isch-

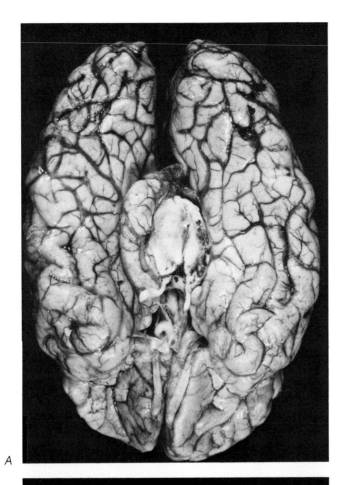

A

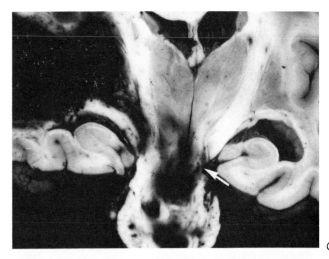

C

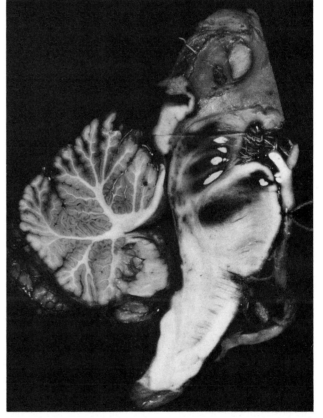

D

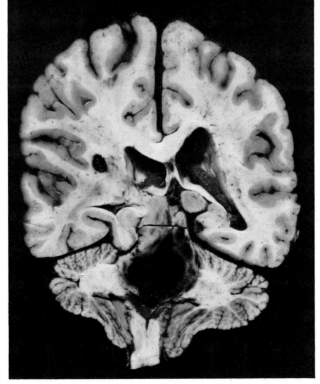

B

Figure 1–52. *A* and *B,* Chronic herniation of left mesial temporal lobe caudally beyond left free edge of tentorium (not shown), with pronounced distortion of rostral brainstem, leading terminally to massive secondary hemorrhages in a patient with organized left frontal subdural hematoma. *C,* Massive left intracerebral hemorrhage from ruptured aneurysm, causing right cerebral peduncle to be jammed against free edge of right tentorial leaflet (not shown but represented by *arrow*) and resulting in Kernohan's notch. *D,* Midsagittal section of brainstem, showing secondary hemorrhages in midbrain and pons. White patches of barium sulfate within hemorrhages represent evidence of leakage from outstretched perforating arteries during limited postmortem angiographic study of

(Continued)

83

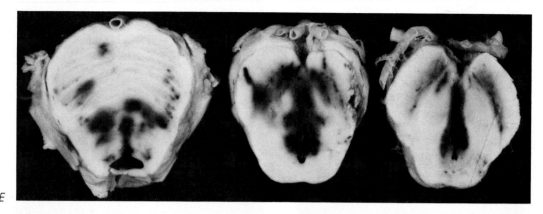

E

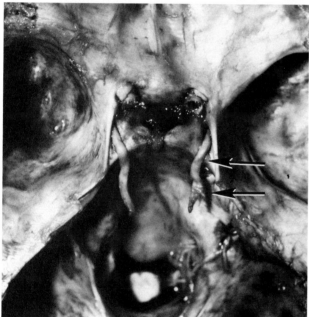

F

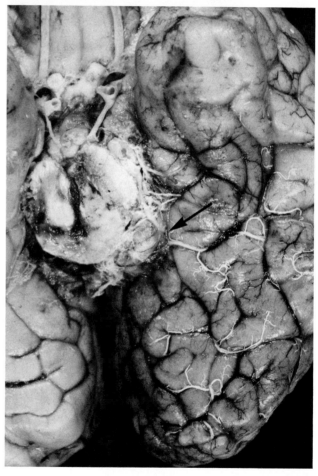

G

(Continued)

rostral basilar artery. E, Typical distribution pattern of secondary hemorrhages in midbrain and pons in early stage; mild right Kernohan's notch is evident in middle slice. F, Isolated oculomotor nerves with two focal points of compression incident to caudal displacement of rostral brainstem: (1) anterior kink (distal in relation to origin of nerve), caused by plica retroclinoidea medialis (*upper arrow*), and (2) posterior (proximal) notch, caused by posterior cerebral artery, more evident on right (*lower arrow*). G, Compression of left posterior cerebral artery by free edge of left tentorial leaflet (not shown) at point indicated by *arrow*, incident to astrocytoma

emic necrosis of the underlying cortex, usually mild and patchy, and edema of the white matter may result. The edema adds to the mass effect on the brainstem.

Herniation of the swollen brain tissue through a craniectomy defect (as in head trauma or recurrent neoplasm), jamming the herniated tissue against the bony edge, causes ischemic necrosis (infarction) of the tissue, in a manner similar to an incarcerated intestinal hernia. Probably, both venous and arterial factors contribute. This type of herniation, particularly that of the chronic type as in recurrent brain tumor, was referred to as "fungus cerebri."

Infratentorial mass lesions such as a cerebellar hemorrhage directly compress the medulla. It must, however, be realized that the medulla can tolerate a considerable degree of compression and deformity when these occur over a prolonged period.

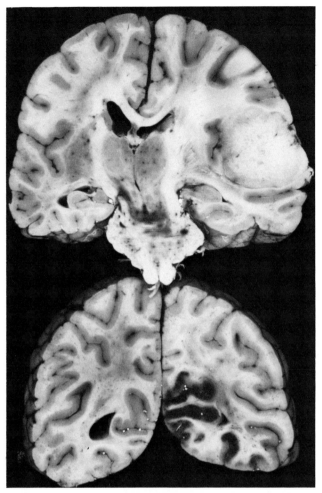

H

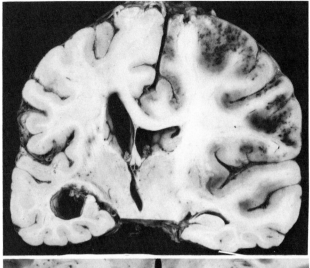

I

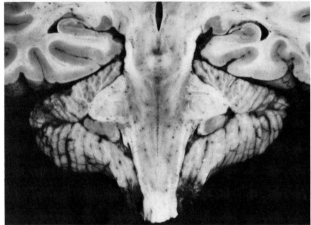

J

of right thalamus. *H*, Recent hemorrhagic infarction in distribution of compressed right posterior cerebral artery in patient with large metastatic carcinoma of lung in ipsilateral hemisphere (postmortem angiography). *I*, Subfalcial herniation of right cingulate gyrus to left due to massive infarction and edema of right cerebral hemisphere as a result of thrombosis of right internal carotid artery. Right uncal herniation and secondary hemorrhage in left thalamus are also evident. *J*, Acute herniation into foramen magnum of cerebellar tonsils, which show evidence of "incarceration" (hemorrhagic necrosis), in a patient with diffuse anoxic cerebral edema.

REFERENCES

Adams H: The "respirator brain" (letter to the editor). *Arch Neurol* 33:589, 1976.

Adams JH, Brierley JB, Connor RCR, et al: The effects of systemic hypotension upon the human brain: clinical and neuropathological observations in 11 cases. *Brain* 89:235–268, 1966.

Brierley JB: The neuropathology of brain hypoxia. In *Scientific Foundations of Neurology*. Edited by M Critchley, JL O'Leary, B Jennett. Philadelphia, FA Davis Company, 1972, pp 243–252.

Carter AB: *Cerebral Infarction*. Oxford, Pergamon Press, 1964, pp 115–122.

Fisher CM: Pathological observations in hypertensive cerebral hemorrhage. *J Neuropathol Exp Neurol* 30:536–550, 1971.

Fisher CM: Cerebral miliary aneurysms in hypertension. *Am J Pathol* 66:313–330, 1972.

Jones HR, Millikan CH: Temporal profile (clinical course) of acute carotid system cerebral infarction. *Stroke* 7:64–71, 1976.

Millikan CH, Bauer RB, Goldschmidt J, et al: A classification and outline of cerebrovascular diseases II. *Stroke* 6:564–616, 1975.

Millikan CH, Moersch FP: Factors that influence prognosis in acute focal cerebrovascular lesions. *Arch Neurol Psychiatry* 70:558–562, 1953.

Pearson J, Korein J, Harris JH, et al: Brain death: II. Neuropathological correlation with the radioisotopic bolus technique for evaluation of critical deficit of cerebral blood flow. *Ann Neurol* 2:206–210, 1977.

Riggs HE, Rupp C: Variation in form of circle of Willis: the relation of the variations to collateral circulation; anatomic analysis. *Arch Neurol* 8:8–14, 1963.

Walker AE: The "respirator brain" (reply to letter to the editor). *Arch Neurol* 33:589–590, 1976.

Whisnant JP, Fitzgibbons JP, Kurland LT, et al: Natural history of stroke in Rochester, Minnesota, 1945 through 1954. *Stroke* 2:11–22, 1971.

Zülch KJ: *Cerebral Circulation and Stroke*. Berlin, Springer-Verlag, 1971, pp 106–122.

2. *Traumatic Lesions of the Nervous System*

2.0 MECHANISMS AND TYPES OF CRANIAL INJURY

The mechanism by which force is applied to the head determines the peculiar effects of injury, and the intensity of the force determines the extent of the lesion(s). *Mechanisms* may be classified as follows (Fig. 2–1):

I. Mechanisms

A. Direct injury
1. Compression of the head by some relatively unyielding object (birth injuries, crushing injuries) (Fig. 2–1 *A*)
2. Head struck by objects in motion
    a. Penetration of the skull by small missiles at high velocity (bullet wounds) (Fig. 2–1 *B*)
    b. Penetration by edged weapons with moderate force and low velocity (stab wounds) (Fig. 2–1 *C*)
    c. Blows by larger objects at relatively low velocity (falling objects, flying fragments of machines or machine products, and so on) (Fig. 2–1 *D*)
    d. Repeated sharp blows or jars to the head ("punch drunk") (Fig. 2–1 *E*)
3. Head in motion striking a relatively immobile solid object (traffic injuries, falls) (Fig. 2–1 *F*)

B. Indirect injury
1. Falls on feet or buttocks

II. Types

With respect to *types* of craniocerebral injuries, an essential distinction must be made among the following types of injury because of the different effects they have on the brain parenchyma:

A. Penetrating (open) injury occurs when the dura is broken through. In addition to causing skull (or spinal) fractures, it exposes the brain (or spinal cord) to the outside. Lacerations or wounds of the brain by foreign objects, including in-driven bone fragments, are the rule.

B. In nonpenetrating (closed) injury, the dura is intact. Even though there may be skull fracture, the brain is shielded from the outside. Cerebral damage includes contusions or hemorrhages due to mechanical stress within the cerebral tissue or to its movements relative to the skull. This type is far more important in civilian accidents. Although there is often relatively minor external evidence of trauma, the brain may have been severely injured.

2.1 SKULL FRACTURES

By themselves, skull fractures may not be of serious clinical consequence, but they may be responsible for various types of damage to the intracranial contents, as will be described below.

A. Skull fractures can be classified by their morphologic features, as follows:
1. Depressed fractures
    These are largely due to the local impact of a moving object or to falling or running into a sharp object. They are likely to tear the dura (open trauma), with or without in-driven fragments.
2. Linear fractures
    These are usually due to the impact of the moving head with a solid object.
3. Special types
    a. Radiating and circumferential fractures associated with the depressed fractures of a gunshot or incised wound
    b. Fractures by diastasis—that is, the opening up of suture lines, usually of children
    c. Meridional fractures—that is, those occurring at a distance from the point of impact because of bending of the skull as a whole
    d. Bursting fractures
    These are incident to gross crushing injuries from compression of the head

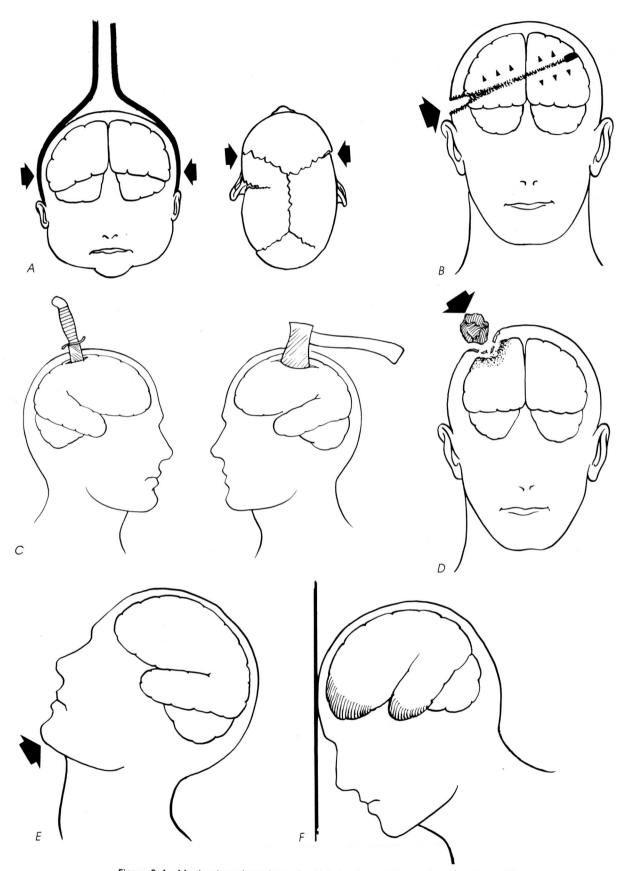

Figure 2–1. Mechanism of craniocerebral injuries. See text for explanation (page 87).

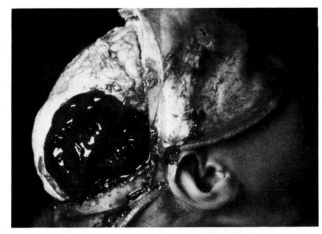

A

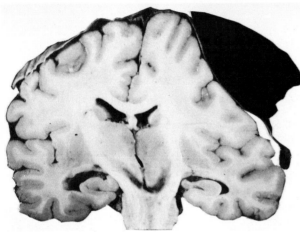

B

Figure 2–2. Cranial epidural hemorrhage. *A,* Acute fatal right temporal lesion in a young child (with scalp reflected and portion of cranial bone removed). *B,* Extensive lesion on right side compressing underlying brain (lower portion of hematoma is not shown). (*A* and *B* courtesy of Kings County Hospital, Brooklyn, New York.)

B. The following anatomic features are noted, depending on the location of the fractures:

1. Fractures of the cranial vault

The fracture lines are usually found between the bony ridges (buttresses) of the skull.

2. Fractures of the base of the skull

The fracture lines tend to follow the line of direction of the applied forces.

3. Vascular tear

This involves mainly the branches of the middle meningeal artery, which runs along the inner surface of the skull.

4. Cerebral lacerations or contusions by depressed fractures

C. Consequences of skull fractures

1. No serious effects

This is especially true when the dura is intact. Conversely, roughly a quarter of fatal head injuries are associated with no evidence of skull fractures.

2. Communications between the intracranial space and septic cavities, such as the nasal and paranasal cavities or the external auditory meatus. This creates the special risk of intracranial infection. Associated meningeal tear will result in cerebrospinal fluid (CSF) leaks (e.g., CSF rhinorrhea).

3. Damage to cranial nerves as they emerge at the base of the skull

2.2 MENINGEAL HEMORRHAGE

There are three types of meningeal hemorrhage to be considered:

A. Epidural or extradural hemorrhage (or hematoma) (Fig. 2–2)
B. Subdural hemorrhage (or hematoma) (Fig. 2–3 and 2–4)
C. Subarachnoid hemorrhage

The first two are of greatest clinical significance. The *epidural* hemorrhage lies between the cranial periosteum and the bone, since the dura proper and the periosteum are inseparable within the cranial cavity—unlike the situation in the spinal canal, where these two membranes are separated by a fatty epidural tissue. The *subdural* hemorrhage collects in the space between the dura and the leptomeninges. In the normal situation, this is largely a potential space. These two types of hemorrhage tend to form a localized accumulation, which exerts a mass effect on the underlying brain, and they are therefore often referred to as hematomas.

The *subarachnoid* hemorrhage, in contrast, tends to diffuse within the subarachnoid space and rarely causes a mass effect. The leptomeninges (arachnoid) may be torn, however, and CSF and subarachnoid blood may accumulate in the subdural space.

Because of the contrasting pathogenesis and effects on the brain, the epidural and subdural hemorrhages are discussed side-by-side in Table 2–1.

Because of the clinical importance of subdural hemorrhage, further explanatory notes will be given below.

1. Elderly persons are considered to be more vulnerable to the tearing force on bridging veins because of the cerebral atrophy that increases the "free traveling distance" of these veins. On the other hand, the increased "free space" between the skull and the brain in the elderly allows them to tolerate a greater volume of blood in this space than a young person would without experiencing symptoms. This also applies to epidural hematomas. We have seen examples of roentgenographically (e.g., by computed tomography scan) "insignificant" acute subdural hematomas in young persons ultimately leading to a significant brain compression. Signs of ventricular compression or midline shift appear to be more reliable indicators of the life-threatening nature of the lesion than its thickness.

2. The organization of a large subdural hemorrhage takes place along the inner surface of the dura in contact with the blood, by activation of previously dormant dural cells. It

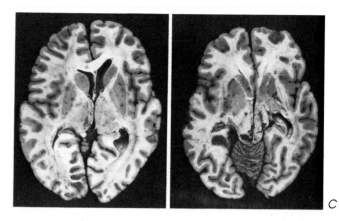

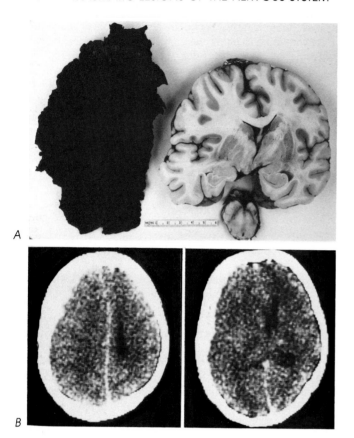

Figure 2–3. Acute cranial subdural hemorrhage. A, Large hemorrhage on left laid flat on side of compressed brain slice. B and C, Computed tomography images (B) of left-sided hemorrhage considered too small to require surgical evacuation (note shift of ventricular system) and gross appearance (C) of compressed brain 21 days after injury (note midbrain compression and secondary hemorrhages).

proceeds along the lateral edge of the hematoma over the inner surface of the blood toward the center. The leptomeninges as a rule remain indifferent and do not participate in the organization.

3. The mechanisms for the characteristically delayed development of clinical symptoms of encapsulated chronic subdural hematomas are not completely understood. Two major factors must be considered:

 a. The possible expansion of the encapsulated fluid

 Since the measured protein contents of hematomas show a general decline as the time between the known head trauma and the evacuation lengthens, it was thought likely that the initially protein-rich fluid that was derived from breakdown of blood attracted plasma osmotically from thin-walled sinusoids, which are numerous in the neomembrane, particularly in the outer one in direct contact with the dura. A similar osmotic mechanism across the thin outer neomembrane (facing the arachnoid) has also been invoked in explanation. Another possible cause for a continued expansion is bleeding into the cyst from these sinusoids. This time-honored concept of continued expansive potential of a chronic subdural hematoma has been at least in part challenged by more recent observations.

 b. The edematous expansion of the compressed underlying brain, largely secondary to venous stagnation

 This appears to take place even if the chronic sub-

dural hematoma remains constant in size. Once the edema sets in, a vicious cycle of further vascular compromise and anoxia leading to more edema can be established. It should also be noted here that the compressed and ''molded'' brain tissue makes a slow recovery to its normal contour after surgical evacuation of the hematoma, and the adverse secondary compressive effects on the rostral brainstem and other structures are not immediately relieved.

4. It has long been assumed that a subdural hemorrhage originally assumes (on anteroposterior view) a convex-concave cross-sectional contour and becomes biconvex later. New radiologic evidence (Radcliffe et al., 1972) suggests that the biconvex hematomas are seen predominantly in the older age group at any time after known traumatic events (after 10 days in this series), and cerebral atrophy is considered a likely underlying factor to account for this configuration.

C. Subarachnoid hemorrhage

This type of bleeding occurs in two main forms: (1) as a constant accompaniment of cerebral contusions, to be described below, or (2) as an independent lesion. It is either focal and limited (commonly) or diffuse (rarely) in extent. It is seldom of clinical significance by itself. Blood tends to accumulate in the sulci and cisterns but rarely to an extent to cause compressive manifestations. Bleeding vessels are rarely identified at autopsy.

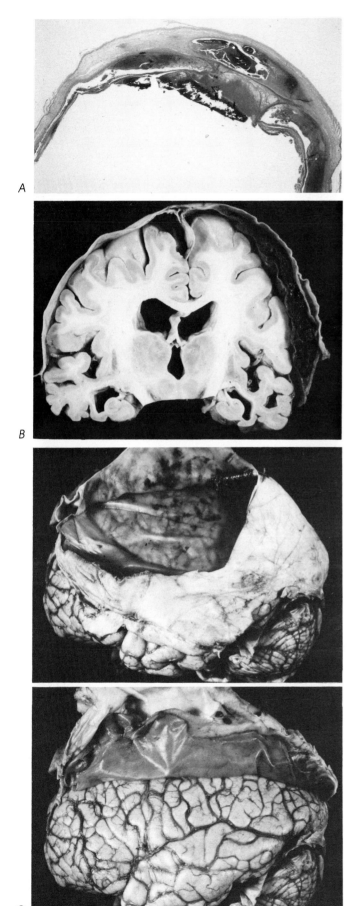

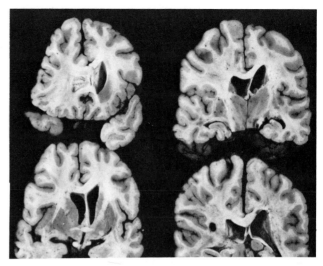

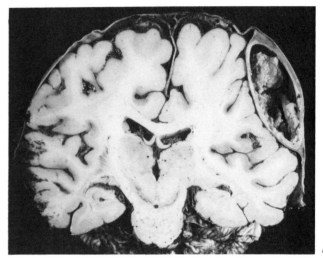

Figure 2–4. Chronic (organized) cranial subdural hemorrhage. *A*, Photomicrograph of multilayered subdural hemorrhages in different stages of organization as seen in a patient with chronic alcoholism (H&E). *B*, Large organized lesion over atrophic brain, which shows little evidence of compressive effects in an aged patient. *C*, Outside (through reflected dural window) and inside (after being reflected up) views of "inner membrane," after removal of liquefied blood. *D*, Persistent ("molded") compression of brain with left-sided chronic lesion surgically evacuated only after catastrophic deterioration (due to brainstem decompensation), too late to save the patient's life (same case as in Figure 1–52 *A* and *B*). *E*, Chronic, partially calcified lesion still containing debris in a patient from a psychiatric institution. The opposite temporal lobe shows recent superficial contusion. (*A*, *C*, and *E* courtesy of Kings County Hospital, Brooklyn, New York.)

TABLE 2–1. Comparison of Epidural and Subdural Hemorrhage

	Epidural Hemorrhage	Subdural Hemorrhage
Incidence	In unselected cases, 0.4% In selected trauma cases, 3.0% In fatal trauma cases, 20%	In unselected cases, 1 to 2% In selected cases, 17% (Munro, 1936) In state hospital cases, 8% In the newborn, 2 to 3%
Type of injury	Almost invariably associated with skull fractures, mainly temporal on the same side	With or without skull fractures; often trivial injury in elderly patients *Note:* Subdural hemorrhage may be seen without a history of trauma. 1. "Nontraumatic," e.g., in blood dyscrasias in which increased bleeding tendency exists 2. "Idiopathic" or "spontaneous" without above causes. Some probably occur after a minor trauma that has been forgotten.
Source of bleeding	1. Arterial. Due to tear of the middle meningeal artery or its branches 2. Dural sinus tear. In roughly 15% of cases (mainly from the sagittal and lateral sinuses)	1. Venous. Due to tear of bridging veins. When the arachnoid is also torn, the CSF leakage will create a variable mixture of blood and CSF in the subdural space which resembles tincture of iodine.

Type of bleeding	All are acute in development, often combined with cerebral contusions or lacerations. Blood appears dark red and is jellylike in consistency.	1. Acute type
		  a. Usually found in association with severe injuries to the brain as a less significant clinical problem
		  b. Exceptionally, clinically significant acute subdural hemorrhage may occur without severe cerebral injuries. This is particularly true among patients with poorly controlled anticoagulant therapy.
		2. Chronic, encapsulated type, often after trivial trauma with delayed onset of symptoms

Location	Lower, mainly over the temporal region (on the middle third) Atypical locations: frontal, subfrontal, subtemporal, occipital, and in the posterior fossa Rarely bilateral	Over the convexity, higher than the epidural, near the vertex and mainly in the middle third Atypical locations: subfrontal, interhemispheric, and in the posterior fossa Bilateral in 15% of cases
Outcome	Arterial bleeding tends to continue, with expansion of the hematoma, leading to increasing compression of the brain which often proves fatal unless evacuated surgically	1. Extensive acute bleeding may rapidly compress the brain tissue in a manner similar to that of epidural hemorrhage. 2. Complete organization and absorption of the blood occurs when the bleeding is limited in volume. The resulting new membrane gives the false impression that the hemorrhage occurred within the dura. This picture was also considered in the past to be inflammatory in origin and was referred to as "pachymeningitis hemorrhagica interna." A large amount of blood (if not acutely fatal) would be encapsulated but not completely absorbed. Breakdown of blood, however, continues within the cavity to a varying degree. This state is known as chronic (encapsulated) subdural hematoma (see note in text). More than two layers of organized hematoma are not uncommon among those who are prone to repeated falls and subdural bleeding (e.g., alcoholics).
Clinical significance	The epidural hemorrhage endangers the patient's life by its rapid, continued expansion from the time of accident.	The subdural hemorrhage tends to go unrecognized until much later after the trauma (which may have been very trivial and has been forgotten, particularly among the elderly), when slow accumulation has reached a sufficient size (subacute, usually not encapsulated) or when the encapsulated hematoma has enlarged (believed to be a result of osmosis from numerous dilated capillary "sinusoids" in the newly formed membranes). It is also very important to realize that the development of symptoms may be insidious and vague. However, a fatal "decompensation" of the brain can occur with alarming rapidity.

2.3 FOCAL CEREBRAL PARENCHYMAL DAMAGE

Several interrelated focal forms of traumatic parenchymal lesions will be considered here, exclusive of deep penetrating wounds, which will be described later. These may be divided into four forms:

A. Contusions, including petechiae
B. Lacerations
C. Hemorrhages
D. Cerebral concussion

A. Contusions

Contusions are "bruises" that are caused by physical distortion of the tissue and are characterized by petechial hemorrhages secondary to tears of capillaries. Evidence for mechanical damage to other elements such as neurons is more subtle and is difficult to discern in the early phase. In longer-surviving cases, an ischemic factor may play a significant role in the production and appearance of the lesion. Contusions tend to involve the ridges of the convolutions and characteristically have an overall wedge-shaped configuration with the apex toward the depth of the brain on cross section (Fig. 2–5 to 2–8).

There are two main mechanisms by which lesions are encountered:

1. With a depressed fracture, with or without penetration of the dura by foreign bodies (including in-driven bone fragments), directly damaging the underlying brain tissue. This

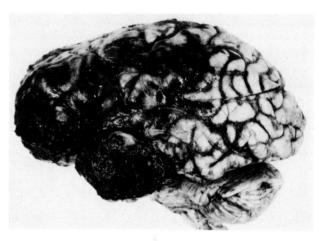

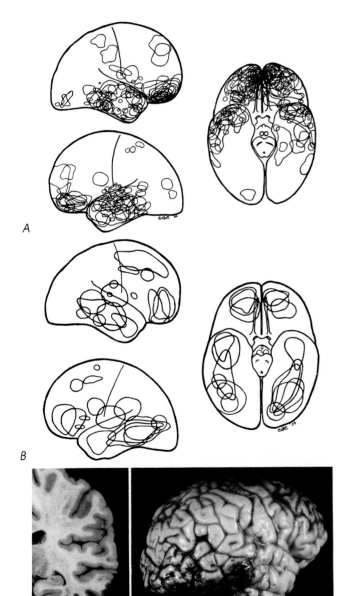

Figure 2–5. Contusions. A and B, Diagrams of distributional patterns of contusions (A) and hematomas (B) derived from composite overlaying of many lesions. C, External and cross-sectional appearance of recent superficial contusion in right lateral temporal lobe. D, Extensive acute contusions in anterior left frontal and temporal lobes, with subarachnoid hemorrhage extending more posteriorly. (A and B from Courville CB: Pathology of the Central Nervous System. Third edition. Mountain View, CA, Pacific Press Publishing Association, 1950. By permission.)

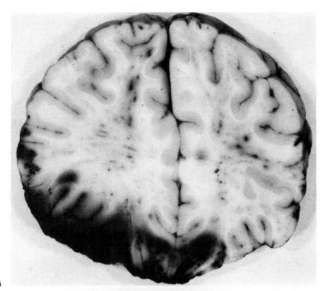

A

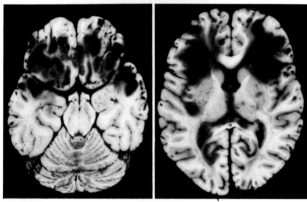

B

Figure 2-6. Contusions. *A,* Recent extensive but asymmetric contusions of frontal lobes. *B,* Bilateral basal frontal and anterior temporal contusions demonstrated in horizontal cuts.

phenomenon is known as "coup" effect and occurs mainly as a result of an object impacting on the stationary head.

2. With or without a depressed fracture, more likely occurring when the head is in motion at the moment of impact and resulting in coup and "contre-coup" lesions of the brain. These lesions occur mainly as a result of the moving head hitting a broad stationary object, for example the dashboard of a car (deceleration injury) (Fig. 2–5 *A*). Less commonly, they occur when an object hits the unsupported head, as in boxing (acceleration injury).

Although many theories have been proposed to explain the precise physical mechanisms involved, none is completely satisfactory. It is, however, generally accepted that the relative movements of the skull and the brain inside it are of paramount importance. The acceleration and deceleration of the skull and delayed movements of the brain tissue may be linear, but, probably more importantly, they are often angular and create rotatory forces of shear strain within the brain substance.

When the locations of contusions in many individual cases are superimposed, a pattern of predilection emerges regardless of the sites of impact (mainly with deceleration injuries), as illustrated in Fig. 2–5 *A*.

It is clear from the diagram that both coup and contre-coup lesions are localized largely in those portions of the frontal and temporal lobes where rough bony structures such as the roof of the orbit and crista galli, the wing of the sphenoid bone, or the petrous ridges are in contact with the soft brain tissue. The sharp ridges of the tentorium and falx also serve as unyielding objects against which the brain is battered.

The cerebellar cortex can also be contused; such a lesion is almost invariably associated with a fracture over it, representing a coup lesion. The smooth surface of the posterior fossa appears to protect the cerebellum from the contre-coup effect.

Small foci of petechiae (contusions) are also known to occur in the dorsal brainstem structures and are thought to be due to rotational effects of the brain movement within the skull. Similarly, the parasagittal cortex and white matter show contusions, usually bilaterally, in addition to those explained by coup and contre-coup effects. A certain shearing effect is known to take place along the line of this type of contusion as the brain moves inside the skull. Some refer to these as "gliding contusions."

More or less diffuse *petechial hemorrhages* in the white matter may be considered here as another form of internal contusion associated with capillary damage, which is believed to be due to a shearing force arising from the rotational movements set up within the brain substance.

These may be subdivided into the following patterns: (1) along the plane of "gliding contusions," as described above; (2) in the corpus callosum and the adjacent white matter in the linear path of a traumatic force (i.e., between the surface coup and contre-coup lesions); (3) evenly scattered throughout the white matter.

Note: Diffuse patchy disruption of nerve fibers in the white matter with little other damage is recorded in some cases. This is presumably caused by a similar mechanism. These lesions may heal as minute foci of necrosis with microglial reaction.

The *morphologic evolution* of the contused brain tissue is explained in three phases:

1. The phase of acute damage

The tissue necrosis is almost invariably associated with petechiae due to capillary disruption and occasional thrombosis. Edema of the damaged and surrounding tissue, particularly in the white matter, is often extensive. The general histologic appearance is somewhat similar to that of hemorrhagic infarction. However, the molecular layer of the cortex, which is regularly spared in an infarct, is often disrupted at the crown of the contused gyri.

2. The phase of clearing

This process is similar to that seen in liquefaction of a hemorrhagic infarct by the activities of phagocytes.

3. The phase of repair

In addition to proliferation of fibrous astrocytes at the margin (as in an infarct), a collagenous repair process takes

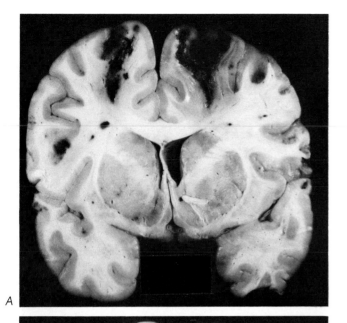

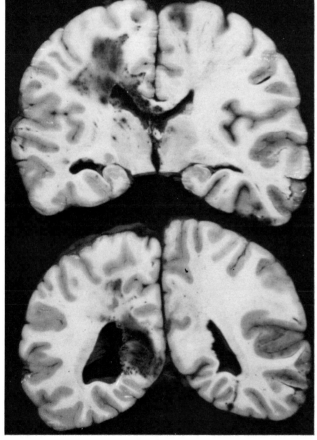

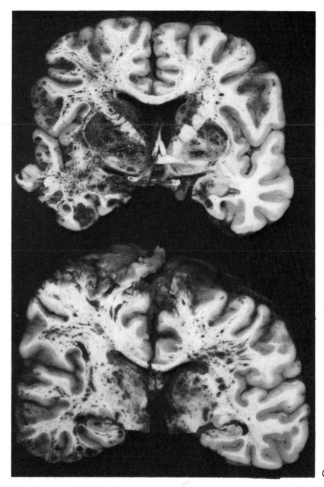

Figure 2–7. "Internal" cerebral contusions. *A*, Recent "gliding" type of contusions in the frontal parasagittal plane. *B*, Petechial hemorrhages in corpus callosum and adjacent white matter. *C*, Diffuse petechial lesions associated with lacerations of dorsal left posterior frontal lobe which were caused by a depressed fracture resulting from a fall on top of the head.

part to a varying degree; its fibroblastic proliferation is due to the reaction of the local blood vessels and the leptomeninges (which are in contact with the cerebral wound) and the dura. Thus, the surface of a healed cerebral contusion is often adherent to the dura. These lesions are characterized

as "fibroglial scars" and are held responsible for a higher incidence of epileptic seizures after contusions than after cerebral infarcts, which heal almost entirely by gliosis. Chronic posttraumatic scars run along the crests of one or more gyri (état vermoulu) and differ from small infarctive

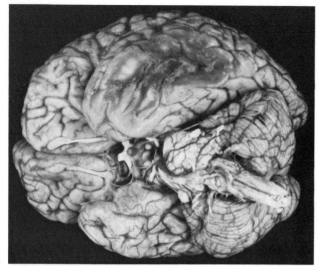

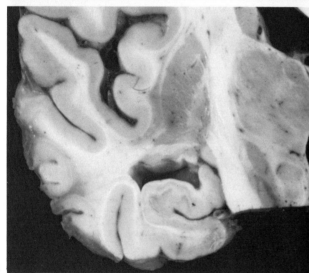

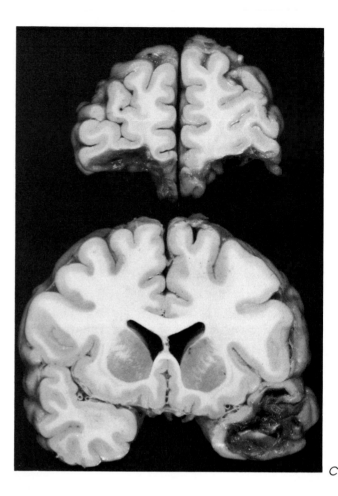

Figure 2–8. Old cerebral contusions. *A* and *B*, External (lateral) and cross-sectional views of superficial left temporal contusion involving crests of adjacent convolutions. *C*, Cross-sectional views of more extensive (deep-reaching) contusions of frontal and temporal lobes.

scars, which tend to favor the depth of the sulci. Some of the large traumatic scars expose a wide area of cerebral white matter.

B. Lacerations

These are tears, that is, outright ruptures of the tissue, and as such they are generally seen at the sites of open wounds where foreign bodies or bone fragments penetrate into the brain for some distance. Lacerations are naturally associated with varying degrees of bleeding if the death of the patient is not instantaneous. Clinically significant lacerations are usually found in the dorsal and lateral aspects of the cerebral hemispheres. The structures at the base of the brain, including the brainstem and cerebellum, may be lacerated when fracture-dislocation occurs in the basal region of the skull. Such lesions are instantaneously fatal and are of forensic and not clinical interest.

C. Hemorrhages (Fig. 2–9)

Petechiae or punctate hemorrhages are a nearly inevitable component of contusions and lacerations. Larger hem-

orrhages (hematomas) may be seen which are more or less independent of them, but truly isolated intracerebral hematomas are infrequent. Their sites of predilection correspond largely to those of contusions.

Hematomas are probably due to disruption of larger blood vessels (as in some cases of laceration) and are generally associated with surface contusions and lacerations seen in severe head injuries. Not infrequently, however, the basal ganglia and thalamus also contain clinically significant hematomas detached from the surface lesions.

Figure 2–9. Traumatic intracerebral hemorrhage. *A*, Brain slices showing recent contusion-hematomas in left basal frontal and anterior temporal regions. *B*, Right frontoparietal hemorrhages associated with local skull fracture caused by boom hitting head at construction site. *C*, Large recent left temporal hemorrhage. *D*, Resolving hematomas in frontal lobes. *E*, Multiple small hemorrhages in basal ganglia (bilateral) and thalamus (right). *F*, Recent hemorrhage in right thalamus through pons.

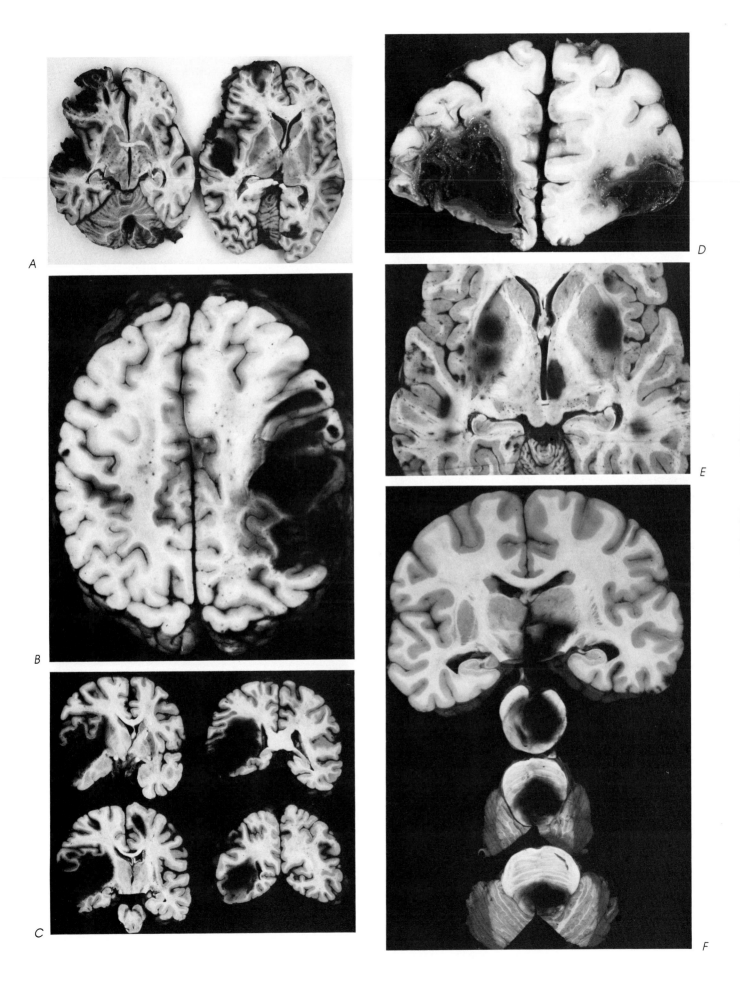

A

B

C

D

E

F

D. Cerebral concussion

By definition, cerebral concussion is a traumatic condition with transient loss of consciousness due to functional disturbance of the brain without demonstrable structural alterations. None of the pathogenetic theories proposed so far appears to provide a satisfactory explanation.

Among the minor structural alterations proposed as being responsible for the clinical picture are (1) nerve cell damage in the reticular formation, (2) tearing of the nerve fibers in the cerebral white matter (see above), and (3) petechial hemorrhages along the floor of the third and fourth ventricles. These hemorrhages are, however, seen occasionally among the unselected nontraumatic autopsy cases.

Duret (1878) conducted animal experiments in which he injected a large amount of fluid into the cranial epidural space and produced petechiae in the periventricular brainstem areas. He theorized that the force of the CSF driven down into the fourth ventricle by the temporarily indented skull was responsible for these petechiae, which in turn were responsible for the immediately paralyzing effect. Berner (1930, 1935) tried to revive the theory. Today, the term ''Duret's hemorrhages'' is used (more correctly) in connection with the secondary brainstem hemorrhages seen in any expanding supratentorial mass (see section 1.9).

No firm anatomic correlate for the immediate paralysis of brain functions has yet been accepted universally. It is not uncommon to see small contusions years later at autopsy after a complete recovery from head trauma (clinical concussion). These small lesions are in all likelihood not the correlates of concussion as such.

2.4 DEEP PENETRATING WOUNDS OF THE BRAIN (FIG. 2–10)

Mainly gunshot wounds are considered in this section. Sufficient blows from blunt instruments with slower velocity result in superficial coup lesions associated mostly with an open fracture, as described in the previous sections.

A. The following missile factors must be considered in assessing their effect on the skull and brain:

1. Composition

A soft-lead bullet usually becomes fragmented and broken up in its passage through the skull; the steel-jacketed one penetrates the bone with its shape unaltered.

2. Size

Other factors being equal, the larger the missile is, the more damage it will cause.

3. Shape

A modern elongated missile turning end over end will create a greater lacerating effect than a round ball of old vintage.

4. Velocity

The velocity of the bullet is the most important of all factors. A bullet injures the brain tissue not only by destruction of tissue along its course through the tissue but also by

its explosive effect, which is proportional to the velocity of the bullet at the time of impact (see below).

5. The line of flight in relation to the surface of the skull

This often determines the type of skull fracture and the nature and extent of intracranial damage. A right-angle entry will cause a round or oval, fairly sharply outlined opening of the skull. As the entry becomes less perpendicular, the lines of fracture radiating about the opening tend to increase in number and length. The exit wound is larger, more irregular than that of entrance, and the radiating fractures are longer and more numerous. A tangential wound, when superficial, may produce only gutter fracture, with little or no depression. When perforating, a tangential wound often causes considerable splintering of the inner table.

B. The traumatic effects of a bullet on the brain are due to the following factors:

1. Explosive and expansile effect

This depends essentially on the velocity of the missile and, to some extent perhaps, on the angle of its penetration. This effect is produced by the expansile force of the gases displaced by the bullet. The cerebral tissues act en masse much as any solid object would. Any profound explosive or shocking effect on the vital centers in the brainstem results in immediate death. Contusions found over the orbital surface of the brain or petechiae in the ventral aspect of the cerebellar hemispheres and distant from the passage of a bullet are testimonial to this force, even though the medulla itself may not display any evidence of tissue damage. The high-velocity bullet from a high-power rifle can literally blow up the skull vault.

2. Lacerating effect

This depends on the size, composition, and degree of penetration of the bullet. The bullet tract is represented by (1) a central channel filled with necrotic tissue that was destroyed by the missile in its passage and (2) a narrow circumferential zone in which death of cells and fibers becomes evident only after a sufficient interval. A secondary tract may result from ricochet of the bullet from the inner table of the skull. With time, the necrotic material becomes phagocytized and removed; this leaves an irregular, partially collapsed canal filled with fluid and surrounded by an irregular glial scar. A variably sized connective tissue plug, adherent to the dura, extends for a variable distance into the wound (as in other penetrating wounds).

3. Hemorrhage

This results from laceration of blood vessels by the bullet or in-driven fragments of bone. Generally, it is seldom excessive, unless one of the larger cerebral arteries or dural sinuses is lacerated. The immediately fatal nature of more severe cerebral damage may preclude the development of massive hemorrhages.

4. Cerebral edema

This plays a considerable part in the fatal outcome in those who survive the initial shock of injury. Both the reaction to the tissue destruction itself and the generalized cerebral anoxia from vasomotor paralysis due to the shocking (expansile) effect of the bullet appear to be important in

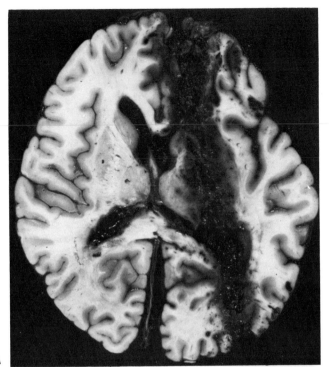

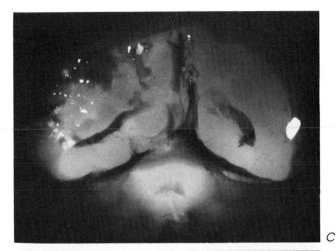

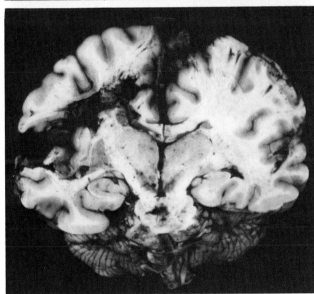

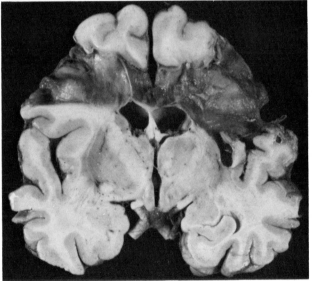

Figure 2–10. Gunshot wound of brain. *A*, Recent anterior-posterior wound tract in right cerebral hemisphere. *B* and *C*, Right-to-left (anteroposterior view) ricocheted bullet tracts in gross specimen (*B*) and on x-ray film (*C*), showing bullet and bone fragments near entry zone and resting bullet in left lateral temporal lobe. *D*, Large side-to-side defect in cerebral hemispheres as end result of small-caliber (.22) bullet wound self-inflicted 10 years previously. (*D* courtesy of Dr. Bruno Volk.)

causing edema. The systemic factors discussed in section 2.5 must also be considered.

2.5 DELAYED VASCULAR COMPLICATIONS

A. Traumatic cerebral edema

It is important to separate two forms: (1) the localized and (2) the diffuse. The combination of the two is not infrequent.

1. *Localized* traumatic cerebral edema

This is an inevitable consequence of tissue destruction such as contusions and hemorrhages and is proportional to the extent of such lesions. When localized edematous changes are visualized clinically, as by computed tomography scan, an underlying contusion should be suspected since the usual petechial hemorrhages of a cerebral contusion often cannot be demonstrated by this means at present.

2. *Diffuse* "traumatic" cerebral edema

This form, unassociated with focal lesions, is more likely to be an expression of cerebral anoxia (hypoxia) due to observed or unrecognized traumatic shock, either immediate or delayed, and to respiratory insufficiency incident to airway obstruction, frail chest, and so on. This occurrence often explains cases with a clinical diagnosis of severe head injury which at autopsy show no focal traumatic cerebral lesions.

B. Evacuation of epidural, subdural, and intracerebral hemorrhage may be followed by *rebleeding*.

C. Cervical arteries may be traumatized concomitantly with head injuries and develop *true* or *false* (or *dissecting*) *aneurysm* or *thrombotic occlusion*.

Rarely, cerebral arteries are involved by similar lesions (Fig. 2–11), at times associated with relatively mild forms of head trauma. Angiographic demonstration of spasm of arteries before thrombosis has been reported. Other lesions show mechanical disruption of the vascular wall, whether due to direct injury or produced indirectly by overstretching. Both the circle of Willis with its major branches and the vertebral-basilar system can be affected. Delayed hemorrhage or infarction will follow.

D. Fat embolism (Fig. 2–12) (see also section 1.10 C)

Although fat embolism is not directly related to head injury, the brain, along with the lungs, is one of the most significant target organs of this systemic phenomenon. Multiple petechiae occur and small infarcts develop as a result of fat droplets plugging up small arteries and capillaries, primarily in the white matter of the brain, although the gray matter is not immune.

2.6 SPINAL CORD INJURIES

The several different modes of insult affecting the spinal column and its contents are described below.

A. Indirect (closed) injuries (Fig. 2–13)

Indirect injuries are due to fracture-dislocation or acute jar to the bone, whose effect is transmitted to the spinal cord.

1. Crush injuries due to direct violence on the spine, resulting from, for instance, falls from a height, striking a beam transversely, or being pinned beneath some collapsing structure or an overturned automobile. These lesions are uncommon, and even when they occur, the spinal cord and its roots may escape serious damage.

2. Indirect injuries by rapid acceleration or deceleration with exaggeration of the normal movements, either hyperflexion or hyperextension, resulting in a fracture or fracture-dislocation of the spine with secondary damage to the spinal cord

a. Hyperflexion of the spine often results in fracture-dislocation of the vertebrae. When it involves the cervical space, it is a result either of falls on the head or, characteristically, of dives into shallow water or sudden forward jerking of the neck, as in a car accident. The site of predilection for fracture-dislocation is the interspace between the C-5 and C-6 vertebrae. Falling objects or heavy weights on the shoulders or upper back (as in mine cave-ins) characteristically result in fracture-dislocation of the T-11, T-12 interspace. Other mecha-

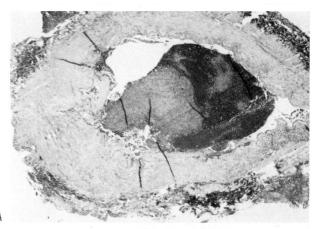

A

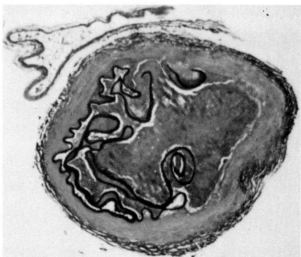

B

Figure 2–11. Indirect (nonpenetrating) traumatic vascular damage. *A*, Traumatic thrombosis of internal carotid artery (cavernous portion), caused by transverse basal fractures across sella and petrous bones. Partially torn segment of internal carotid artery with recent thrombosis (H&E). *B*, Traumatic dissecting aneurysm of middle cerebral artery. Cross section of affected segment of right middle cerebral artery (just proximal to trifurcation).

nisms of cord injuries include compression fracture (teardrop type) with protrusion of the posterior fragments or displaced laminar fragment(s) and tear of the ligaments of the vertebrae and anulus fibrosus with an acute posterior disk protrusion.

b. Hyperextension of the spine, particularly of the cervical spine, typically results from a person's being thrown out of a moving vehicle and landing on the forehead, with the whole body jackknifing backward. This results in forward bulging of the ligamenta flava posteriorly. The bony spurs of degenerative osteoarthritis anteriorly in elderly patients accentuate compression of the cord. An acute posterior disk protrusion can also occur. Posterior dislocation of a vertebra, however, is usually prevented by the long spinal ligaments.

3. Forms of medullary or extramedullary lesions

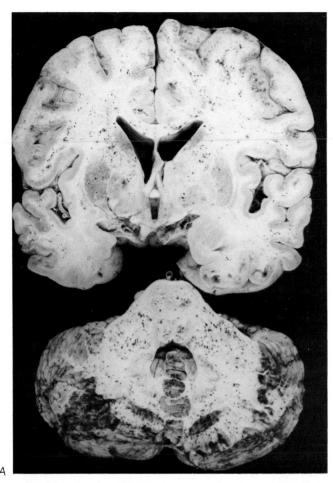

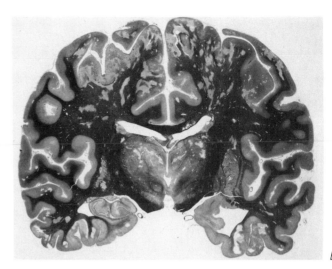

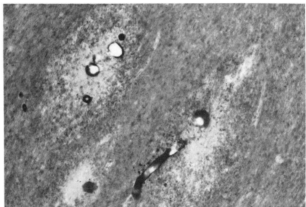

Figure 2–12. Fat embolism. *A,* Gross appearance of cerebral and cerebellar hemispheres with multiple petechiae. *B,* Celloidin section of cerebral hemispheres better delineating small infarcts as pale areas (LFB/CV). *C,* Fat globules obstructing capillaries in the white matter (frozen section, fat stain).

Injuries to the spinal cord parenchyma are caused chiefly at the time of an accident by sudden mechanical stresses to which the nerve tissue is subjected, whether there is a fracture-dislocation or not. When there is dislocation with pressure on the cord or with continued stretching of the cord over a bony or cartilaginous protrusion, ischemia will produce additional tissue damage or at least hinder recovery. Several forms of medullary damage may be distinguished, as follows.

a. Spinal concussion

This is associated with only temporary sensory or motor dysfunction (comparable to cerebral concussion). It requires a force generally greater than that which causes cerebral contusion. Although it is generally assumed that this is a purely functional condition, structural changes may occur at the point of impact and also at some distance from it; milder forms of those structural changes that are described below have been reported.

b. Spinal contusion

This injury may be divided into simple contusion and contusion-compression.

• *Simple contusion* is a rather uncommon lesion; it often involves only the immediate portion of the cord which has been impacted by the bony structure.

• *Contusion-compression* is, in essence, cord crush (Fig. 2–14) and is usually seen as a result of severe fracture-dislocation but can also be due to temporary compression between the bulged ligamenta flava and anterior bony spurs during hyperextension of the cervical spine. The tissue damage is characterized by edematous softening (necrosis) intermingled with small hemorrhages which may be called "hemorrhagic pulping." The lesion may be transversely partial or complete. In most severe instances, the cord is actually transected. However, a thin shell of leptomeninges may retain the anatomic continuity in the absence of the parenchyma.

B. Direct, penetrating injuries (Fig. 2–15)

1. Stab wounds (Fig. 2–15 *A*)

Blades usually penetrate between the vertebrae without bony damage. Hemisection or modified hemisection of the spinal cord will result.

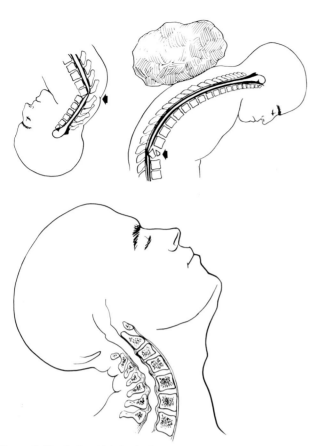

Figure 2–13. Indirect injuries to the spinal cord. See text for details. (*Top* modified from Courville CB: *Pathology of the Central Nervous System.* Third edition. Mountain View, CA, Pacific Press Publishing Association, 1950.)

2. Gunshot and other missile wounds (Fig. 2–15 *B*)

Although damage to the vertebra(e) is the rule, occasionally a missile passes between the vertebral laminae without bony damage and inflicts serious damage to the cord parenchyma. The tissue changes are a combination of initial mechanical damage and damage caused by subsequent hemorrhage, which is often considerable. With high-velocity bullets, the neural tissue may be disintegrated over one or more segments above and below the level of entry in association with considerable bleeding into epidural and subdural spaces. Even when the bullet does not touch the dura or spinal cord. by giving a severe jar to the spinal column it may cause complete or almost complete softening of the cord tissue at the level of impact and minor lesions for a distance of several segments above and below.

3. Combination of direct and indirect violence as in (1) wounds caused by high-velocity bullets and (2) fracture-dislocation with laceration or piercing of the cord by spicules of bone. The tissue damage characteristically extends for several segments above and below the point of impact, not unlike the pattern seen in a spinal cord infarction.

Subsequent evolution of the lesion is similar to that of

an infarct—that is, liquefaction and removal of debris by macrophages, cavitation, and marginal gliosis. The leptomeninges become fibrotic and adherent to the dura to varying degrees. Resprouting of posterior root nerves accompanied by proliferation of Schwann cells within the cavitary segments is a CNS equivalent of the peripheral traumatic neuroma.

C. Traumatic hematomyelia

Although small hemorrhages are an almost invariable accompaniment of the crushed spinal cord, a limited hemorrhage in the central gray matter has been reported, usually after flexion injuries to the spine. Clinical signs and symp-

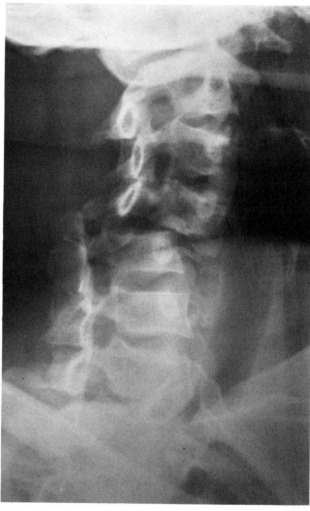

A

Figure 2–14. Spinal contusion. *A* and *B,* Fracture-dislocation of cervical spine (C-4 on C-5) on x-ray film (*A*) and extensive spinal cord contusions in longitudinal gross specimen (*B*). *C,* Recent cervical spinal contusion maximal at C-5 segment on cross section. *D,* Long-standing contusive lesion of cervical cord, resulting in collapsed cavity surrounded by leptomeninges. *E,* Twenty-year-old cervical cord contusion with less complete tissue damage resulting not in a cavity but in thin, contracted gliotic segments, which can be transilluminated.

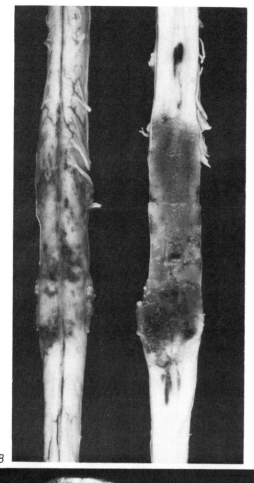

B

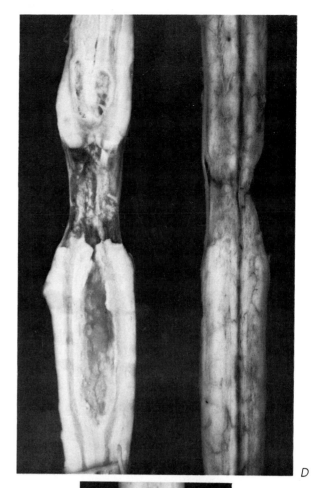

D

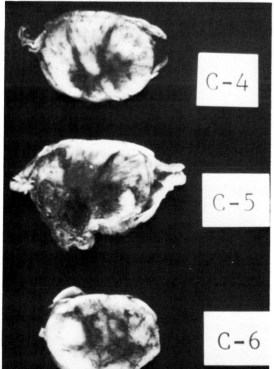

C-4

C-5

C-6

C

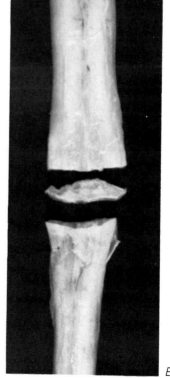

E

103

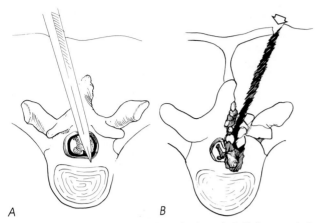

Figure 2–15. Direct injuries to the spinal cord. *A,* Stab wound. *B,* Bullet wound. (Modified from Courville CB: *Pathology of the Central Nervous System.* Third edition. Mountain View, CA, Pacific Press Publishing Association, 1950.)

toms are similar to those seen in syringomyelia. The precise mechanism or reason for this lesion is not known.

D. Subarachnoid hemorrhage is often lacking, even with spinal cord contusion, unlike the situation with the brain.

When it is present, eventual organization may cause constriction of the cord and spinal roots by "chronic adhesive arachnoiditis."

E. Subdural and epidural hemorrhages are rarely of practical importance.

It may be noted that epidural bleeding is due to venous damage (compare intracranial epidural hemorrhage).

2.7 CHRONIC OR SUBACUTE COMPRESSIVE MYELOPATHIES (FIG. 2–16)

The spinal cord and its roots may be compressed by various subacute or chronic conditions of the spinal column, among

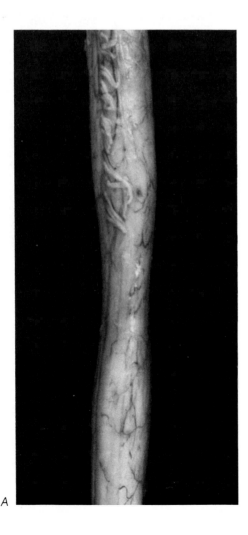

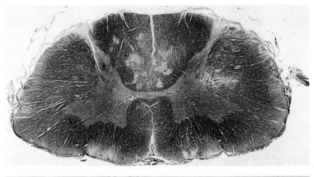

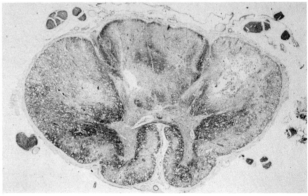

Figure 2–16. Compressive myelopathy. *A* and *B,* Lateral view (*A*) of focally compressed cervical spinal cord as a result of a metastatic lesion of the spine and an LFB/PAS/H-stained section (*B*) of affected segment, showing early damage to long tracts. *C,* Stained section (LFB/CV) of thoracic spinal cord surgically relieved of compression from metastatic spinal tumor but not until extensive damage had been sustained, mainly to long tracts, including foci of cavitary necrosis.

which metastatic lesions and protruded intervertebral disks are the most common and important. In earlier years, tuberculous spondylitis with vertebral compression was one of the most important conditions.

The changes found are attributed to direct mechanical pressure on the structures and to vascular compression, primarily of veins, which cause venous stagnation and edema. Arterial compression or spasm may play a part in some instances. Myelin sheaths appear more vulnerable to the effects of mechanical pressure and to minor degrees of anoxia than are neurons and axons in the spinal cord.

The earliest change is vacuolar degeneration of the white columns, which is due to the presence of distended myelin sheaths, some containing swollen axons, initially in the lateral columns (the posterior portion) and the dorsal columns. Wider areas of the white matter become involved and the older lesions appear more frankly necrotic, with additional involvement of the astroglial scaffolding. The ventral horn may become softened, particularly at the base.

In more rapidly developing lesions, there may be frankly necrotic changes from the onset, involving the entire cross-sectional area or part of it. In such cases, a vascular cause is more strongly suspected, although rarely local arteries show thrombosis or other occlusive changes. Compression of an important radicular artery at or close to the intervertebral foramen is postulated.

It must be emphasized that somewhat like the situation involving an intracranial subepidural hematoma, once symptoms of cord compression have emerged, the cord can be irreversibly damaged in a relatively short time, despite chronicity of the offending condition. As with a chronic subdural hemorrhage, spinal compressive lesions often present a medical emergency.

2.8 PERIPHERAL NERVE INJURIES (FIG. 2–17)

The principles of peripheral nerve injuries are discussed in section 0.3.

When a nerve is severed, the gap between the cut ends is filled with blood and plasma and later becomes organized by invading fibroblasts. If the gap is small, the proximal end is united by fibroblastic granulation tissue, through which regenerating axonal sprouts from the proximal end try to reach the distal end. Because of the tendency of the axonal sprouts to run along the fibroblasts (which form collagenous tubules) and the tendency of the fibroblasts to be oriented in varying directions, the axons grow in haphazard directions and form a bulge of varying size. If the gap is too large to be bridged, a gross stump composed of proliferated axons, fibroblasts, and Schwann cells arranged in a haphazard pattern of interlacing bundles is formed at the proximal end. This is called a "traumatic" or "amputation" neuroma. A few axons may reach the distal end even in this situation.

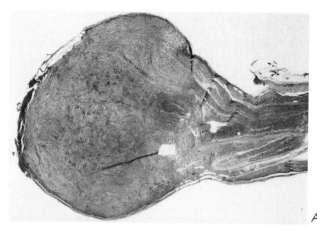

A

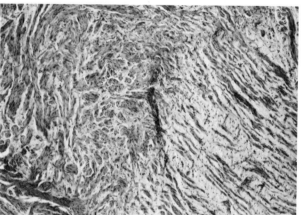

B

Figure 2–17. Traumatic neuroma of peripheral nerve. *A,* Low-power photomicrograph of proximal stump of severed nerve (in longitudinal section) with bulblike enlargement at the end (H&E). *B,* Closer view of transitional zone with relatively orderly arrangement of residual nerve fibers and disorderly bundles of sprouting nerve fibers accompanied by Schwann cell proliferation.

Controversy exists whether proliferation of columns of Schwann cells precedes or follows the growth of regenerating axons. Few if any of these axons become myelinated.

REFERENCES

Berner O: Über kleine, aber tödlich verlaufende traumatische Gehirnblutungen, die sog: "Duretschen Läsionen"; eine rechtsmedizinische Studie. *Virchows Arch [Pathol Anat]* 277:386–419, 1930.

Berner O: Concussion of the brain. *Am J Surg* 29:273–281, 1935.

Duret H: Cited by Berner O (1930).

Munro D, Merritt HH: Surgical pathology of subdural hematoma: based on a study of one hundred and five cases. *Arch Neurol* 35:64–78, 1936.

Radcliffe WB, Guinto FC Jr, Adcock DF, et al: Subdural hematoma shape: a new look at an old concept. *Am J Roentgenol* 115:72–77, 1972.

3. *Infectious Disease*

3.1 SUPPURATIVE BACTERIAL INFECTIONS OF THE INTRACRANIAL AND INTRASPINAL CONTENTS

A. Suppurative dural lesions

These infectious lesions are relatively infrequent in modern medical practice. There are two anatomic forms, epidural and subdural abscess, which are presented below in tabular form for comparison (Table 3–1).

B. Suppurative (or purulent) leptomeningitis (Fig. 3–1)

This form of infection is characterized by extensive polymorphonuclear leukocytes and a varying amount of fibrin exudation in the leptomeningeal space in response to invasion of this space by pyogenic bacteria. Appropriate bacterial staining will demonstrate the offending organisms free in the space or engulfed by phagocytic leukocytes.

The pus tends to accumulate along blood vessels and in the sulci but eventually becomes confluent. The cellular infiltrates are diffuse in fully developed cases, but fibrin exudates are often seen emanating from thin-walled veins. Subintimal cellular infiltration of varying degrees is present in arteries; this change may be severe with some pathogens (endarteritis obliterans). Both arteries and veins may become thrombosed. Necrotizing vasculitis may be seen in some instances.

The underlying cortex may show extension of inflammatory changes along the Virchow-Robin space of penetrating vessels. Small cortical (and even subcortical) infarcts or hemorrhages may also result from vascular changes de-

TABLE 3–1. Comparison of Epidural and Subdural Abscess

Epidural Abscess	Subdural Abscess (or Empyema)
Etiology	
This form almost always results from an extension of some infectious process of the bones of the skull or the spine (e.g., otitis media, mastoiditis, trauma, metastatic osteomyelitis). It occasionally results from adjacent soft-tissue suppuration via a venous route.	This form is also often secondary to foci of suppuration involving the bone or sinuses (e.g., otitis media, mastoiditis, paranasal sinus empyema). The extension of suppuration across the dura occurs most commonly as a result of thrombophlebitis of the emissary veins. This accounts for the development of an abscess distant from the original focus of infection. A direct transdural extension of infection may occur in some instances.
It may be secondary to direct suppuration after a bone fracture.	An isolated traumatic form occurring after a penetrating wound of the skull is rare.
It may be metastatic from a distant focus of suppuration, especially in the spinal epidural space, which is rich in fatty connective tissue.	A metastatic form is rarely seen.
Note: As was already discussed in section 2.2, the cranial "epidural" space is actually beneath the periosteum, inasmuch as the latter and the dura proper are inseparably fused here.	
Evolution	
The *intracranial* form is usually a circumscribed lesion. It may on occasion become sufficiently large to compress the brain and cause increased intracranial pressure. The infection may progress through the dura to produce a subdural abscess, leptomeningitis, or brain abscess.	The *intracranial* form is usually seen over the dorsolateral aspects of the cerebral hemispheres, over the frontal polar regions or in the interhemispheric fissure. Partial organization and loculation is common, with the formation of granulation tissue, which fuses the dura and the leptomeninges (compare with subdural hematoma, see section 2.2). This is more readily symptomatic as a result of compression of the underlying brain and the development of increased intracranial pressure. The complications include thrombosis of superficial cerebral veins and venous sinuses (see section 1.6), leptomeningitis, or brain abscess.
The *spinal* form is most commonly seen in the thoracic area. The pus accumulates predominantly dorsal to the spinal cord and usually spreads over several segments and may extend down to the lumbar space. Often there is a rapid development of neurologic deficit and pain due to compression of the spinal cord and nerve roots.	*Spinal* subdural empyema is rare.

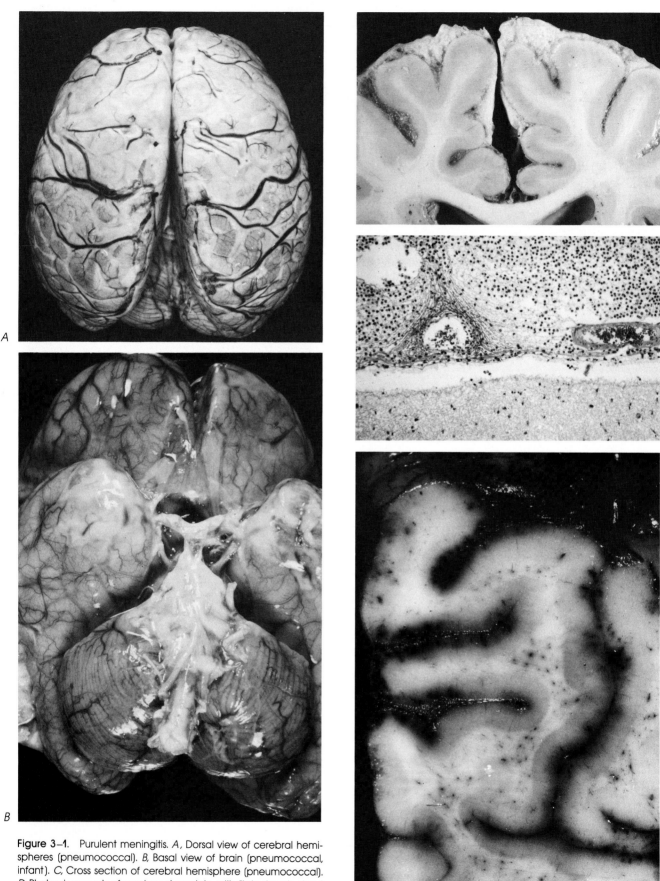

Figure 3–1. Purulent meningitis. *A*, Dorsal view of cerebral hemispheres (pneumococcal). *B*, Basal view of brain (pneumococcal, infant). *C*, Cross section of cerebral hemisphere (pneumococcal). *D*, Photomicrograph of meningeal exudate, with fibrin strands about vein (H&E). *E*, Pneumococcal meningitis with patches of subarach-

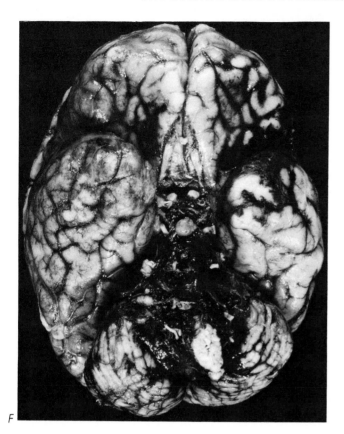

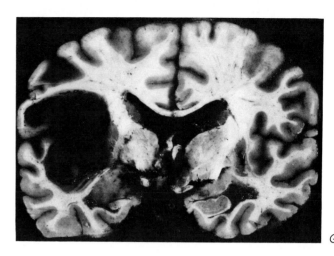

noid hemorrhage and perivascular hemorrhages in cortex. F and G, Hemorrhagic meningitis due to *Pseudomonas* infection. View of base of brain (F) and hemorrhagic infarction about left sylvian fissure (G). (B, C, and E courtesy of Kings County Hospital, Brooklyn, New York.)

scribed above. Occasionally, there is a "wide front" infiltration of leukocytes in the superficial cortex.

Inflammation may extend into the ventricular cavity (purulent ependymitis or ventriculitis or pyoventricle) (Fig. 3–2). The cellular exudate is formed over the surface of the ependymal lining and in and outside of the choroid plexus. In fact, the choroid plexus is regarded as the port of entry for some blood-borne pathogens. The ependymal lining often becomes disrupted, and there is local proliferation of subependymal astrocytes. Small subependymal veins have a tendency to show changes of necrotizing venulitis.

The pathogen may reach the leptomeninges by one of the following routes:

1. Directly as a result of a penetrating wound

2. After an infection of the neighboring structures, such as otitis media, mastoiditis, paranasal sinusitis, or, less often, cranial osteomyelitis, facial cellulitis, or erysipelas, either by direct extension or by retrograde thrombophlebitis

3. By blood-borne dissemination from an infectious focus elsewhere in the body (e.g., suppurative lesions of the lungs).

Various pathogens are involved. In approximately 70% of cases, diffuse purulent meningitis is due to pneumococci or meningococci. Some of the more commonly seen forms are shown in Table 3–2.

Healing of purulent meningitis is accompanied by connective tissue proliferation in the subarachnoid space which may lead to leptomeningeal fibrosis of varying degree. A

significant obstruction of the CSF outflow passage by this process will result in internal hydrocephalus. Pronounced subependymal glial proliferation in the aqueduct can cause obstructive hydrocephalus.

C. Brain abscess (Fig. 3–3)

Brain abscess is a localized suppuration within the brain substance. Pyogenic pathogens reach the brain by the routes outlined under "purulent leptomeningitis." In recent years, the blood-borne dissemination from distant sources, as in sepsis secondary to visceral suppuration or septic embolism from the heart, has assumed greater importance as uncontrolled infections in the tissues contiguous or adjacent to the brain have become infrequent. In the latter situation, staphylococci and pneumococci are the most frequent pathogens.

Streptococci, both aerobic and anaerobic, and staphylococci are the most frequently isolated organisms, the former usually from distant sources and the latter commonly through direct (open) traumatic lesions. Gram-negative aerobic and anaerobic organisms are recovered with increasing frequency from patients with a variety of primary foci of infection. More than one organism was isolated from the brain abscesses of 32% of the surgically treated patients (overall figure after 1970, 58%) in a Mayo Clinic series, 1961 to 1973 (Brewer et al., 1975). Some 20% of clinical cases have no identifiable primary sources.

Histologic evolution of an abscess is outlined in the flow sheet on p. 111.

TABLE 3–2. Pathogens Commonly Causing Leptomeningitis

Pathogens	Routes	Lesions
Pneumococcal	Hematogenous Otitis, sinusitis Penetrating wound Unknown (¼)	Fibrin-rich, thick exudate, which is more evident over the vertex
Meningococcal	Nearly all hematogenous	Relatively thin exudate (more pronounced at the base) is the rule, with or without petechial hemorrhages, focal softening, or even small abscesses (septic embolism of smaller vessels). In Friederichsen-Waterhouse syndrome, overt meningitis is often absent.
Influenzal	*Children:* Primary (after a respiratory infection) *Adults:* Secondary to infection elsewhere (pneumonia)	Exudate is thicker over the vertex; there is a tendency to gross cortical softening or venous thrombosis.
Streptococcal	Otitis, mastoiditis, sinusitis	Thin exudate more evident over the vertex
Staphylococcal	Rare; embolic, venous (especially cavernous sinus) thrombosis, contiguously through traumatic or surgical cranial defects	Thick exudate
Gram-negative organisms (*Escherichia coli, Pseudomonas, Proteus*)	Mainly among neonates	Hemorrhagic exudate. With necrotizing arteritis, there is a tendency toward cerebral tissue necrosis, especially in perivascular white matter.
Listeria	Often among debilitated persons or patients with malignancies	Often associated with microabscesses (*Listeria* nodules), particularly in the brainstem

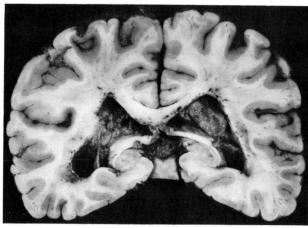
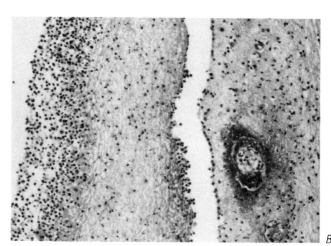

Figure 3–2. Purulent ependymitis. *A,* Patient who was on long-term steroid therapy for systemic lupus erythematosus. *B,* Ventricular exudate (fibrin and neutrophils) and "necrotizing" vasculitis of subependymal vein (H&E).

Histologic Evolution of an Abscess

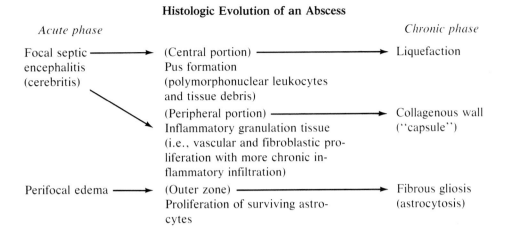

Although multiplicity is thought to be the rule for hematogenous (metastatic) brain abscesses, nearly half of clinically significant cases involve a solitary lesion.

The damaging effects of cerebritis and early abscess on the brain are caused by (1) local tissue destruction and irritation and (2) a volumetric increase of the lesion (including its peripheral edema), acting as a rapidly expanding mass and increasing intracranial pressure. Chronic, well-encapsulated abscess is less likely to cause a mass effect.

The following forms of secondary involvement of the neighboring tissue may occur: (1) formation of a "daughter" abscess by rupture of a poorly developed capsule and extension of the inflammatory process under pressure into the surrounding parenchyma; (2) purulent ependymitis (and pyoventricle or pyocephalus) as a result of ventricular extension of the abscess; and (3) purulent leptomeningitis due to the cortical surface extension of the abscess (with or without actual rupture), focal at first and then diffuse at later stages (if the patient survives long enough).
Note: Either (2) or (3) can lead to the other or they may occur simultaneously.

Suppurative disease of the spinal cord parenchyma is extremely rare and may take the forms of (1) suppurative myelitis, which is a diffuse infection of certain portions of the spinal cord and is equivalent to focal cerebritis, and (2) spinal abscess, whose mode of development is similar to that of brain abscess.

D. Septic embolism

An occlusion of an artery by a septic (i.e., infected) embolus, usually from infected heart valves (bacterial endocarditis), has two major consequences (Fig. 3–4 *A*):

1. Occlusive effect
There will be an *infarction* in the territory of the affected artery.

2. Infective effect
The arterial wall in contact with the embolus becomes involved in *focal arteritis*. Further extension into the adventitial aspect will result in focal infection of the adjacent tissue, either *focal meningitis* or focal *brain abscess*. When there is a significant weakening of the vascular wall by the inflammatory destruction (particularly of the muscularis), a segmental ballooning of the wall occurs and results in the picture of a *septic aneurysm*. This lesion may heal, but it may also eventually rupture and result in a *hemorrhage,* either subarachnoid or intracerebral (or both). The hemorrhage may be relatively limited (perivascular extravasation) or massive (and fatal). Breaking up of infected emboli into the already infarcted area or area to be infarcted will create a *septic infarct* (i.e., infected infarction). These changes are diagrammatically illustrated in Figure 3–4.

Although these two factors are always at work, certain types of pathologic changes predominate in certain situations; they are largely dependent on the size of the arteries involved and perhaps on the virulence of the pathogens (Fig. 3–4 *B*). Illustrative cases are presented in Figures 3–5 to 3–7.

Note: In *septicemia,* in which there are much smaller clumps of bacteria circulating in the blood, smaller parenchymal capillaries are more likely to be the initial site of CNS infection. Therefore, multiple or single abscesses are the principal lesions in this situation.

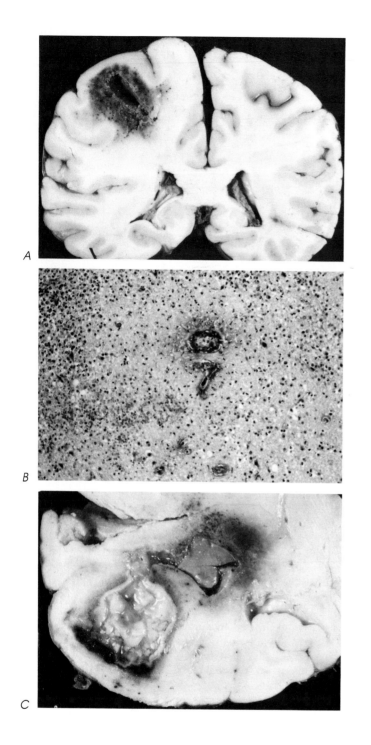

A

B

C

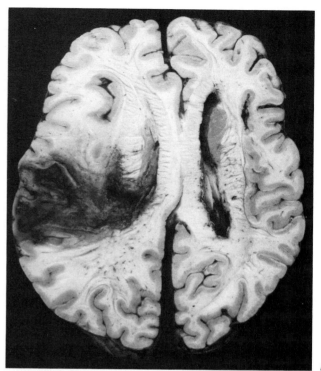

D

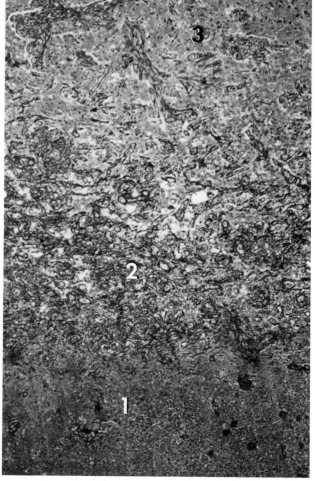

3

2

1

E

Figure 3–3. Brain abscess. *A* and *B,* Acute cerebritis with early central tissue breakdown in left parietal lobe, secondary to septic abortion—gross (*A*) and microscopic (H&E) (*B*) views. *C,* Early abscess in left temporal lobe with "daughter" abscess formation (upper right in photograph). *D* and *E,* Large, early encapsulated abscess in left temporoparietal region but rupturing into left lateral ventricle seen in gross (*D*) and microscopic (*E,* reticulin) views. Note three

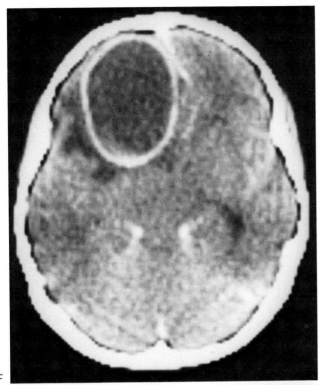

F

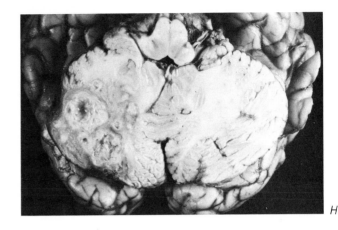

H

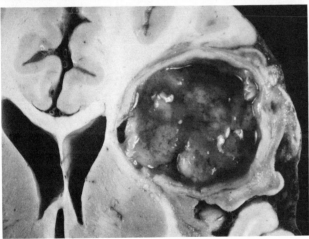

G

zones: (1) necrotic center, (2) inflammatory granulation tissue with pronounced proliferation of blood vessels, and (3) gliotic peripheral zone. *F,* Computed tomography scan images after contrast injection in early, encapsulated left frontal lobe abscess. *G,* Well-encapsulated chronic brain abscess in right frontal lobe. *H,* Multiple chronic cerebellar abscesses secondary to otitis media. (*A, B, C, G,* and *H,* courtesy of Kings County Hospital, Brooklyn, New York.)

3.2 TUBERCULOUS AND SYPHILITIC INFECTIONS AND SARCOIDOSIS

A. Tuberculous infection of the nervous system

Several clinicopathologic forms are recognized.

1. Epidural infection

This form is almost entirely limited to spinal epidural tuberculosis due to extension of vertebral tuberculosis (Pott's disease). Both of these conditions, alone or in combination, can cause compression of the spinal cord. Rarely, this form of tuberculosis gives rise to tuberculous meningitis.

2. Subdural infection

This rare disorder takes the form of either miliary lesions on the floor of the cranium, in cases of tuberculous leptomeningitis, or widespread lesions (tuberculoma-enplaque), which usually show some spread into the leptomeninges and farther to the cerebral cortex.

3. Tuberculomas (Fig. 3–8)

Tuberculomas of the brain parenchyma (and of the leptomeninges and choroid plexus) usually form as a result of primary dissemination and histologically are granulomas with central caseous necrosis. The cellular infiltrate includes lymphocytes and histiocytes in the form of epithelioid and giant

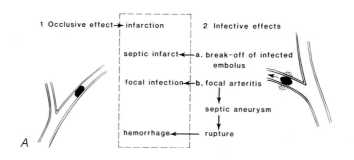

1. Large arteries at the base of the brain (Fig. 3–4 *B1*)
   a. Obstruction ⟶ Distal infarction (often massive)
      (immediate)   (shaded area)
   b. Septic aneurysm ⟶ Focal leptomeningitis (dotted
      (delayed)   area)
                            Focal subarachnoid hemor-
                            rhage (occasionally massive)
                            with or without parenchymal
                            extension

2. Smaller leptomeningeal branches (Fig. 3–4 *B2*)
   Obstruction
        +   Septic infarct with focal lepto-
   septic arteritis ⟶ meningitis and hemorrhage in
   (nearly simultaneous) overlying leptomeninges

3. Small parenchymal arteries (Fig. 3–4 *B3*)
   a. Minimal or no infarctive consequence
   b. Microabscesses ⟶ large abscesses
                            (single or multiple)
                  or
   petechial hemorrhages (solid area) ⟶ massive hemorrhages
                                         (single or multiple)

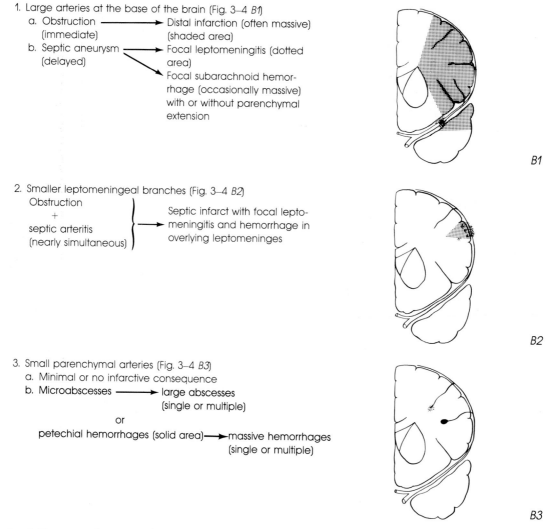

B1

B2

B3

Figure 3–4. *A,* Diagrammatic representation of different conse- quences of septic embolization to cerebral arteries. See p. 111 for details. *B,* Various combined tissue effects of septic embolism as related to size of the affected vessel.

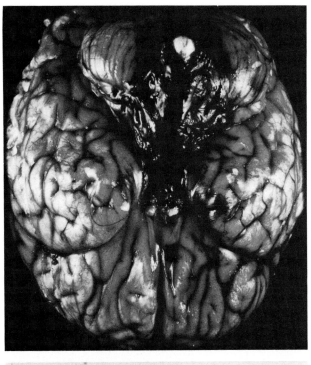

A

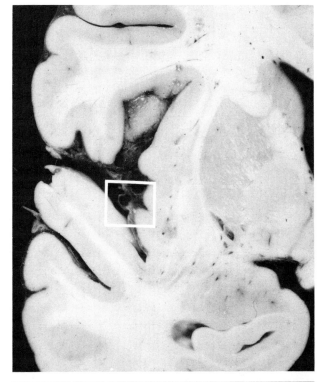

C

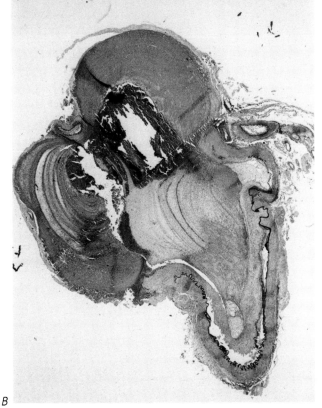

B

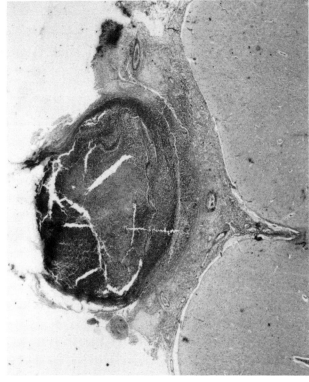

D

Figure 3–5. Septic embolism to a major cerebral artery. *A* and *B,* Subarachnoid hemorrhage at base of brain, due to ruptured septic aneurysm of anterior communicating artery. *A,* Basal view of brain. *B,* Histologic section of primary lesion (EvG). *C* to *E,* Septic emboli- zation to left middle cerebral artery branch in sylvian fissure, with distal infarction and focal arteritis and leptomeningitis but without rupture of artery. *C,* Left sylvian fissure. *D,* Histologic appearance of occluded artery from area shown by box in *C* (cross section, H&E).

(Continued on p. 117)

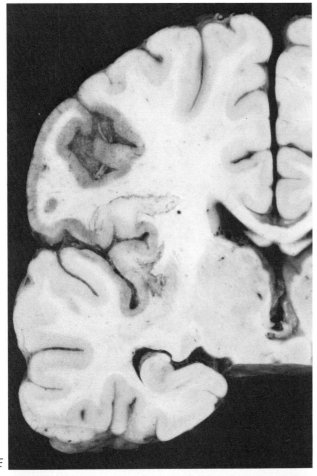

E

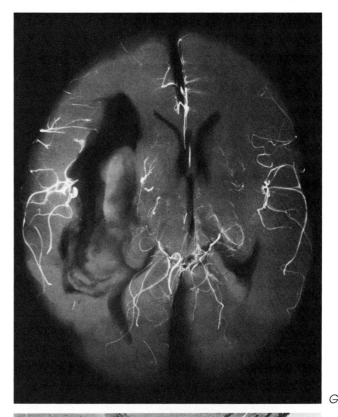

G

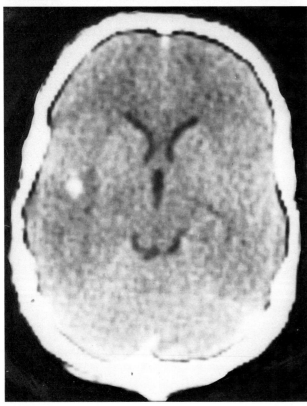

F

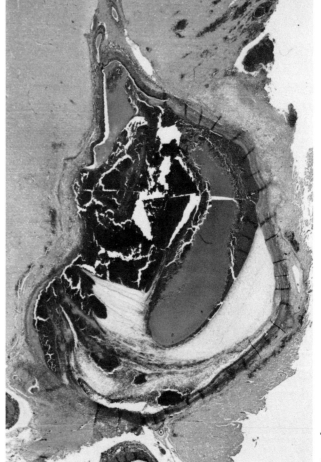

H

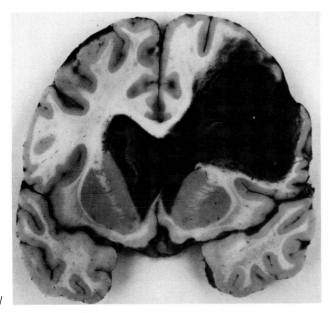

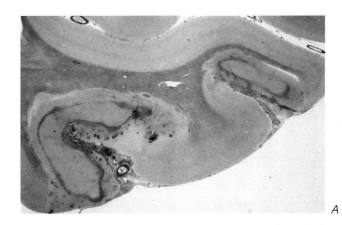

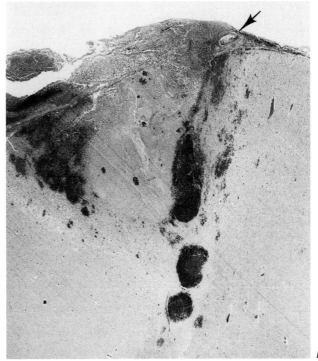

Figure 3–5. *E,* Distribution of infarct. *F* to *H,* Septic embolic occlusion of left middle cerebral artery branch in sylvian fissure, first resulting in distal infarction and then in local aneurysmal dilatation that subsequently ruptured and caused massive left cerebral hemorrhage. *F,* Contrast-enhanced computed tomography scan. *G,* Postmortem angiogram of slice containing septic aneurysm but with blood removed. *H,* Histologic appearance of septic aneurysm (EvG). *I,* Large frontal hemorrhage due to ruptured septic aneurysm. (*B* from Siekert RG: Neurologic manifestations of infective endocarditis [subacute bacterial endocarditis]. *In* Handbook of Clinical Neurology. Vol. 33, Pt. 1. Edited by PJ Vinken, GW Bruyn. Amsterdam, Elsevier/North-Holland Biomedical Press, 1978, pp 469–477. By permission.)

Figure 3–6. Septic embolism to leptomeningeal artery. *A,* Low-power histologic appearance of septic infarcts largely in sulcal portions of gyri (LFB/PAS/H). *B,* Low-power histologic appearance of septic infarct at crest of cortex, showing hemorrhagic leptomeningitis and hemorrhagic infarct containing bacterial colonies. *Arrow* points to affected artery (H&E).

cells. They are usually small and multiple. In certain underdeveloped countries, large tuberculomas acting as mass lesions constitute a large portion of neurosurgical lesions. In the United States, this form is rarely encountered.

4. Leptomeningeal infection

This appears in two somewhat distinct forms:

a. Leptomeningeal tuberculosis (Fig. 3–9)

This form consists of isolated tuberculomas (as described above) of varying size. In most cases it is associated with tuberculomas of similar size within the

brain tissue. This does not invariably result in the second form (b) described below.

b. Generalized tuberculous meningitis (Fig. 3–10)

This form is characterized by grayish, gelatinous, thick exudate predominantly at the base of the brain and cisterns. Microscopically, the exudate consists of polymorphonuclear cell infiltration, fibrin exudation, endarteritis, hemorrhages, and pronounced caseous necrosis, in addition to small chronic granulomas, which are often obscure. Perivascular parenchymal extension

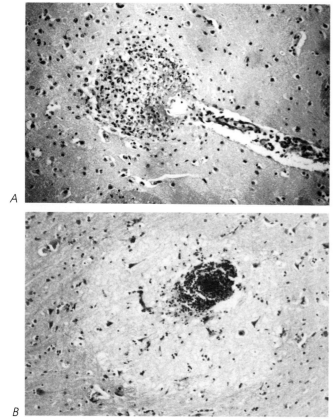

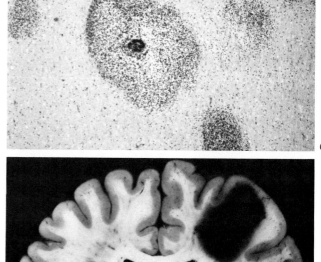

Figure 3–7. Septic embolism to small parenchymal arteries. *A,* Cortical artery with focal necrotizing arteritis and acute inflammatory reaction extending into parenchyma (H&E). *B,* Cortical microabscess with clump of bacteria in center surrounded by narrow zone of acute infarction (H&E). *C,* Multiple small abscesses in white matter with clump of bacteria in the center in one of them (H&E). *D,* Larger hemorrhage in right frontal white matter.

of the inflammatory process and hemorrhagic cerebral infarcts of varying size are frequent.

The leptomeningeal type of reaction is thought to be primarily a hypersensitive reaction due to discharge of bacilli into the leptomeningeal space from small cortical, meningeal, or choroid plexus tuberculomas. It is most often seen in young children (peak at 1 to 3 years of age) as part of a generalized miliary tuberculosis. In adults, it is often secondary to an active extrapulmonary tuberculosis, which gives rise to repeated hematogenous dissemination. It is less commonly associated with primary dissemination and rarely with the active primary complex in adults.

B. Sarcoidosis (Fig. 3–11)

Although sarcoidosis has not been proved to be of infectious etiology, it is convenient to discuss this disease here because of its morphologic similarity to chronic tuberculous forms of infection.

Typical lesions are noncaseating granulomas closely related to blood vessels in the leptomeninges, most often around the base of the brain and in the posterior fossa. Varying degrees of extension into the cerebral parenchyma via the

Virchow-Robin spaces are also seen, and cranial nerves, including the optic chiasm and optic nerves, often become involved. Less often, lesions within the brain such as in the basal ganglia or the pons may exist, with little evidence of leptomeningeal involvement. The infundibulum and hypothalamus may be affected in this fashion.

The course of the intracranial disease is usually slow, with or without clinical remissions or arrest; but in other cases, it may be fatal within a matter of weeks. Hydrocephalus and cranial nerve palsies including visual defects, diabetes insipidus, or other signs of hypothalamic damage are the usual clinical symptoms. Facial nerve palsies occur and may be due to uveoparotitis, in which sarcoidosis is the most common cause. In a few cases, the intracranial disease occurs with no apparent systemic involvement.

C. Syphilis (lues) (*Treponema pallidum* infection) (Fig. 3–12)

Three major types of pathologic changes of syphilis are recognized, mainly in relation to the stage of infection.

1. Subacute secondary meningitis

In the pre-penicillin period, 30 to 60% of patients with the secondary stage of syphilis showed evidence of mild

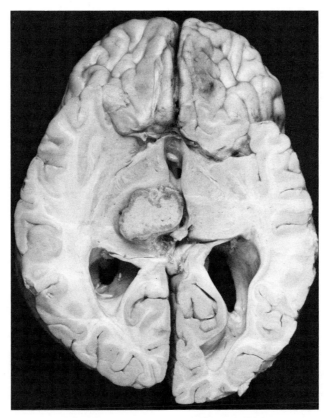

Figure 3–8. Large tuberculoma in thalamus.

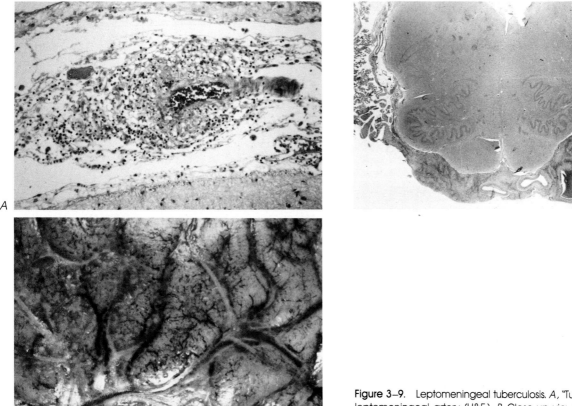

Figure 3–9. Leptomeningeal tuberculosis. *A,* "Tubercle" about small leptomeningeal artery (H&E). *B,* Close-up view of multiple miliary tubercles in cerebral leptomeninges. *C,* Leptomeningeal tuberculoma with central caseous necrosis in front of medulla.

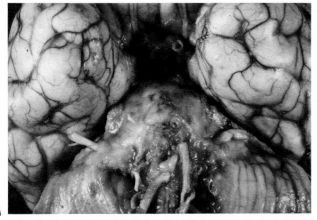

A

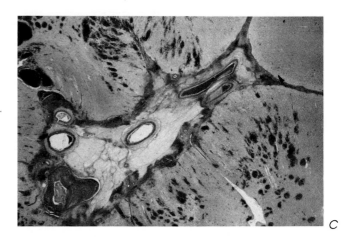

C

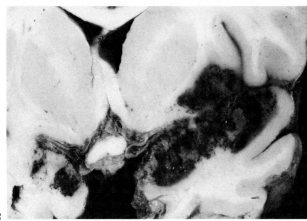

B

Figure 3–10. Generalized tuberculous meningitis. *A*, Thick exudate at base of brain, particularly over pons. *B* and *C*, Leptomeningeal exudate in sylvian fissures and hemorrhagic infarction of surrounding cortices. *B*, Gross specimen. *C*, Histologic section (H&E). (Courtesy of Kings County Hospital, Brooklyn, New York.)

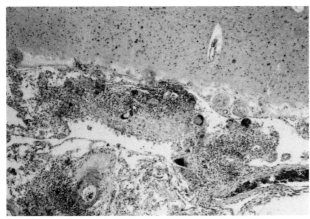

A

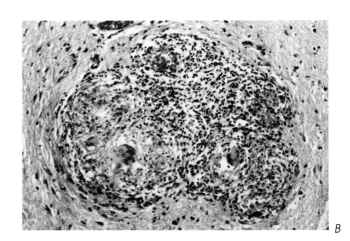

B

Figure 3–11. Sarcoidosis. *A*, Leptomeningeal noncaseating granuloma (H&E). *B*, Perivascular extension of leptomeningeal process into parenchyma of gyrus rectus (H&E).

120

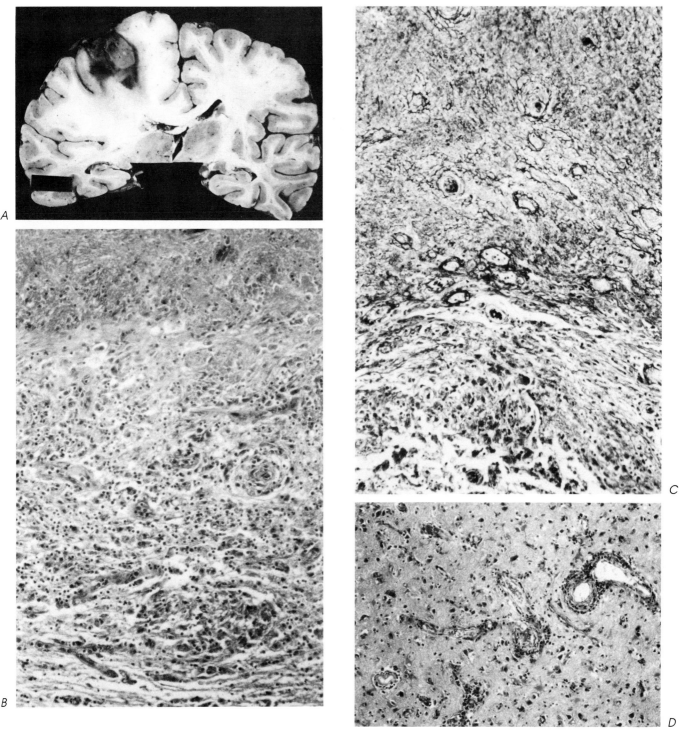

Figure 3–12. Syphilis. *A*, Gumma of left parietal region. *B* and *C*, Histologic appearance at edge of gumma (necrosis at top of pic-

tures) (*B*, H&E; *C*, reticulin). *D*, Low-power histologic view of cerebral cortex in general paresis (H&E). *E*, "Rod cells" (*arrows*) containing

(Continued on next page)

121

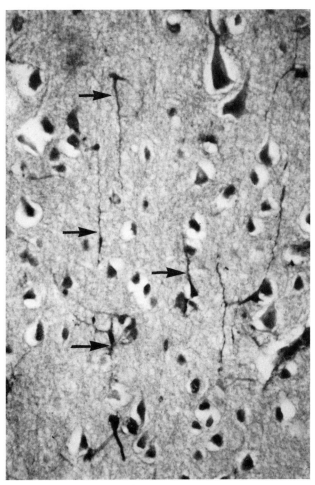

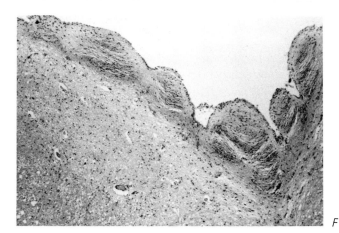

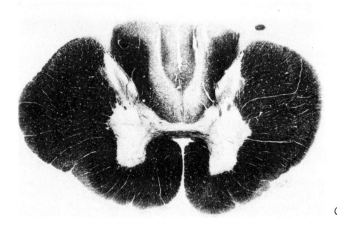

E

F

G

iron in cortex in general paresis (iron stain). *F,* Granular ependymitis in floor of fourth ventricle in general paresis (H&E). *G,* Tabes dorsalis affecting cervical cord (Weigert). (*A* courtesy of Dr. Juan Olvera-Rabiela.)

meningeal inflammation, which was usually clinically silent. Rare postmortem cases show diffuse, mainly lymphocytic meningitis, which is greatest over the base.

2. Meningovascular syphilis

In the tertiary stage, 20 to 25% of all untreated patients show tertiary lesions of some kind. Roughly 5 to 10% of these patients show the meningovascular type of CNS lesion, as compared with cardiovascular involvement, which is seen in 80 to 85%. There is lymphocytic and plasmacytic infiltration of the leptomeninges, with or without miliary granulomas (gummata). Perivascular parenchymal extension may also be present. Concomitant arteritis with mural lymphocytic and plasma cell infiltration and subintimal connective tissue proliferation frequently results in cerebral infarcts of varying size, which often determine the clinical manifestation of this form of CNS involvement. Heubner's endarteritis obliterans represents a healed end stage. A rare special form is pachymeningitis cervicalis hypertrophicans (in reality arachnoiditis as well), in which the dura, arachnoid, and pia together form a dense fibrous adhesion, sometimes with focal calcification (or ossification) in the cervical region. Secondary degenerative changes occur, usually greater in the white matter, presumably as a result of vascular stasis and mechanical compression of the cord.

3. Parenchymatous syphilis

a. General paresis

This takes the form of subacute encephalitis due to invasion of the brain by *T. pallidum.* The presence of this organism in the brain after a long asymptomatic interval, along with histologic changes elsewhere resembling those of the secondary stage, may be considered as evidence of prolongation of the secondary stage of infection. This occurrence is thought to be due either to failure of the patient to produce neutralizing or destructive antibodies or to failure of the antibodies to reach the spirochetes.

In early stages the brain may be entirely normal grossly. In the late stage, it shows pronounced atrophy, particularly in the frontal lobes. The diffusely affected cortex shows dropping out of neurons with chronic atrophic changes of remaining neurons and proliferation of plump and fibrous astrocytes, creating a picture of a disorganized cortical pattern. Additionally, hypertrophy and proliferation of small capillary vessels occur, associated with perivascular lymphocytic and plasmacytic infiltration and diffuse rod cell proliferation. The long axis of the rod cells is usually perpendicular to the cortical surface, and staining for iron demonstrates iron granules in these cells; this finding is helpful in diagnosis (although not entirely pathognomonic). *T. pallidum* organisms are demonstrated with difficulty and appear in variable numbers. The leptomeninges show mild infiltration by lymphocytes and plasma cells but none of the vascular changes characteristic of the meningovascular syphilis described above. If the condition goes untreated, death will follow within 3 years.

A variant of this disorder is Lissauer's dementia paralytica, a rare form of general paresis characterized clinically by epileptic or apoplectiform attacks followed by focal signs (e.g., hemiplegia or aphasia) and a more prolonged course (7.9 years on the average). The greatest atrophy occurs in the temporal lobes, asymmetrically, with pseudolaminar degeneration of the cortex. The usual exudative changes are found in the less atrophic cortex. Iron granules are often absent.

b. Tabes dorsalis

This form is characterized by degeneration of the spinal dorsal roots and column, particularly at the lumbosacral and lower thoracic levels. The dorsal root ganglia, in contrast, usually show little change. Although the dural entry zone of the posterior roots is thought to be the primary site of involvement, no theories have gained general acceptance. Spirochetes are demonstrable less often than in general paresis.

A variant of tabes dorsalis is taboparesis, in which the usual pathologic substrate combination is actually tabes and meningovascular syphilis rather than tabes and general paresis.

c. Syphilitic optic atrophy

In syphilitic optic atrophy there is chronic pial inflammation in the intracranial portion of the optic nerve and chiasm and degeneration of nerve fibers; this change is often eccentric or irregular but is greatest at the periphery. Spirochetes have been demonstrated in the nerve sheath and optic nerves in a large proportion of cases. This type of lesion is more often than not associated with tabes dorsalis and is occasionally seen with

chronic meningovascular syphilis. The chronic phase of the disease is accompanied by considerable fibrous thickening of the pia arachnoid in the intraorbital portions, with adhesions to the dura.

4. Congenital syphilis

This disorder may take the form of (1) meningovascular syphilis with obstructive hydrocephalus early in infancy; (2) general paresis with clinical manifestations at the end of the first or during the second decade and with a more diffuse brain involvement, the cerebellar cortex being often severely affected; or (3) tabes dorsalis, which is rarely encountered.

3.3 FUNGAL INFECTIONS

Fungal infections of the CNS and its covering are relatively infrequent, yet they have become an increasing problem in clinical practice in recent years. This development is largely due to the increased longevity of persons with somatic malignancies or other diseases that were previously more rapidly fatal, because of chemical or immunosuppressive therapy. Despite their increased chances for survival, these patients are rendered more susceptible to fungal infection than the general population.

Almost invariably, the infections become established elsewhere in the body before the nervous system is affected, although in some instances (as in cryptococcosis), the primary site of involvement may be clinically silent or inconspicuous. Their primary mode of CNS invasion is hematogenous, and contiguous spread from the adjacent tissues is infrequent (as in mucormycosis).

As was the case with pyogenic bacterial infections (section 3.1), various types of tissue alteration are seen, including septic or nonseptic infarct, abscess, hemorrhage of varying size, and, rarely, septic aneurysm with subsequent rupture. Additionally, granuloma formation is common with this class of infection either by itself or in combination with abscess formation (which is usually seen in the central portion); in such cases, the designation "granuloma-abscess" is appropriate.

The principal types of fungal infection of the CNS are listed below in tabular form.

Pathogen and Morphology in Tissue	*Portal of Entry and Types of Somatic Infection*	*Primary Forms of Involvement of CNS and Its Coverings*
A. Cryptococcosis (Fig. 3–13) *Cryptococcus neoformans,* which is widely distributed in nature. The most important source of infection is exposure to pigeon excrement. Yeastlike budding cells with a thick mucopolysaccharide (therefore metachromatic) capsule are seen.	1. Pulmonary infection 2. Cutaneous infection (less frequent) The primary target of hematogenous dissemination is the CNS.	Chronic leptomeningitis with pleomorphic expressions including: (1) gelatinous "bubbly" exudate with limited lymphocytic reaction, (2) granulomatous reaction with macrophages containing fungi, later accompanied by fibrosis, and (3) granulomas ("torulomas") of varying size (infrequent) There is frequent perivascular extension of the infection into the cortex and basal ganglia.

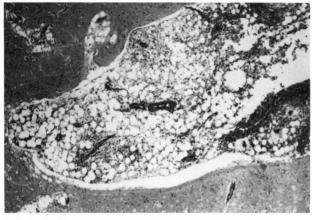

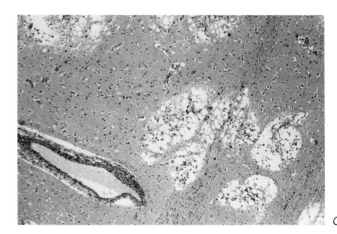

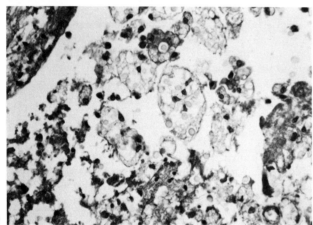

Figure 3–13. Cryptococcosis. *A*, Low-power view of leptomeningeal inflammatory reaction with limited parenchymal extension along cortical blood vessels. *B*, Close-up view of exudate, showing yeasts (with their capsules recognized as halo in this H&E preparation), many of which are engulfed by macrophages. *C*, Extensive perivascular invasion of yeasts and inflammatory reaction to them in basal ganglia (H&E).

B. Candidiasis (Fig. 3–14)
Candida albicans, a common saprophyte of the skin and mucous membrane of man
Yeastlike budding cells and branching filaments are found.

Mainly surface (skin and gastrointestinal mucosa) infections with rare dissemination
CNS involvement occurs chiefly as part of systemic candidiasis or secondary to candidal endocarditis (natural valves or prostheses).

1. Chronic granulomas are uncommon because the infection is usually a terminal event.
2. Microabscesses to larger granuloma-abscesses occur. Acute arteritis, often necrotizing, may accompany these lesions but is less striking than with aspergillosis or mucormycosis.
3. Basal leptomeningitis resembling a pyogenic infection may occur infrequently.

C. Aspergillosis (Fig. 3–15)
Aspergillus fumigatus, a common saprophyte on decaying vegetation
Dichotomously branching septate hyphae are seen.

Airborne infection of the lungs, followed by hematogenous dissemination. Nearly all patients have underlying debilitating conditions.
CNS dissemination is infrequent. This may be secondary to *Aspergillus* endocarditis of implanted valve prostheses.

1. Granuloma-abscesses, with or without basal meningitis, which take the form of purulent exudation with small granulomas
2. Septic infarcts, when larger leptomeningeal or basal arteries are affected. The fungi often penetrate through the vascular wall into the surrounding tissue and elicit a polymorphonuclear cell reaction. Hemorrhage, often extensive, may accompany infarction.

D. Mucormycosis (phycomycosis) (Fig. 3–16)

Mucor and *Rhizopus*
Broad, branching nonseptate hyphae (10 to 15 μm wide) appear as hollow tubes.

1. Nasal and paranasal sinus infection with characteristic dark bloody crusts in debilitated persons
2. Direct extension into the orbit and cranial cavity, occasionally by way of fifth cranial nerves
3. Aspiration into the lung (pulmonary mucormycosis), then to the CNS by hematogenous dissemination

1. Large areas of acute meningeal inflammation and hemorrhagic coagulative necrosis of underlying brain tissue, usually the ventral aspect by contiguous invasion from the extracranial tissue. A characteristic pattern of vascular luminal and mural invasion and proliferation associated with thrombosis is the major microscopic feature. Fungi may lie free in the necrotic brain tissue, but intense polymorphonuclear cell reaction is also not uncommon.
2. Septic embolism to cerebral arteries with subsequent septic infarct of varying size, similar to aspergillosis

E. Coccidioidomycosis (Fig. 3–17)

Coccidioides immitis
Yeastlike cells with double-contoured refractile capsules and endospores are found.

Primarily a self-limited respiratory infection
Only 0.05% of cases result in hematogenous dissemination resembling miliary tuberculosis.
The CNS is affected in 10 to 25% of disseminated cases; it appears not uncommonly as a primary disease with apparent exclusion of all other tissue lesions.

Leptomeningitis, primarily basilar, with polymorphonuclear cells and fibrous exudation in acute phase and later with small granulomatous nodules or large plaques accompanied by slowly evolving fibrosis.
Cranial osteomyelitis is frequently associated.
Parenchymal granulomas are unusual.

The following pathogens are now classified as higher forms of bacteria. They will be discussed here, as traditionally, because of the similarity between these organisms and true fungi discussed above, in terms of their morphologic features and the tissue reactions evoked by them.

F. Actinomycosis (Fig. 3–18)

Actinomyces israelii, a natural inhabitant of the body of man and animals, saprophytic and parasitic in behavior
Thin (<1 μm pseudohyphae) filaments are gram-positive but acid-fast-negative and have a tendency to form "sulfur granules" (a dense tangled mass of threads).

Cervicofacial (the most frequent), abdominal, and thoracic forms of primary actinomycosis are recognized.
CNS involvement is by direct extension or by the hematogenous route.

1. Granuloma-abscess of varying size, generally multiple
2. Meningitis, predominantly basilar, may occur.

G. Nocardiosis (Fig. 3–19)

Nocardia asteroides, which is ubiquitous in soil, grass, and grains
Very similar to *Actinomyces.* They are thin filaments, which are gram-positive and variably (partially) acid fast; they do not form sulfur granules.

Primary lung lesions through inhalation
Hematogenous dissemination may cause CNS lesions; these may be the only detectable lesions in the body in some cases.

Granuloma, often multiple and rarely large

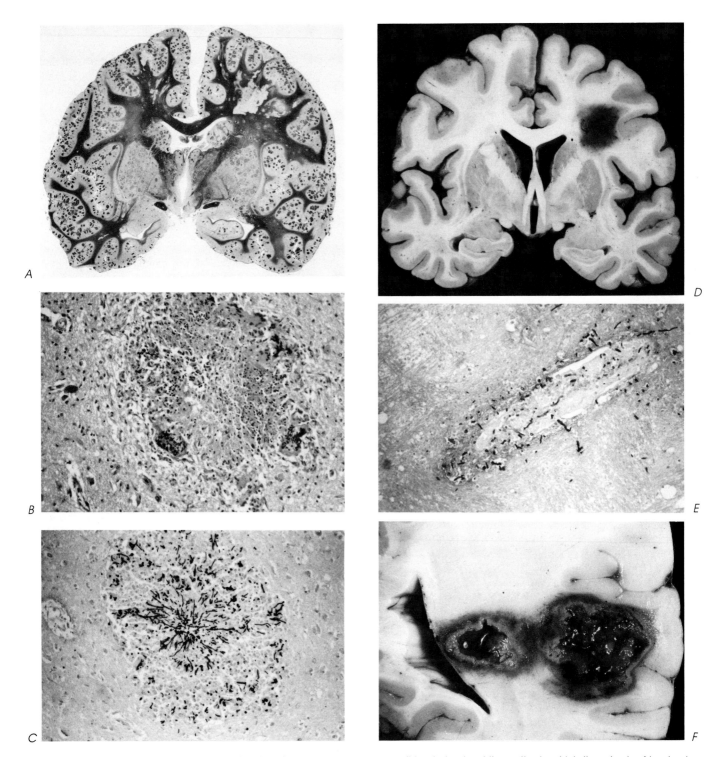

Figure 3–14. Candidiasis. *A* and *B,* Multiple microabscesses, predominantly in cortex, in a child with disseminated candidiasis after severe burn. *A,* Photomacrograph (LFB/CV). *B,* Photomicrograph of single microabscess with giant cells at periphery (H&E). *C,* Acute microabscess stained with silver fungal stain. *D* and *E,* Hemorrhagic necrotizing lesion in white matter in which thrombosis of involved arterioles and perivascular inflammatory reaction parallel the presence of fungi. *D,* Gross appearance. *E,* Silver fungal. *F,* Larger chronic granuloma-abscesses in temporal lobe. (*F* courtesy of Kings County Hospital, Brooklyn, New York.)

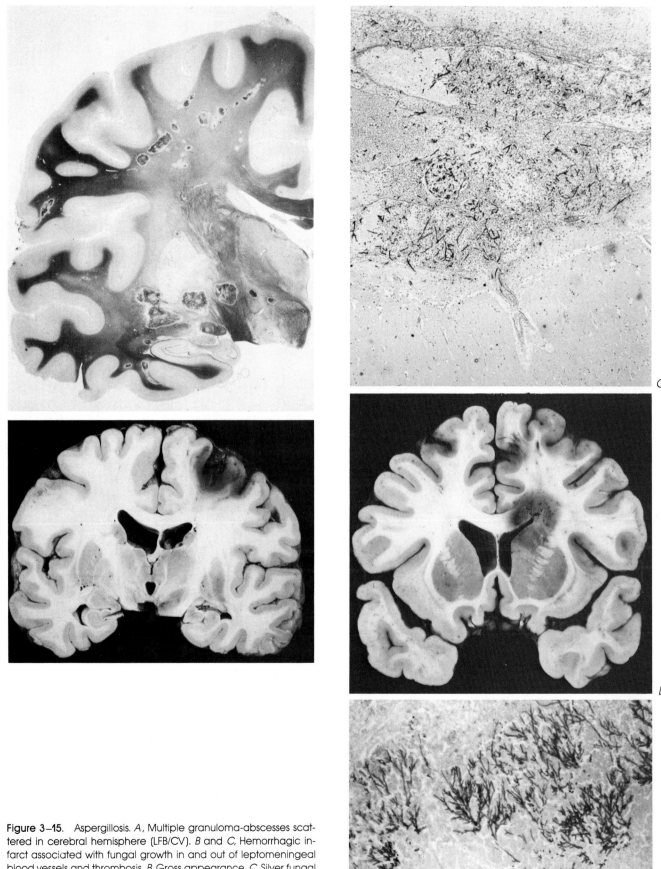

Figure 3–15. Aspergillosis. *A*, Multiple granuloma-abscesses scattered in cerebral hemisphere (LFB/CV). *B* and *C*, Hemorrhagic infarct associated with fungal growth in and out of leptomeningeal blood vessels and thrombosis. *B*, Gross appearance. *C*, Silver fungal stain of meningeal vessels. *D*, Hemorrhagic infarct of white matter. *E*, Typical branching pattern of fungi as seen in small embolic lesion (silver fungal).

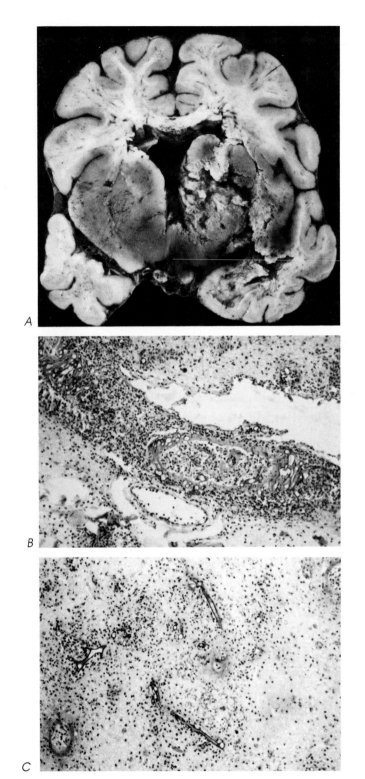

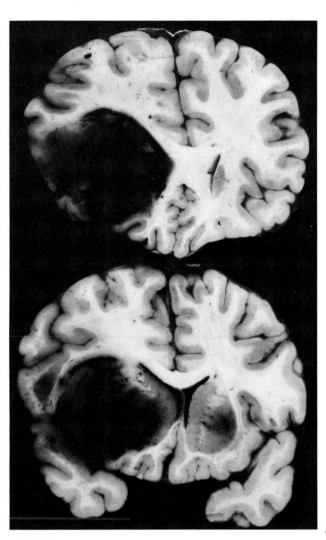

Figure 3–16. Mucormycosis (phycomycosis). *A* and *B,* Acute basal leptomeningeal inflammation, vascular thrombosis, and fungal invasion of parenchyma through vascular wall, leading to a large area of hemorrhagic coagulative necrosis. *A,* Gross appearance. *B,* Histologic section of basal meninges (H&E). *C,* Close-up view of involved cerebral white matter, showing broad nonseptate hyphae and inflammatory reaction. *D,* Gross appearance of hemorrhagic infarct in the territory of the artery caused by occlusion of left middle cerebral artery segment by fungal hyphae and thrombus.

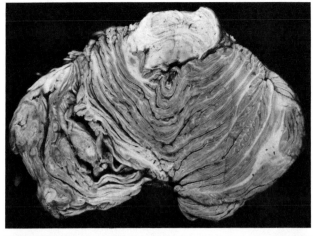

A

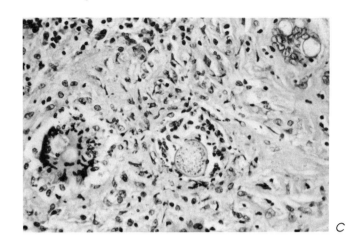

C

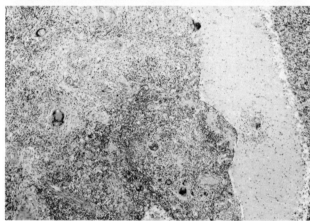

B

Figure 3–17. Coccidioidomycosis. *A,* Granulomatous leptomeningitis of cerebellar hemisphere (predominantly on left). *B* and *C,* Low-power (*B*) and high-power (*C*) views of granulomatous reaction and endospores (H&E).

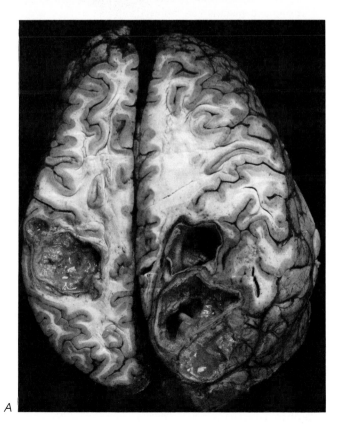

A

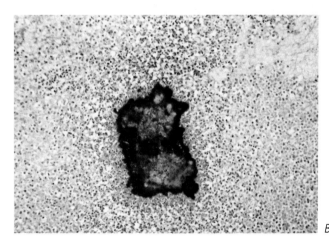

B

Figure 3–18. Actinomycosis. *A,* Multiple abscesses in parieto-occipital regions. *B,* "Sulfur granules" (Gram).

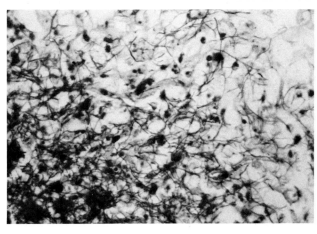

Figure 3–19. Nocardiosis. *A*, Multiple granuloma-abscesses in cerebral hemispheres. *B*, High-power microscopic view of filaments (Gram).

3.4 VIRAL INFECTIONS

I. Dissemination, Morphology, and Histopathology

A. There are three principal routes of spread of viruses into the nervous system.

1. By hematogenous dissemination. This is the most important route. It occurs after virus multiplication at the initial point of entry, such as the pharynx and gastrointestinal mucosa for poliovirus and the subcutaneous tissue and vascular endothelium at the site of insect bite in cases of arboviruses.

2. Through peripheral nerves, by replication and extracellular diffusion, as with rabies virus

3. Through the olfactory mucosa and the olfactory or trigeminal nerves, probably as with herpes simplex virus

B. The general morphologic characteristics of CNS virus infection are as follows:

1. Little or no distinctive gross alterations, with some notable exceptions, such as herpes simplex encephalitis

2. Diffuse distribution of lesions. Although some viruses show a predilection for certain neuronal groups, as in poliomyelitis and herpes zoster, the majority show inconstant overlapping patterns of distribution which are of limited help in histologic diagnosis.

3. Primary neuronal involvement in most cases and occasional primary glial involvement

C. Common features of histopathology

1. Nerve cell alterations, which are by no means always characteristic although they are important in diagnosis

    a. Degeneration (chromatolysis, eosinophilia, and nuclear changes) leading to the appearance of a "ghost cell" and to eventual disappearance, associated with a variable degree of neuronophagia (first by neutrophils and later by monocytes)

    b. Eosinophilic (and occasionally amphophilic) inclusions. Type A intranuclear inclusions are characteristic of viral disease; they are spherical, are surrounded by a halo, and displace nucleoli, as in herpes simplex encephalitis and subacute sclerosing encephalitis. Type B inclusions are small and occasionally multiple without causing displacement of the nuclear contents, and they are not limited to viral disease. Other viral infections have intracytoplasmic inclusions, such as subacute sclerosing encephalitis and rabies.

2. Tissue necrosis, varying in extent from that limited to involved individual neurons and their immediate vicinity (e.g., polio) to areas of pannecrosis (e.g., herpes simplex encephalitis)

3. Inflammatory cellular exudation, which is usually an outstanding feature, although variable in cell type and extent. Neutrophils, microglial cells, macrophages, lymphocytes, and plasma cells (less frequently) in various mixtures can be observed. Microglial proliferation, usually in the form of "rod cells" or angular cells, is a fairly constant feature, particularly in subacute to chronic forms. It may be diffuse, as in subacute sclerosing encephalitis, or focal. Focal forms have neuronophagia (around dying neurons as in polio), glial nodules (without a dying neuron in the center), glial shrubs (in the molecular layer of the cerebellum, along the dendrites of a dying Purkinje cell), or glial stars (a loose collection of 10 or more microglial cells, sometimes related to small vessels).

II. Principal Forms of CNS Viral Infection

A. Picornaviruses

1. Poliovirus
Polio(encephalo)myelitis
(Fig. 3–20)
An acute febrile disease with often asymmetric pa-

The virus preferentially attacks large motor neurons, such as anterior horn cells, motor neurons of cranial nerves, and Betz cells.

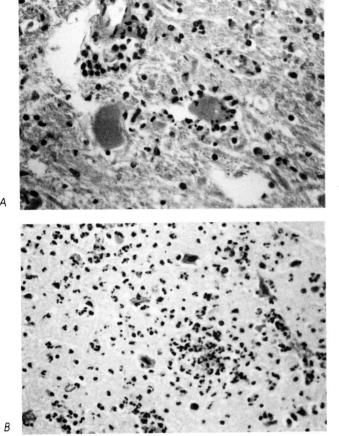

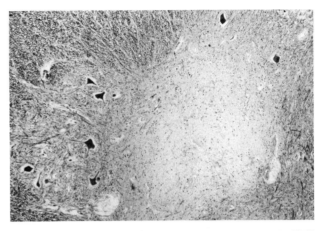

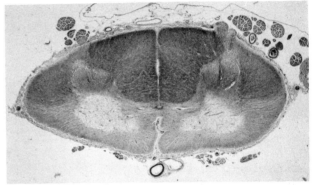

Figure 3–20. Poliomyelitis, anterior. *A*, Two affected anterior horn cells, with neuronophagia in one (H&E). *B*, Acute inflammatory changes in motor cortex (H&E). *C*, Residual state of mild poliomyelitis, with focal neuronal loss in lumbar segment (LFB/PAS/H). *D*, Old (20 years) lesion with extensive bilateral anterior horn destruction of upper lumbar spinal cord (LFB/PAS/H).

ralysis (usually predominantly involving legs, arms, and trunk, in that order) of limbs and cranial motor nerves (10 to 15%) which persists after the febrile phase

Mortality is 5% overall but is higher in adolescents and adults.

Chromatolysis, necrosis, and phagocytosis of affected neurons occur, accompanied by lymphocytic perivascular and leptomeningeal infiltration, not necessarily at the sites of most severe cell necrosis.

When the infection is severe, the anterior horn as a whole undergoes necrosis. More widespread lesions of less intensity are found scattered in the brain and spinal cord. Focal gliosis (astrocytosis), which is often patchy and focal, follows recovery.

2. Coxsackievirus
Aseptic meningitis (group A or B)
Clinically this is a nonparalytic poliomyelitis. Occasionally, paralytic illness or encephalitis is observed.

3. Echovirus
   a. *Aseptic meningitis*
   b. *Acute cerebellar ataxia*
In children, with benign course

B. Arboviruses (Fig. 3–21)
Group A

1. *Eastern equine encephalitis*

Few autopsy reports are available.

As above.

Widespread neuronal degeneration, arteritis with mural

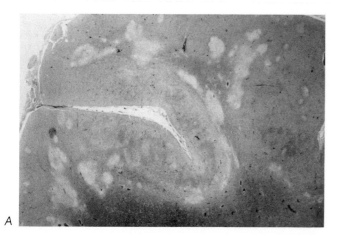

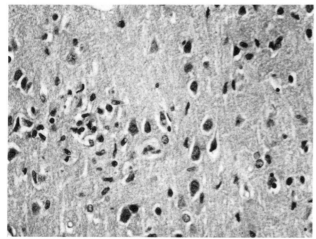

Figure 3–21. Arbovirus encephalitides. *A*, Low-power view of patchy cortical and subcortical areas of necrosis (LFB/PAS/H). *B*, Loosely arranged microglial nodules in cortex.

3. *Venezuelan equine encephalitis*
An even less severe disease, seen in the southeast, mainly in Florida.

The changes are correspondingly milder.

Group B

4. *St. Louis encephalitis*
The most common arbovirus disease in the United States. Inapparent infection is frequent, and the mortality is low (2 to 12%). Three-fourths of clinical cases show encephalitis and one-fourth aseptic meningitis or nonspecific symptoms.

Neuronal degeneration and glial nodules, with slight perivascular and meningeal mononuclear infiltration.

5. *Japanese B encephalitis*
Mainly children are affected. Mortality is as high as 60% in moderate and severe cases.

Neuronal degeneration and glial nodules, focal necrosis, and perivascular and meningeal mononuclear infiltration

6. *California virus encephalitis*
An important cause of encephalitis in the United States, affecting mainly children. Fatality is low.

Neuronal degeneration and patchy foci of inflammation. The white matter and cerebellum are usually spared.

C. Myxovirus
1. Influenzavirus
Influenza encephalitis

Neuronal degeneration and the usual inflammatory reaction are described. More often, the CNS symptoms may be considered due to febrile reaction (especially in children) and anoxia from extensive pulmonary infection.

D. Paramyxovirus
1. Measles virus
 a. *Measles encephalitis*
 Young (under age 10) children are primarily affected. Fatality is low.

Perivascular mononuclear infiltration and demyelination have been described in a few autopsied cases.

This appears to represent a form of postinfectious encephalomyelopathy (see section 4.1) of presumed allergic origin. Multinucleated giant cells and intranuclear and intracytoplasmic inclusions (as seen in the lungs) are also described.

 b. *Subacute sclerosing panencephalitis* (Fig. 3–22)
 Children less than 12 years old are affected predominantly. The

The gray matter (cortical, basal, and brainstem) shows the picture of subacute encephalitis reminiscent of that of general paresis (see section 4.2), characterized by

Fulminating febrile disease with mortality of more than 50% affecting the younger age group. Survivors often have severe residual deficits.

2. *Western equine encephalitis*
More common in the United States but less severe than the eastern equine form

necrosis and fibrin deposition, and intense neutrophilic/round cell infiltration often leading to microabscesses underlie the severe clinical picture. Both gray and white matter are affected, and the white matter may show focal necrosis.

Pathologic changes are milder than those with the form above, with a relative paucity of neuronal changes and less inflammatory reaction. Patchy demyelination of the white matter is more extensive and petechiae are more frequent. Numerous cystic cavities may be seen in the chronic stage.

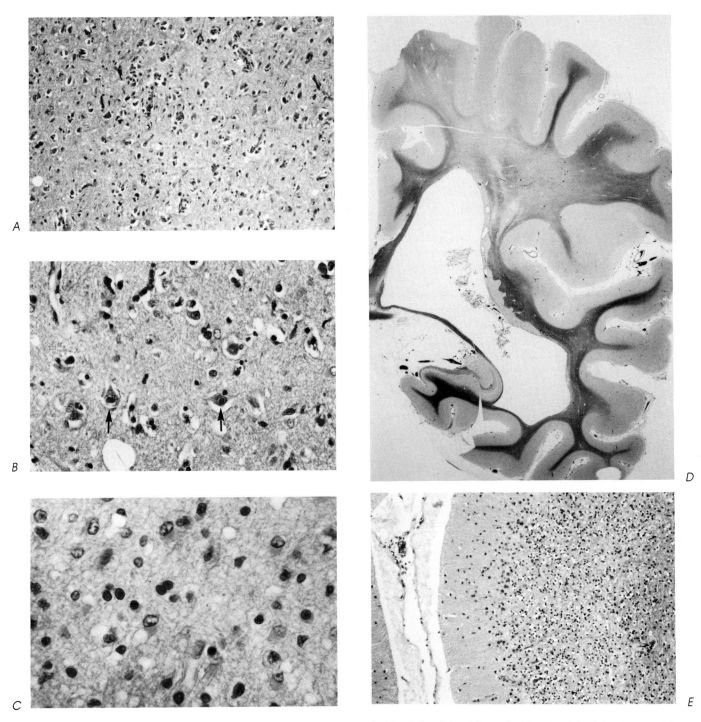

Figure 3–22. Subacute sclerosing panencephalitis. A and B, Low-power (A) and higher-power (B) views of involved cerebral cortex with neuronal inclusions (*arrows*), chronic inflammatory reaction, and astrocytosis (H&E). C, Intranuclear inclusion bodies in oligo-dendroglial cells in white matter (Lendrum's inclusion body stain). D, Diffuse demyelination of cerebral white matter (Loyez). E, Devastated cerebellar cortical layers in chronic case.

course runs from a few months to a few years and is almost invariably progressive and fatal.

2. Mumps virus
Neurologic complications are reported 2 to 10 days after the onset of parotitis. Mortality is low.

E. Rhabdovirus
Rabies virus
Rabies (Fig. 3–23)

eosinophilic intranuclear and intracytoplasmic inclusions of neurons, neuronal loss, microglial (rod cell) proliferation, and astrocytosis—giving rise to a disorganized laminar pattern—and perivascular and meningeal lymphocytic infiltration.

The white matter shows patchy and diffuse demyelination, intranuclear inclusions in oligodendroglial cells and their eventual loss, and reactive astrocytosis.

The relative severity of cortical versus white matter involvement varies from case to case. Pronounced cerebral atrophy, sometimes associated with Alzheimer's neurofibrillary tangles, is seen in long-standing cases.

The CNS pathology has not been elucidated. Perivenous demyelinating encephalomyelitis (see section 4.1) occurs 7 to 14 days after mumps parotitis.

A generalized encephalomyelitis with particular involvement of the brainstem is characteristic. Perivascular (more lymphocytic than neutrophilic) infiltration and neuronal degeneration occur.

F. Herpes
1. Herpesvirus hominis
Herpes simplex encephalitis (Fig. 3–24)
This is the most important cause of sporadic, often fatal (up to 70%) encephalitis in the United States. No seasonal incidence is noted. In the adult form, no obvious cutaneous or visceral lesions are associated with the fulminating febrile disease of the brain.

Apparently independently of the above changes, infrequent glial nodules are seen in the brainstem.

Characteristic Negri bodies are present. These are single or multiple acidophilic (eosinophilic) cytoplasmic inclusions with basophilic "inner formation" (containing virus particles) in neurons in the areas not involved by inflammation, especially in the hippocampus and cerebellum. These bodies are often absent in fatal human cases. Inclusions without inner formation are often called "lyssa" bodies.

In premature infants, who contract the disease from genital lesions of their mothers during delivery, there is acute encephalitis with disseminated visceral lesions ("hepatorenal necrosis").

In other age groups, mostly adults, the disease takes the form of acute hemorrhagic necrotizing encephalitis, characterized by massive tissue necrosis with petechial and some confluent hemorrhages with a predilection for the "limbic lobe" (basal frontal, cingulate, and temporal gyri, and the insula). The lesion is then converted into masses of lipid-laden macrophages, and later a collapsed gliotic scar, the evolutional pattern of which is similar to that of an infarct. In early stages (as seen in biopsy), focal necrotizing vasculitis (with petechiae), focal tissue necrosis, and eosinophilic intranuclear inclusions in glial cells (mainly oligodendroglial cells and occasionally astrocytes) and neurons are seen. The neurons often show eosinophilic degeneration. Perivascular and meningeal infiltration by lymphocytes is also seen in this stage.

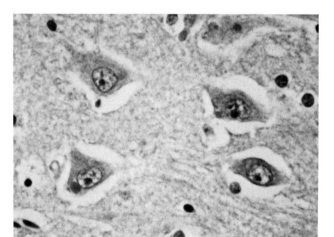

Figure 3–23. Rabies. Negri bodies are seen in cytoplasm of pyramidal neurons of hippocampus (H&E).

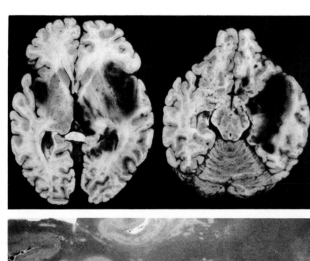

A

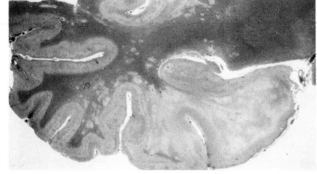

B

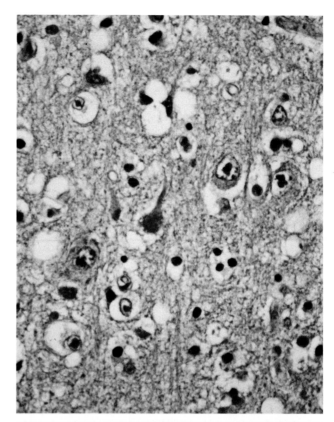

C

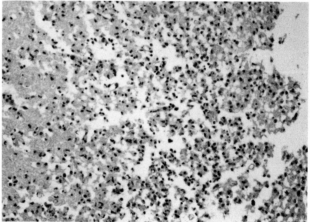

D

Figure 3–24. Herpes simplex encephalitis. *A,* Gross appearance of hemorrhagic necrotizing lesions in orbital-temporal, insular, and hippocampal regions bilaterally. *B,* Patchy, partially confluent pattern of tissue necrosis as demonstrated in ventral region of temporal lobe (H&E). *C,* Early nonnecrotic lesion containing neurons and glial cells with type A intranuclear inclusion bodies. *D,* More advanced stage of necrosis in cortex largely replaced by macrophages.

Aseptic meningitis
Two percent of viral meningitides are said to be due to herpesvirus.

2. Varicella-herpes zoster virus
Herpes zoster (Fig. 3–25)

The dorsal ganglia are primarily affected and show acute round cell infiltration, petechiae, and swollen and degenerating neurons. Eosinophilic intranuclear inclusions are seen in some neurons and satellite cells.

3. Cytomegalovirus
Cytomegalovirus encephalitis (Fig. 3–26)
   a. In infants, the encephalitis, as part of

Extension of inflammation into the leptomeninges and the posterior entry zone of the spinal cord (or into the brainstem in cases of trigeminal ganglion involvement) may occur in some instances.

In infants, there is widespread multifocal necrosis with intranuclear inclusion bodies in enlarged affected cells, which often fuse to form

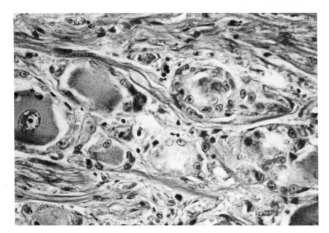

Figure 3–25. Herpes zoster with ganglion cell degeneration and intranuclear inclusion bodies in nearly all of the capsular cells.

disseminated infection, is due to transplacental transmission, which often results in stillbirth, prematurity, or neonatal death.

b. In adults, this disorder is rare and less extensive and is usually associated with lymphoreticular malignancy or immunosuppressive therapy.

G. Papovavirus
Progressive multifocal leukoencephalopathy (Fig. 3–27)

giant cells. Vascular endothelial cells, neurons, astrocytes, oligodendroglial cells, and ependymal cells are all affected. Chorioretinitis is also common. The end stage of the process in survivors is characterized by cortical and subependymal foci of gliosis and calcification associated with hydrocephalus, hydranencephaly, microcephaly, and so on.

The basic lesions consist of multifocal, often confluent areas of demyelination in the cerebral white matter (and infrequently elsewhere). Microscopically, the affected foci show amphophilic intranuclear inclusion bodies in oligodendroglia which eventually disappear as demyelination and phagocytosis progress. Also characteristic, as part of the gliosis, is the development of large astrocytes with bizarre nuclei, simulating anaplastic tumor cells. Inflammatory reactions are conspicuously absent even during the actively demyelinating phase.

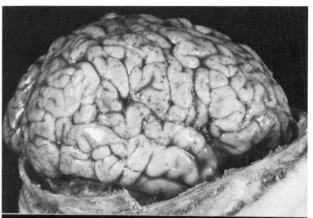

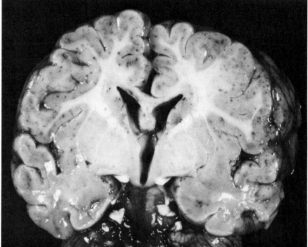

A

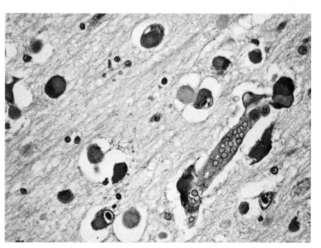

B

Figure 3–26. Cytomegalovirus encephalitis. *A,* Gross external and cross-sectional appearance of multiple petechiae. *B,* High-power view of white matter with numerous enlarged cells with intranuclear inclusions in a fatal neonatal case (H&E).

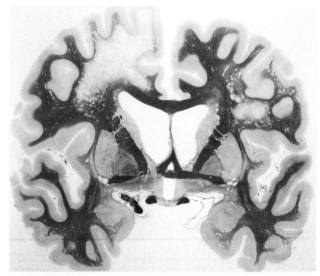

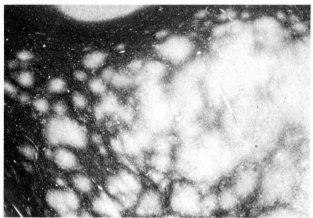

A

B

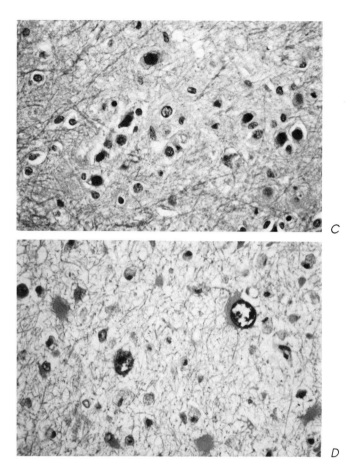

C

D

Figure 3–27. Progressive multifocal leukoencephalopathy. *A*, Section of cerebral hemispheres with bilateral white matter lesions (LFB/CV). *B*, Close-up view of white matter, showing multiple, small focal demyelinating lesions with a tendency to coalesce (LFB/CV). *C*, Early individual lesion with oligodendroglial nuclei filled with inclusion bodies and early hypertrophic change in astrocytes (H&E). *D*, Two large bizarre astrocytes in area of completed demyelination.

H. Suspected viral disease in which the etiologic agent has escaped detection

Encephalitis lethargica or epidemic encephalitis (of von Economo) (1916–1921) Today, this disease is significant as a cause of parkinsonism in some survivors, often many years after the acute febrile illness.

The pathologic changes are similar to those of primary viral encephalitis, with predilection for the basal ganglia, midbrain, and hypothalamus.

In cases of postencephalitic parkinsonism, the substantia nigra shows destruction of pigmented cells, pigment-laden macrophages, and gliosis (see section 5.2). Alzheimer's neurofibrillary tangles are often found here, even in middle-aged persons.

I. Transmissible encephalopathies suspected of being slow virus infections in man

1. *Creutzfeldt-Jakob disease* (Fig. 3–28)
A subacute, fatal disease of late adulthood characterized by progressive dementia with various focal neurologic deficits (e.g., cortical blindness, aphasia) and evidence of cerebellar, pyramidal, extrapyramidal, and even lower motor neuron involvement. The disease has been successfully transmitted to animals and in-

The very characteristic changes consist of a widespread microcystic appearance of the gray matter (status spongiosus), mild nonspecific neuronal degenerative change and eventual neuronal loss, and reactive astrocytosis, often with clustering of hypertrophic astrocytes in the total absence of inflammatory cellular infiltration. This appearance permitted the traditional classification of this disease among so-called degenerative

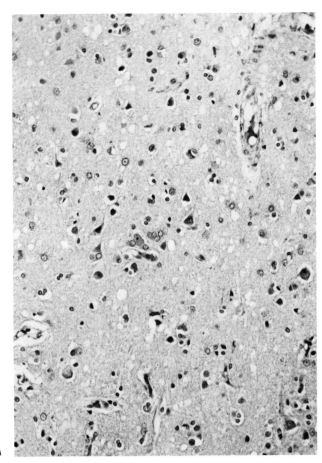

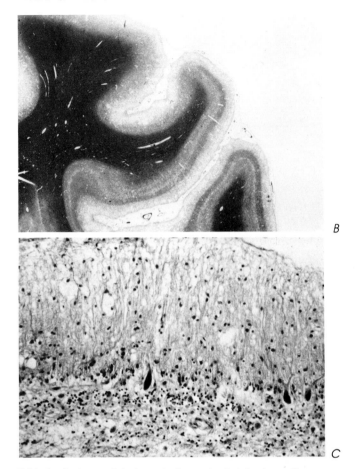

Figure 3–28. Creutzfeldt-Jakob disease. *A,* Cerebral cortex with spongy degeneration and mild astrocytosis (H&E). *B,* Cerebral cortex with pronounced spongy change, particularly in upper layers (Weil).

C, Markedly depopulated cerebellar cortex in late stage. (*B* courtesy of Kings County Hospital, Brooklyn, New York.)

advertently to other humans through organ transplantation (e.g., cornea). (Also see Section 5.1 D.)

2. *Kuru*
A disease endemic in part of New Guinea, thought to be transmitted among tribe members by ritualistic cannibalism, particularly of the brain of deceased relatives. It is now nearly extinct.

diseases. These features resemble those of some slow virus diseases in animals, such as scrapie of sheep and mink encephalopathy.

The features are very similar to those of Creutzfeldt-Jakob disease, and they are collectively referred to as subacute spongiform encephalopathies. Amyloid plaques ("kuru" plaques) in the cerebellar cortex are more characteristic of kuru but are occasionally observed in Creutzfeldt-Jakob disease.

3.5 RICKETTSIAL INFECTIONS

Involvement of the CNS occurs often in epidemic typhus (*Rickettsia prowazekii,* transmitted by louse), Rocky Mountain spotted fever (*R. rickettsii,* transmitted by tick), and

scrub typhus (*R. tsutsugamushi,* transmitted by mite). The rickettsial lesions, which are seen scattered diffusely throughout the brain and spinal cord, are primarily those of small blood vessels with swelling of the endothelial cells and mural thrombosis, which is followed by perivascular infiltration by leukocytes and microglial cells to form a type of microglial nodule known as a "typhus nodule" (Fig. 3–29). Microinfarction may follow. Recovery is associated with formation of small glial scars (astrocytosis).

3.6 PARASITIC INFECTIONS

A. Protozoal infection
1. Toxoplasmosis (Fig. 3–30)

Although toxoplasma infection is widespread, as evidenced by a high incidence of positive serologic tests among adults, clinically evident cases are rare.

Congenital infection results when the mother happens to be pregnant at the time of her initial asymptomatic infection. It causes devastating damage to the neonatal brain (20% are born prematurely). There are numerous miliary granulomas throughout the brain, and focal and confluent zones

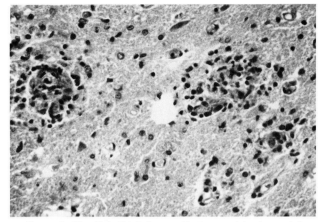

Figure 3–29. Rickettsial disease. Typhus nodules in medulla.

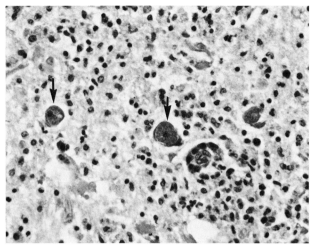

Figure 3–31. Cerebral amebiasis. Acanthamoeba organisms (*arrows*) in acute encephalitic lesion (H&E).

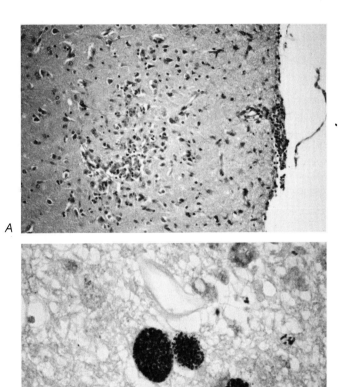

A

B

Figure 3–30. Toxoplasmosis. *A,* Microscopic granuloma in cerebral cortex in acquired adult case (H&E). *B,* Toxoplasma organisms in cyst (silver stain).

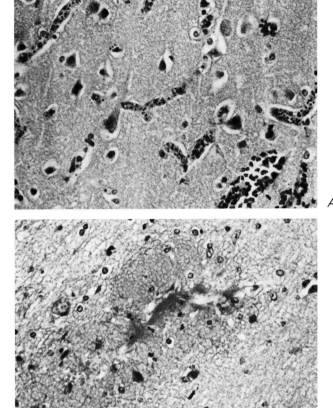

A

B

Figure 3–32. Malaria. *A,* Cerebral cortical capillaries filled with sludging red cells with "malaria pigments." *B,* Petechiae from white matter capillary.

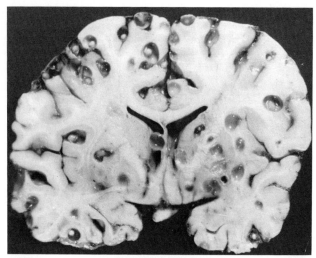

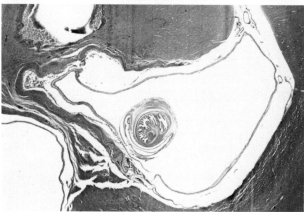

Figure 3–33. Cysticercosis. A, Gross appearance of multiple cysts. B, Close-up view of one of them (H&E). (A courtesy of Dr. Juan Olvera-Rabiela.)

of tissue necrosis are seen. The changes are more extensive in the cortex and periventricular zones, and early calcification occurs in them. The leptomeninges show inflammatory reaction. Chorioretinitis of similar nature coexists regularly.

In rare clinical childhood or adult disease, disseminated miliary toxoplasmosis may occur in the brain (toxoplasmosis meningoencephalitis). A localized toxoplasmic granuloma may act as a space-occupying lesion. Acquired toxoplasmosis occurs more often in patients who have been extensively treated with immunosuppressive agents for malignancy, renal transplantation, collagen disease, and the like. In such cases, the brain shows scattered necrotic foci associated with free and encysted *Toxoplasma gondii*. Rarely, large confluent areas of necrosis behave like a mass lesion.

2. Cerebral amebiasis (Fig. 3–31)

The CNS is rarely invaded by *Entamoeba histolytica* or *Iodamoeba buetschlii*.

In contrast, primary amebic meningoencephalitis caused by free-living amebae of the genera *Naegleria* and *Acanthamoeba* is gaining recognition as a serious, often fatal, disease. The organisms enter into the intracranial cavity through the nose during swimming in contaminated water. *Naegleria* infection is characterized by purulent meningitis of rapid evolution, whereas *Acanthamoeba* causes a diffuse necrotizing granulomatous encephalitis that may be slower in evolution.

3. Cerebral malaria (Fig. 3–32)

This often rapidly fatal disease is seen in about 2% of cases of infection by *Plasmodium falciparum*. Capillaries are filled with sludging red cells infected with malarial parasites, which cause capillary hemorrhages and small foci of ischemic necrosis surrounded by microglial reaction (Dürck's nodes) and more diffuse edema. Grossly, petechiae are more evident in the white matter.

B. Metazoal infections

1. Cysticercosis (Fig. 3–33)

This is the larval or intermediate stage of infection with the pork tapeworm, *Taenia solium*. The larvae (*Cysticercus cellulosae*), which gain entrance to the general circulation through the intestinal mucosa, may encyst in the brain substance, in multiplicity, and provoke local inflammatory reaction and then granuloma formation. Blockage of the ventricular system, leading to hydrocephalus, may occur. The lesions often become calcified as the larvae die.

2. Schistosomiasis

The ova of trematodes seldom involve the nervous system. *Schistosoma japonicum* has a tendency to localize in the cerebral hemispheres and *S. mansoni* and *S. hematobium* in the spinal cord. A necrotizing parenchymal focus infiltrated by polymorphonuclear cells, particularly eosinophils and giant cells, is the characteristic lesion. Healing by fibrosis and calcification follows the death of the ova.

REFERENCE

Brewer NS, MacCarty CS, Wellman WE: Brain abscess: a review of recent experience. *Ann Intern Med* 82:571–576, 1975.

4. *Demyelinating Disease*

4.0 INTRODUCTION

The term "demyelinating disease" is traditionally applied to a group of CNS diseases that chiefly affect the myelin sheath and largely spare the axon. They are obviously a heterogeneous group, of diverse causes; and they usually exclude those cases of known metabolic defects which involve other elements of the nervous system and those due to such exogenous factors as ischemia, toxins, and infective agents.

The two major conceptual subgroups of demyelinating disease (in the broader sense) are as follows:

I. Demyelinating disease (in the narrower sense) or myelinoclastic disease, in which a disease process of some exogenous origin affects and destroys the normally constituted myelin sheath. Myelin breakdown proceeds along the usual pathway down to sudanophilic products (triglycerides and cholesterol esters) as would occur in any myelin destructive process.

II. Dysmyelinating disease, in which defective formation of myelin exists as the main feature of the disease as a result of a proved or suspected inborn error of metabolism—that is, a genetically determined enzymatic disturbance. When this process of defective myelination is only part of a more widespread metabolic disturbance, as in the lipidoses (see section 6–1) or in some of the aminoacidopathies (e.g., phenylketonuria, maple syrup urine disease), the disease is not included here. Conversely, however, many of those traditionally included here are being found to have minor but widespread abnormalities involving other visceral organs.

It is apparent that the decision to include or exclude a disease is largely a matter of convention and convenience.

4.1 MYELINOCLASTIC DISEASES

In the absence of an established cause of these diseases, the current (and tentative) separation of disease entities is based largely on morphologic features and clinical characteristics (Fig. 4–1).

A. Pattern of disseminated perivascular demyelination
1. Acute disseminated encephalomyelitis (or encephalomyelopathy) (ADEM) (Fig. 4–2).
Clinical Features: The disease may occur (1) shortly after a specific infection, in particular, exanthematous viral disease of childhood, for example measles, German measles, chickenpox, or smallpox (postexanthematous, post- or para-infectious encephalomyelitis), (2) spontaneously or in the course of a nonspecific (viral ?) respiratory infection, and (3) after vaccinations against smallpox, typhoid, tetanus, diphtheria, or rabies ("postvaccinal encephalomyelitis"). The onset is usually abrupt and the course is monophasic, although a few cases with subsequent relapse(s) have also been reported.
Pathology: There is perivascular (mostly perivenular) inflammatory cell infiltration, mainly composed of mononuclear cells (lymphocytes and histiocytes) with an admixture of neutrophils in the early stages, associated with a zone of demyelination which follows the course of affected venules for a long distance. Mononuclear cells soon become lipid-laden macrophages. Perivascular astrocytosis marks the healing stage. The lesions are generally symmetric and involve the entire neuraxis, although the distribution is variable.

2. Acute hemorrhagic leukoencephalitis (AHL) or acute necrotizing hemorrhagic encephalopathy (ANHE)
Clinical Features: The disease, which predominantly affects young adults, occurs spontaneously or develops after an upper respiratory tract infection with abrupt onset, fever, and rapidly developing coma, leading to death within a few days.
Pathology: The lesions consist of fibrinoid necrosis of venules, neutrophilic and later mononuclear infiltration, hemorrhage, and fibrin exudation into the surrounding tissue and perivascular edema (which tend to become confluent) and a zone of perivascular tissue destruction (with some axonal damage).

These two types are considered to represent two extremes of a morphologic spectrum, and various mixtures of these features are often found in any given case. The gross appearance depends, therefore, on variable combinations of faintly yellowish streaks and petechiae associated with edema, which may become confluent.
Note: 1. Experimental allergic encephalomyelitis (EAE), which is produced by sensitizing animals to myelin (myelin basic protein) of the CNS, closely resembles the human conditions listed above. The severity of tissue reactions can be manipulated to simulate either ADEM or ANHE. EAE can be transferred to a healthy animal

Three Basic Distribution Patterns of Lesions in Demyelinating Disease

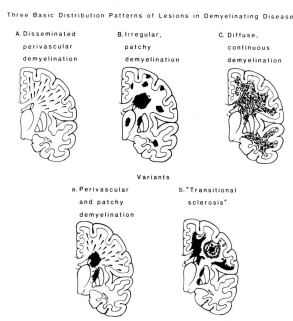

A. Disseminated perivascular demyelination

B. Irregular, patchy demyelination

C. Diffuse, continuous demyelination

Variants

a. Perivascular and patchy demyelination

b. "Transitional sclerosis"

Figure 4–1. Schematic representation of three basic types of "demyelinating disease" and variants. *A,* Disseminated perivascular demyelination. *B,* Irregular, patchy demyelination. *C,* Diffuse, continuous demyelination. *a,* Perivascular and patchy demyelination. *b,* "Transitional sclerosis."

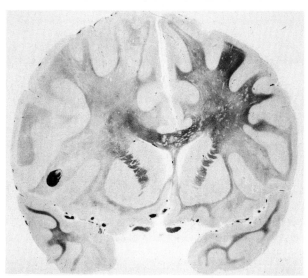

A

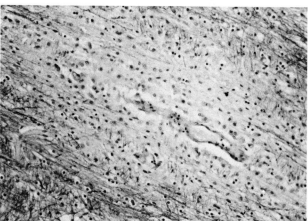

B

Figure 4–2. Acute disseminated encephalomyelitis with mild hemorrhagic component seen in an adult woman after an acute nonspecific upper respiratory infection. *A,* Myelin preparation of frontal lobes, demonstrating scattered perivascular streaks of demyelination (LFB/CV). *B,* Photomicrograph of an individual perivascular focus of demyelination (LFB/PAS/H).

by injection of lymphocytes from an affected animal (cell-mediated hypersensitivity reaction). In humans, it is not known how this apparently cell-mediated hypersensitivity reaction is initiated. In EAE with ANHE-like lesions ("hyperacute EAE"), a circulating antibody is thought to be involved additionally.

2. Although active myelin destruction by monocytes has been stressed as the primary morphologic event in these conditions (and they are classified, therefore, as demyelinating disease), some of the more recent publications point to the primary importance of vascular damage, presumably related to circulating immune complexes and activation of complement. The term "disseminated vasculomyelinopathy" was used by Poser to express this point of view. The picture of AHL or ANHE can also be seen (previously described under the term "brain purpura") as a manifestation of sensitivity to drugs, in association with a generalized Shwartzman reaction complicating gram-negative septicemia or with some of the diseases presumed to be autoallergic. Complement-mediated endothelial damage is postulated to be the final common pathogenetic pathway in all of these vasculopathies. Perivascular demyelination, with or without more extensive tissue damage, is considered a secondary phenomenon.

3. A variant of human ADEM occurs after repeated injections of old antirabies vaccine (prepared from animal spinal cord tissue) (Fig. 4–3)
Clinical Features: The course tends to be chronic and have a multiphasic pattern.

Pathology: Perivascular demyelinating lesions have the tendency to become confluent and form "plaques," particularly near the ventricles, as seen in multiple sclerosis (variant *a* of Fig. 4–1).

4. Guillain-Barré syndrome (acute idiopathic polyneuritis or acute inflammatory neuropathy) (Fig. 4–4)
Clinical Features: Generally, after a vague febrile illness or an upper respiratory infection, and occasionally as a complication of specific viral infections, there is an acute onset and rapid spread (either ascending or descending) of motor weakness and subjective sensory disturbances. The cerebrospinal fluid tends to show elevated protein levels and low cell counts. The disease is self-limiting and leads to spontaneous recovery, unless death occurs from respiratory paralysis.
Pathology: The essential lesion consists of perivascular, segmental demyelination associated with a mononuclear cell

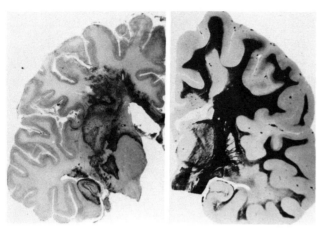

Figure 4–3. Acute demyelinating disease after antirabies vaccination therapy with the old Pasteur method. Nissl stain indicating active cellular infiltration at edges of "plaques" (left). Myelin preparation delineating partially confluent zones of demyelination (right). (From Society of Neuropathology [ed]: *Atlas of Neuropathology.* Tokyo, Igaku-Shoin, 1967. By permission.)

infiltration accompanied to a greater or lesser extent by wallerian degeneration within the substance of peripheral nerves and the spinal and cranial nerve roots. Later, lipid-laden macrophages are formed. The CNS changes are limited to central chromatolysis of lower motor neurons, reflecting the peripheral wallerian degeneration.

Note: As in EAE, injections of foreign peripheral nervous system protein will cause experimental allergic neuritis (EAN), which is regarded as the animal model of this human disease. Activated lymphocytes, which invade the nerve parenchyma, are held responsible for initiating myelin destruction, and the passive cellular transfer of EAN is possible.

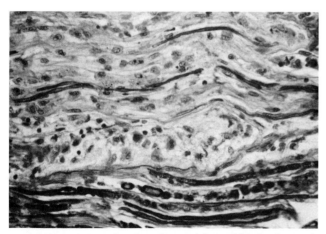

Figure 4–4. Guillain-Barré syndrome. Advanced lesion is seen in cauda equina root with ballooned macrophages, some with a few scattered undigested fragments of myelin sheaths in areas of demyelination (LFB/PAS/H).

B. Pattern of irregular patches of demyelination

1. Multiple sclerosis

a. Chronic relapsing variety or classic multiple sclerosis (Charcot type) (Fig. 4–5)

This is the most common form of demyelinating disease. It affects young adults and is characterized by a slowly progressive course with irregular, fluctuating periods of exacerbation and remission of focal symptoms.

Pathology: The chronic lesions, "plaques," found typically in patients with a prolonged illness, are large, irregular, sharply delineated, discontinuous lesions. They are grossly grayish and soft and tend to retract from the cut surface.

The entire neuraxis may be affected, but the preferential sites are the periventricular cerebral white matter, the optic nerves, the subpial and periventricular regions of the brainstem, and the spinal cord. The gray matter is also involved. Also common are small plaques confined to the cerebral cortex or straddling the junction of the cortex and the white matter. The lesions are found with little regard to anatomic boundaries; that is, they are unsystematic. Roughly, but only roughly, these lesions are symmetric.

The plaques represent a zone of selective demyelination with sparing to a very high degree of axons, associated with subsequent astrocytosis. In large, long-standing lesions or initially more severe lesions, a partial destruction of axons, leading to wallerian degeneration, is common.

Special varieties are (1) shadow plaques, which may be seen independently but more often at the periphery of classic plaques and which are characterized by undiminished numbers of myelin sheaths appearing thin and less intensely stained, and (2) clearing plaques, which appear similar to the above but show partial demyelination; that is, they contain slightly reduced numbers of myelin sheaths with degenerative changes such as focal swelling. Both lesions show mild astrocytosis but contain no myelin breakdown products. The distinction between the two is not always clear-cut, and transitional forms may be recognized. Although they are generally considered to be early lesions, the possibility that they represent partial remyelination in established lesions has been suggested.

b. Acute variety—acute multiple sclerosis (Marburg type) (Fig. 4–6)

This relatively uncommon disease takes a more rapid and often a febrile course, with steady progression of symptoms for several weeks, often leading to death. Young adults are more commonly affected.

Characteristic pathologically are large patches of acute demyelination with intense monocytic (lymphocytic-histiocytic) inflammatory reaction and phagocytosis, more clearly seen at the expanding edge. Axonal damage is more frequent and more severe than in the plaques of usual multiple sclerosis, particularly in the center of the lesions. Astrocytosis is prominent at the margins and in the central portion of the lesions. These

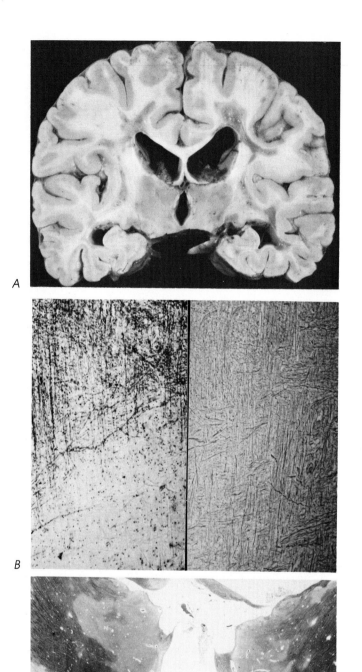

A

B

C

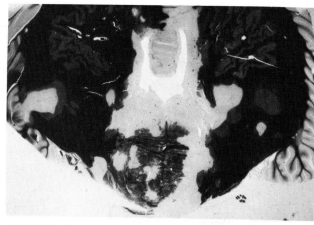

D

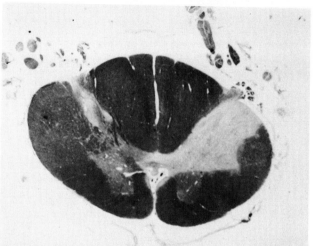

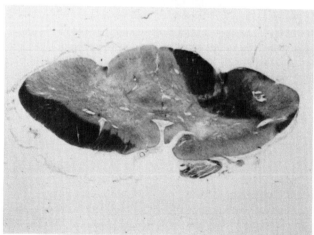

E

Figure 4–5. Multiple sclerosis, chronic type. *A*, Irregular, predominantly periventricular plaques of demyelination appearing darker, semitranslucent, and slightly retracted from cut surface. *B*, Comparison of adjacent myelin (left) and axon (right) preparations at edge of old plaque, demonstrating relative preservation of axons in demyelinated plaque. *C*, Myelin-stained section of thalami with irregular plaques of demyelination. *D*, Myelin-stained section of pons and cerebellum with irregular plaques with periventricular predilection and shadow plaques, some at the periphery of "complete" plaques and others apparently independent of them. *E*, Myelin-

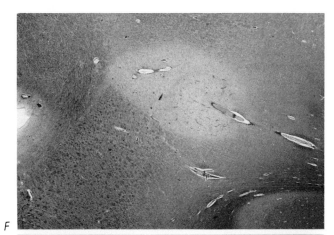

F

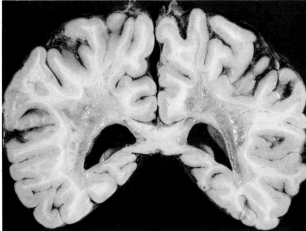

G

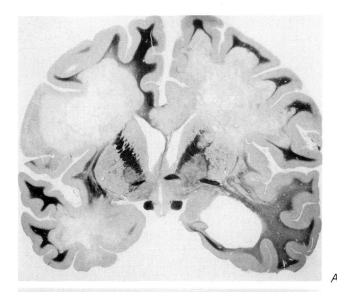

A

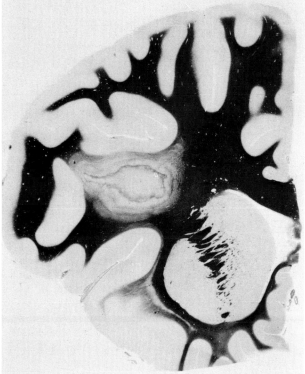

B

stained sections of cervical and thoracic spinal cord segments with irregular and noncontiguous demyelinated plaques. *F,* Incidental, minute multiple sclerosis plaque composed of complete and incomplete zones of demyelination focally about venule (but not following its entire length) in cerebral white matter. *G,* Extensive demyelination of transitional type distribution in otherwise classic recurrent multiple sclerosis. (*A* and *G* courtesy of Kings County Hospital, Brooklyn, New York.)

features often lead to a mistaken tissue diagnosis of infarction or glioma on biopsy. Although there is no consensus as to the cause or mechanism of demyelination, it appears likely that an acute demyelination occurs only in the presence of the cellular infiltrate, as in EAE and human ADEM. However, the perivascular dependence of lesions is not constant in acute multiple sclerosis, and once the lesion has become established it expands along a wide front. These large lesions often assume a "concentric" pattern of demyelination or more irregular wavy or mosaic patterns (Balo's concentric sclerosis).

As stated, smaller patches of similarly acute character may be found in classic chronic multiple sclerosis during a flareup.

Figure 4–6. Multiple sclerosis, acute variety. *A,* End stage of bilateral, extensive foci of "acute demyelination" with more extensive necrotic damage centrally, resulting in cyst formation; wavy pattern is seen at periphery (LFB/CV). *B,* Small acute demyelinating lesion of Balo's concentric type in left frontal lobe.

c. Neuromyelitis optica (Devic's disease) (Fig. 4–7)

This is a clinical syndrome with prominent visual and spinal cord symptoms occurring within a few days or weeks of each other. The consensus is that it represents a form of classic multiple sclerosis with predilection for

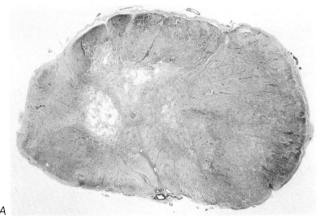

A

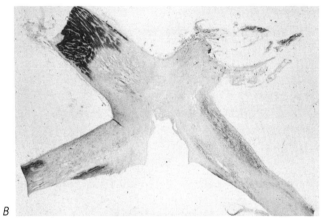

B

Figure 4–7. Devic's disease. *A,* Upper cervical cord segment with demyelination and cystic cavity formation (LFB/PAS/H). *B,* Extensive demyelination of optic nerves, chiasm, and tracts in horizontal section, with cavitary degeneration of optic nerve on one side (Weil).

the optic nerves and spinal cord. The pathologic process tends to be more intense, with resultant areolar (microcystic) or cavitary changes in these sites.

Perivenular demyelinating lesions of ADEM or diffuse sclerosis-like lesions have also been described as other types of anatomic substrate of this clinical syndrome.

C. Diffuse continuous pattern of demyelination

1. Schilder's disease (diffuse cerebral sclerosis) (Fig. 4–8)

Three cases of "encephalitis periaxialis diffusa" which Schilder described are now known to be of different etiology, and only the first (1912) case (which he thought to be a juvenile variant of multiple sclerosis) corresponds to the current usage of the term. The term is restricted to an acutely or subacutely progressive monophasic childhood disease characterized by the presence of usually bilateral but not necessarily symmetric, continuous large patches of demyelination with a relatively clear-cut advancing edge of active monocytic infiltration, myelin breakdown, and phagocytosis. The lesion has a tendency to spare a rim of subcortical white matter. Axonal damage may be severe. Except

for the difference in the pattern of lesions, histologic features of myelin breakdown and phagocytosis are identical to those of multiple sclerosis or ADEM. Unlike multiple sclerosis, however, the brainstem and spinal cord involvement is along the tracts, and haphazardly placed clear-cut patches of demyelination characteristic of multiple sclerosis are not noted here. It is a sporadic disease (unlike neutrophilic leukodystrophy and adrenoleukodystrophy, described below).

Some modern writers believe that there is no further justification for the continued use of the term, declaring that it merely represents multiple sclerosis affecting an immature brain.

D. Combined patchy and diffuse pattern of demyelination (variant *b* of Fig. 4–1)

When this pattern is thought to exist in a given case, the term "transitional sclerosis" is applied by some authors. The existence of such cases is thought to speak for the essential identity of multiple sclerosis and Schilder's disease. The final resolution of this problem calls for the elucidation of the etiologic factors involved.

It should be noted that some of the *chronic* relapsing cases of classic multiple sclerosis have lesions that are less circumscribed or confluent and therefore resemble those of Schilder's disease. This is due in part to wallerian degeneration beyond the confines of the original plaques.

As previously discussed, in *acute* multiple sclerosis, the lesions tend to be large and confluent and less distinct at the margins, but they are still basically multicentric rather than continuous from the onset.

4.2 DYSMYELINATING DISEASES (LEUKODYSTROPHIES)

This category encompasses a number of familial conditions that occur predominantly in infancy and childhood and are characterized by abnormal formation of myelin.

Although the primary defect is considered to be a disturbance in myelinogenesis, the abnormally or incompletely constituted myelin sheath may well be more susceptible to catabolic processes, both normal and abnormal. Therefore, it is to be expected that in some of the dysmyelinating diseases, one may also encounter some myelinoclastic features.

As a whole, this class of disease is very rare, and many of the reported cases occupy nosologically uncertain positions. Only those that have been relatively well defined are discussed here.

Morphologically, they have certain main features in common:

(1) Widespread and often symmetrically bilateral degeneration or failure of myelin formation of the central nervous system (similar to pattern *C* [Fig. 4–1] of the demyelinating group, but often more patchy in severity of involvement)

(2) Absence of inflammatory reactions

(3) Some degree of axonal destruction.

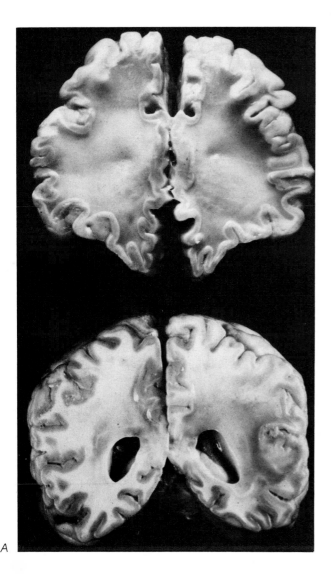

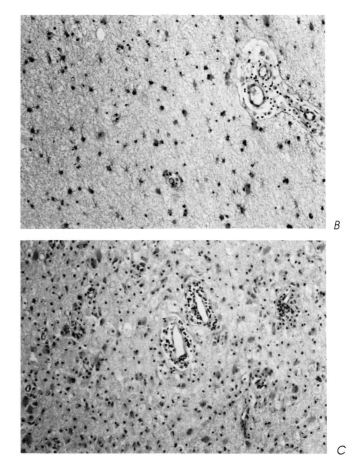

Figure 4–8. Schilder's disease. *A*, Gross appearance of lesion apparently advancing in frontal to occipital direction. *B* and *C*, Old quiescent central (*B*) and more actively demyelinating peripheral (*C*) portions (H&E).

A. Metachromatic leukodystrophy (Fig. 4–9)

Clinical Features

1. The late infantile form is the most common type and is inherited as an autosomal recessive trait. At the onset (12 to 18 months of age), progressive leg weakness and ataxia are present. Upper limb involvement and progressive dementia with regression of speech and intelligence follow. The terminal stage is marked by decortication or decerebration and lack of response to auditory and visual stimuli. Seizures occur in about half of the cases. Death usually occurs by age 7 years.

2. Biochemically, there is a deficiency of aryl sulfatase A, demonstrable in leukocytes, urine, or cultured fibroblasts, which prevents the conversion of sulfatide into the cerebroside and leads to accumulation of the sulfatides (see section 6.1).

3. Other clinical forms, probably genetically distinct, are the juvenile and adolescent or adult types.

Pathology

1. More severely affected are those fibers that myelinate late in ontogenesis. Myelin loss is often incomplete, but U fibers are not spared. Accompanying axonal loss is often severe. Fibrous astrocytosis is moderate.

2. The affected white matter is grossly grayish or ivory white in color with faint striation or granularity.

3. There is accumulation of sulfatides free in the white matter and in phagocytes, oligodendroglial cells, and astrocytes, and even in some neuronal groups (hence the alternate designation of sulfatide lipidosis, or simple storage leukodystrophy). Ultrastructurally, a membrane-bound laminar pattern with dark and light bands, concentric membranes, and granular inclusions constitutes the accumulated substance.

4. The peripheral nervous system shows segmental demyelination with sulfatides in Schwann cells and in phagocytes.

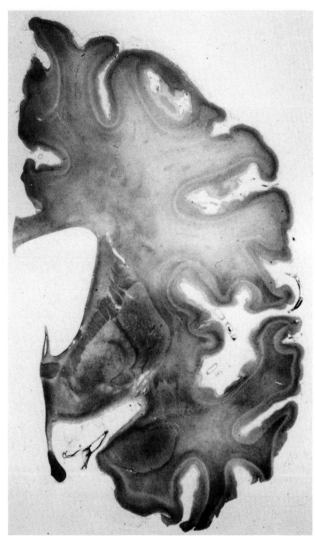

A

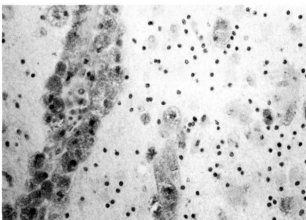

B

Figure 4–9. Metachromatic leukodystrophy. *A,* Myelin-stained preparation of one cerebral hemisphere, demonstrating diffuse pattern of myelin loss. *B,* Cerebral white matter showing ballooned macrophages containing PAS-positive granules scattered randomly and also concentrated about small vessel, along with hypertrophied astrocytes, some with similar granules in their cytoplasm.

5. In the histochemistry of sulfatides, metachromasia by acidified cresyl violet (frozen sections) is diagnostic; the substance is PAS-positive on frozen or paraffin sections.

6. The kidneys, gallbladder, liver (bile ducts), and other visceral organs show accumulation of sulfatides in their cells.

B. Globoid cell leukodystrophy (Krabbe's disease) (Fig. 4–10)

Clinical Features

1. The onset is late infancy (3 to 5 months) or early childhood, with an autosomal recessive mode of inheritance. Retardation or absent mental development, spasticity progressing to total decerebration, and frequent episodes of pyrexia are characteristic.

2. Biochemically, there is a deficiency of galactocerebroside-β-galactosidase, resulting in the accumulation of galactocerebroside.

Pathology

1. The disease has no consistent predilection for certain areas, but remarkably complete myelin loss is seen along some tracts; U fibers are relatively spared.

2. Tissue presence of cerebroside elicits the characteristic phagocytic reaction in the forms of epithelioid cells and multinucleated, multilobulated giant cells (globoid cells). No specific diagnostic histochemical method is known for the substance but it is PAS-positive even on paraffin sections.

Ultrastructurally, hollow tubules with an irregularly crystalloid cross section constitute the accumulated material.

3. Focal neuronal loss may occur in the cerebral cortex, and cerebellar Purkinje and granular cells may be depleted; this is followed by astrocytosis.

4. The peripheral nervous system may show mild segmental demyelination with inclusions (as above) in Schwann cells and phagocytes, which seldom evolve to typical globoid cells.

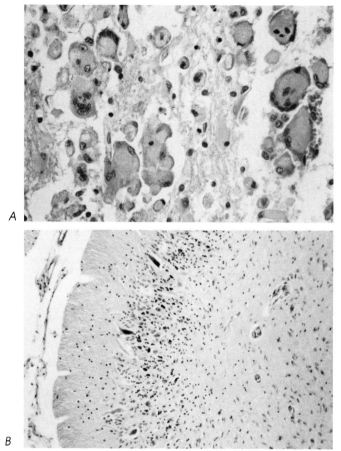

Figure 4–10. Globoid cell leukodystrophy (Krabbe's disease). *A,* Typical globoid cells in well-developed lesion scattered randomly but also concentrated around venules, which show mild perivascular lymphocytic infiltration. *B,* Cerebellar folia in advanced stage, with pronounced loss of granular cells and Purkinje cells.

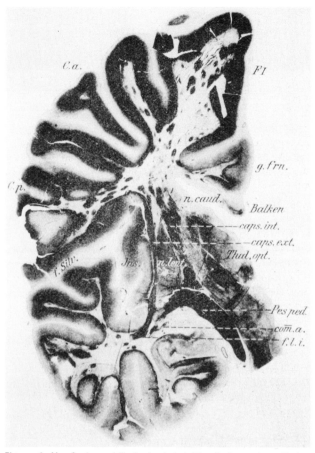

Figure 4–11. Sudanophilic leukodystrophies. Pattern of myelin loss in patient with Pelizaeus-Merzbacher disease. (From Merzbacher L: Eine eigenartige familiär-hereditäre Erkrankungsform [Aplasia axialis extracorticalis congenita]. *Z Gesamte Neurol Psychiatr* 3:1–138, 1910. By permission of Johann Ambrosius Barth.)

C. Sudanophilic (orthochromatic) leukodystrophies (Fig. 4–11)

These are a heterogeneous group of disorders of the myelin sheaths of presumed endogenous origin, sharing as a common feature the sudanophilic character of the lipid material found in the white matter.

C-1. Simple orthochromatic leukodystrophy

Clinical Features	*Pathology*
1. Onset is in infancy, childhood, and adulthood with male preponderance.	1. Pathologic features resemble those of Schilder's disease, with or without mild inflammatory reaction. Demyelination is diffuse and has no sharp borders; it varies in intensity from diffuse myelin pallor to intense and cystic destruction of the white matter. Orthochromatic lipid-laden macrophages are present in the perivascular zone or throughout the affected white matter.
2. Metabolic disturbances have not been identified.	
3. The nosologic identity is often difficult to establish, particularly if the case is sporadic.	
	2. A subtype (mainly in adults) with black-yellow

pigment granules in phagocytes and astrocytes is recognized.

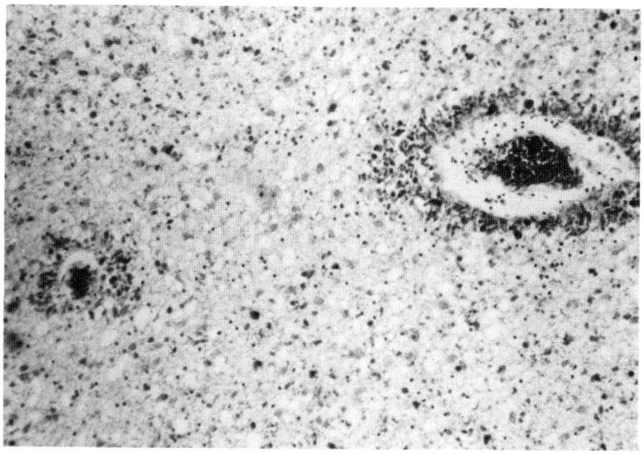

C-2. Adrenoleukodystrophy

Clinical Features

1. This is a childhood disease almost exclusively affecting boys. The average age at onset is 7 years and the course is 2 to 3 years. An adult type with a more prolonged course also occurs.

2. Clinically, there is a nonspecific combination of relentless, progressive deterioration of mental and neurologic functions and evidence of adrenal insufficiency of varying degree.

3. Many of the cases previously diagnosed as belonging to Schilder's disease are now recognized to be examples of adrenoleukodystrophy.

Pathology

1. The pathologic features resemble those of Schilder's disease, often with both sudanophilic and PAS-positive products in macrophages.

2. PAS-positive linear intracytoplasmic inclusions (''spicules'') are seen in white matter macrophages, Schwann cells, and adrenal balloon cells. Ultrastructurally, they are laminar structures made up of two parallel leaflets.

3. Accumulation of cholesterol esters with very long chain fatty acids has been demonstrated in the white matter.

C-3. Pelizaeus-Merzbacher disease

Clinical Features

This is a predominantly sex-linked inherited disease with the onset in the first months of life or later in childhood and with a rather protracted course. A number of other subtypes are described with various ages of onset, types of myelin loss, and hereditary patterns.

Pathology

Myelin deficiency is characteristically in a tigroid pattern with conspicuous zones of preservation about blood vessels. The paucity of lipid-laden macrophages is in striking contrast to the degree of myelin loss. Axons are well preserved.

D. Leukodystrophy with Rosenthal fibers (Alexander's disease) (Fig. 4–12)

Clinical Features

1. This is the rarest of all leukodystrophies, in which mental and neurologic deterioration occur early in infancy and are associated with progressive macrocephaly. Death occurs within a few months to a few years.

Pathology

1. Diffuse myelin deficiency of variable intensity is seen, with disintegration of axons throughout the neuraxis.

2. There is widespread formation of Rosenthal fibers in astrocytes, most

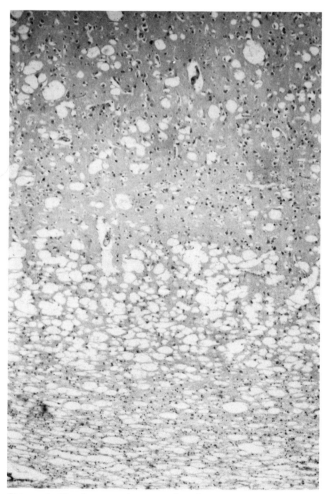

Figure 4–12. Alexander's disease. Medium-power photomicrograph shows affected white matter with Rosenthal fibers particularly about small vessels (H&E).

Figure 4–13. Spongy degeneration. Low-power photomicrograph of cerebral cortex and gyral white matter demonstrates typical spongy appearance. (Courtesy of Dr. Bruno Volk.)

SUMMARY

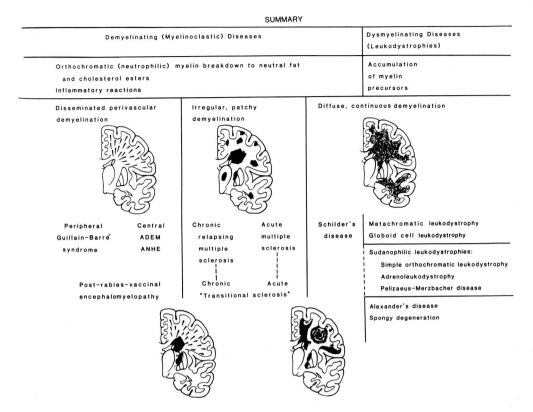

Demyelinating (Myelinoclastic) Diseases	Dysmyelinating Diseases (Leukodystrophies)
Orthochromatic (neutrophilic) myelin breakdown to neutral fat and cholesterol esters Inflammatory reactions	Accumulation of myelin precursors

Figure 4–14. Diagrammatic summary of "demyelinating diseases." ADEM = acute disseminated encephalomyelitis; ANHE = acute necrotizing hemorrhagic encephalopathy.

2. Familial incidence is low (? autosomal recessive).

E. Spongy degeneration of the nervous system (van Bogaert-Bertrand disease, formerly Canavan's spongy sclerosis) (Fig. 4–13)

Clinical Features

1. This is an autosomal recessive disease which is frequent among (but not limited to) Jews. A metabolic basis has not been identified.

Pathology

1. The brain is enlarged. There is reduction of stainable myelin sheaths associated with a spongy state in the subcortical and central white matter; compact prominently in the subpial, perivascular, and subependymal zones.

2. There is an infantile onset with hypotonia followed by spasticity, blindness, and progressive psychomotor deterioration. Death usually occurs before 1 year of age, from intercurrent infection.

tracts are less severely affected (e.g., corpus callosum, internal capsule). Poorly fibrous astrocytosis with Alzheimer type II astrocytes is seen.

2. Ultrastructurally, the sponginess is due to separation of myelin lamellae with rupture into extracellular space and expansion of the astrocytic processes.

The morphologic features of the major demyelinating diseases discussed in this chapter are summarized in Figure 4–14.

5. Degenerative Diseases

The designation "degenerative disease" has historically been conferred on neuropathologic conditions in which etiologic factors are unknown. They are clinically progressive diseases with an insidious onset, often familial in occurrence, sometimes with a definitely established hereditary pattern. Anatomically, they have a tendency to affect certain functionally related neurons and tracts ("systems") preferentially. A subtle biochemical change, determined by a defect of an enzyme or a structural protein, is believed to underlie each of these disorders. Many of the disorders that formerly belonged to this group have now been traced to such etiologic defects, as in the case of cerebral lipidosis, or at least to some definable biochemical abnormality. Others may eventually be linked to extrinsic causes, such as slow virus infection.

At present, our knowledge of these diseases is mainly descriptive, and the diagnosis is largely dependent upon successful exclusion of other etiologically defined conditions. Pathologically, these disorders are characterized by a progressive, more or less symmetric breakdown of cells (primarily neurons) which is marked by rather nonspecific histopathologic changes leading to the eventual disappearance of the cells. Little or no inflammatory reaction or macrophage formation, only subtle fibrillary gliosis (astrocytosis), marks the sites of slow demise of the functioning neural element.

A tentative distinction between many of these disorders is accomplished primarily on the basis of anatomic distribution of lesions but is also aided by certain more specific alterations of cells seen in some of these conditions, such as inclusion bodies of one type or another. Representative examples of these histologic features are listed in Table 5-1.

This chapter is organized in accordance with the traditional classification, based on the anatomic system or systems that are primarily involved, which reflects our current inability to identify etiologic factors involved. This method, however, is of practical convenience, since the clinical symptoms are largely dependent on the anatomic sites of the lesion rather than on the types of lesion or etiologic conditions.

5.1 SENILE AND PRESENILE DEMENTIAS (WITH PREDOMINANT CEREBRAL CORTICAL INVOLVEMENT)

There are several different morphologic substrates in patients with dementia within these vague chronologic boundaries. These different lesions often do not respect the arbitrary chronologic cut-off point (usually age 65 years).

A. Simple (senile or presenile cerebral) atrophy

This disorder is characterized by neuronal loss and nonspecific changes of remaining neurons (simple atrophy or pigmentary atrophy) and astrocytosis in the cerebral cortex, mainly in the frontal and temporal lobes, which grossly show shrinkage of the gyri and widening of the sulci; the ventricles are dilated as a result of loss of cerebral substance (ex vacuo hydrocephalus).

This change is probably a result of "physiologic" or natural demise of neurons, an aging phenomenon. The rapidity of this process naturally varies from person to person, and it is indeed difficult to establish a norm for any given age.

B. Alzheimer's disease (Fig. 5–1)

This disease is characterized by the presence of (1) Alzheimer's neurofibrillary degeneration (tangles) and (2) senile plaques, in addition to the nonspecific neuronal loss, atrophic changes, and reactive astrocytosis described above. The frontal and temporal lobes are again more severely atrophic, and the ventricles show ex vacuo hydrocephalus.

1. Alzheimer's tangles are ultrastructurally composed of a pair of filaments 100 Å thick in double helices. These are different from two normal cell ultrastructures: microtubules and microfilaments (neurofilaments). The cells bearing these abnormal tangles apparently undergo disintegration and leave behind the tangles free in the tissue. Little or no reaction is elicited from other cellular elements in the cortex (see also Fig. 0–6 C).

2. Senile plaques are composed of swollen neurites (dendrites and axons) containing, among other features, the same

TABLE 5-1. Histologic Features of Degenerative Diseases

Types of Neuronal or Axonal Changes	Degenerative Disease/Syndromes*
Pigmentary degeneration, simple atrophy	Simple (pre-)senile atrophy (physiologic aging?)
Pigmentary atrophy	Systemic atrophies ("abiotrophy") e.g., Huntington's chorea Spinocerebellar degeneration Motor system diseases (ALS, etc.)
Alzheimer's neurofibrillary degeneration	Alzheimer's disease Parkinson dementia/ALS complex of Guam Heterogeneous system degeneration Postencephalitic parkinsonism
Pick's argentophilic inclusion	Pick's disease
Lewy body	Idiopathic Parkinson's disease
Eosinophilic inclusions (cytoplasmic)	Familial ALS
Lafora body (amyloid inclusion)	Myoclonus epilepsy
Senile plaque	Presbyophrenic dementia Alzheimer's disease-senile dementia
Axonal dystrophy	Physiologic aging? Infantile neuroaxonal dystrophy Hallervorden-Spatz disease

*ALS = amyotrophic lateral sclerosis.

material that constitutes Alzheimer's tangles and a core of intracellular amyloid fibrils in varying concentration. Occasional microglial cells that also contain amyloid fibrils are seen in the vicinity. These cells are probably phagocytic in their main function, and the origin of amyloid material is uncertain. Because the abnormal neurites are the *sine qua non* of the lesion, the term "neuritic plaque" has been suggested as a better designation. Astrocytosis around the plaques is not an uncommon feature.

3. The following "minor characteristics" are also observed. Simchowicz's granulovacuolar degeneration consists of small basophilic granules surrounded by a halo; it is found almost exclusively in pyramidal neurons of the hippocampus in "normal" elderly persons or in patients with Alzheimer's disease. Alzheimer's tangles and these granules sometimes coexist in some neurons. Hirano's bodies are short, eosinophilic, rodlike structures that are found, usually extracellularly, in the same location under similar circumstances.

In the older literature, elderly patients (over 65) with these characteristic changes were diagnosed as having senile dementia and those with the same histologic changes under age 65 were classified as having presenile dementia or Alzheimer's disease. Implicit in this concept was that Alzheimer's tangles and senile plaques were products of physiologic "aging."

Currently, a view is gaining support that these are not normal concomitants of old age and that they are due to some form of disorder of metabolism, possibly even to slow virus infection. Therefore, regardless of the patient's age, as long as histologic criteria are satisfied, he or she is said to be suffering from Alzheimer's disease.

Many elderly persons with "normal" mental capacities in life are found to have a few tangles or plaques in the cortex, particularly in the hippocampus and neighboring regions of the temporal lobe. This finding, in fact, led to the earlier view that these are physiologic phenomena. Generally speaking, presumably "normal" elderly persons may have more numerous and widespread senile plaques in both paleocortices and neocortices, whereas the tangles tend to be absent or confined to the above-named regions. For clinical dementia associated with the finding of numerous senile plaques and no or only few Alzheimer's tangles, McMenemey (1968) revived the term "presbyophrenic dementia," which was coined by Fischer (1907). Naturally, the precise boundary is difficult to draw, and this may represent only an early phase of Alzheimer's disease.

Conversely, there are only a few, rare conditions in which Alzheimer's tangles are found in the absence of senile plaques, including known and suspected viral encephalitides (subacute sclerosing panencephalitis and postencephalitic parkinsonism). This appears to support the view that the tangles are not a necessary concomitant of old age.

In any event, Alzheimer's disease as defined above is the commonest anatomic substrate of dementia in the elderly. There is no evidence to suggest that the condition is related to vascular insufficiency, a notion that still persists in some quarters.

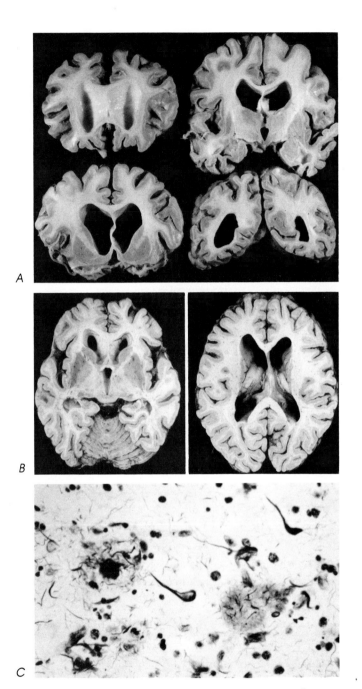

A

B

C

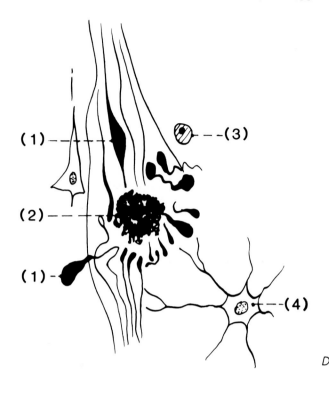

D

Figure 5–1. Alzheimer's disease. *A*, Coronal sections of cerebral hemispheres. Note wide sulci and enlarged ventricles and absence of significant arterial disease and vascular lesions in parenchyma. *B*, Horizontal sections of cerebral hemispheres. *C*, Senile plaques (one with core and the other without) and Alzheimer's tangles as demonstrated by silver impregnation (see also Figure 0–6 *C*). *D*, Diagrammatic illustration of senile (neuritic) plaque. *1*, Swollen neurites filled with abnormal mitochondria, dense bodies of lysosomal type, and double-helical filaments. *2*, Amyloid "core." *3*, Phagocytic cell containing neuritic debris and amyloid material. *4*, Astrocytes and their processes.

C. Pick's disease or lobar atrophy (Fig. 5–2)

In this rare condition, there is severe but relatively well circumscribed atrophy, the frontal and temporal lobes being preferentially affected. Occasionally, basal gray nuclei such as the caudate, putamen, and globus pallidus and also the substantia nigra may show atrophy, with or without clinical correlates.

Histologically, severe loss of neurons and cortical and subcortical astrocytosis (often with spongy appearance, i.e., status spongiosus) underlie the gross atrophy. Two types of characteristic changes are noted (see Fig. 0–6 *D* and *E*):

1. Argentophilic inclusions, a mixture of neurofilaments and microtubules. These are confined largely to large neurons of the hippocampus and adjacent temporal lobes and are not always demonstrable (only in one-third of cases in some series).

2. Pick cells—"balloned cells"—which are pale, globose cells that are found in actively atrophying areas and are more widespread. These cells are considered by some to be evidence of axonal damage distally (retrograde degeneration). Ultrastructurally, they are filled with masses of neurofilaments and microtubules, vesicles, and endoplasmic reticulum.

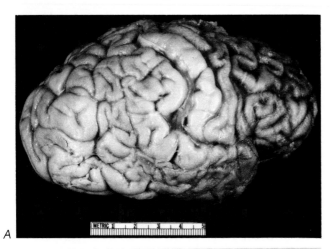

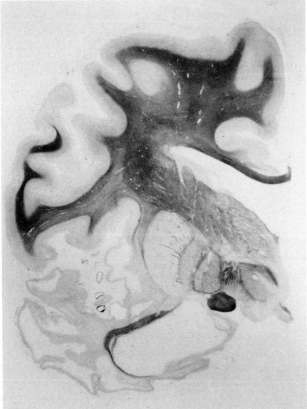

Figure 5-2. Pick's disease. *A,* External view of right cerebral hemisphere, showing pronounced atrophy of frontal and temporal lobes. *B,* Cerebral hemisphere section stained by LFB, showing pronounced atrophy of temporal lobe with preservation of optic radiation.

D. Creutzfeldt-Jakob disease

This condition (in the older literature described under the name "spastic pseudosclerosis" or "cortico-striato-spinal atrophy") is now known to be transmissible to animals and humans. A slow viral infection is suspected, but no agent has been identified to date (see Chapter 3 for details). A low molecular weight protein without demonstrable nucleic acid (unlike viruses), "prion," similar to the scrapie agent recently was postulated as the etiologic agent.

E. Conditions other than primary neuronal degeneration associated with dementia of presenile and senile periods

1. Normal-pressure hydrocephalus

It has been known for more than 25 years that some patients in whom symptomatic hydrocephalus developed had normal cerebrospinal fluid pressure yet improved dramatically after ventricular shunt. The recent interest in this normal-pressure hydrocephalus was brought about by a series of articles in the mid 1960's describing middle-aged or elderly persons who had a clinical triad of dementia, gait disturbance, and urinary incontinence associated with pronounced ventricular dilatation without cortical atrophy and who showed dramatic symptomatic relief after shunting.

The mechanism (and associated structural alterations, if any) by which this reversible dementia occurs remains unexplained, and controversy exists as to the precise criteria for the selection of patients for shunting, particularly in view of the limited success rates in most recent series.

On the other hand, some patients who satisfy the pneumoencephalographic and radioisotope cisternographic criteria for normal-pressure hydrocephalus may have structural lesions such as cortical atrophy (often with changes of Alzheimer's disease) and multiple small infarcts. No significant improvement would be expected by shunting in these patients, but paradoxically some do improve despite these organic lesions and this further complicates the mystery surrounding normal-pressure hydrocephalus.

Note: Although it is generally accepted that the ventricles tend to enlarge and the brain tends to atrophy with age, it has been pointed out that the ventricles enlarge independently of the development of cortical atrophy. This may suggest that the increase in ventricular size in normal persons is related to shrinkage of the white matter rather than to cortical atrophy.

It must be remembered that ventricular size at autopsy is often significantly reduced from that in the living state. Multiple factors of terminal illness and the agonal period contribute to brain anoxia and edema. Formalin fixation produces brain tissue swelling, and postmortem tissue changes when autopsy is delayed also contribute to apparent reduction of the ventricular size.

2. Multi-infarct dementia

Although there is no pathologic evidence to support the notion that cerebrovascular disease contributes to diffuse degenerative change of neurons leading to clinical dementia in old age, multiple small infarcts resulting from diverse forms of vascular disease can cause gradual mental deterioration without signs of the focal and episodic nature of the lesions. The term "multi-infarct dementia" has been popularized to cover this situation. The most common underlying vascular lesions are atherosclerosis and arteriolar sclerosis, both of which are aggravated by hypertension and diabetes, as discussed in Chapter 1. Lacunar state and Binswanger's encephalopathy are special forms of multiple small infarction underlying multi-infarct dementia. It must be remembered that the effects of large infarcts that result only in higher psychomotor and cognitive disorders, such as apraxia and aphasia, unaccompanied by overt motor deficit, may be confused with manifestations of dementia.

A special form of senile and presenile vascular disorder is *primary cerebral amyloid angiopathy* (Fig. 5–3). This disorder usually occurs independently of systemic vascular amyloid deposition, but it is almost always coexistent with senile plaques. Mild changes are relatively common in elderly persons and cause no parenchymal damage. Although they are not mutually exclusive, two general types have been recognized relative to the size of vessels:

a. Lesions affecting cortical arterioles and capillaries (micro-angiopathy) have been known as "plaque-like angiopathy" (or "drusige Entartung") of Scholz. Amyloid often infiltrates the adjacent cerebral tissue (perivascular plaques). No hemorrhage or ischemic changes are noted in relation to these.

b. Lesions affecting leptomeningeal or superficial cortical perforating arteries have been known as congophilic angiopathy (of Pantelakis), in which the amyloid deposit is largely confined to the vascular wall. The lumen of these larger affected vessels tends to become narrow as a result of an increase in subintimal connective tissue. These changes are most pronounced in the posterior dorsal region of the cerebral hemispheres.

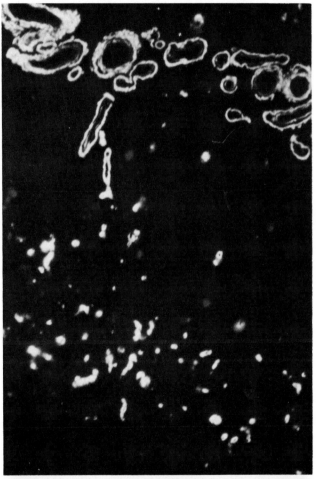

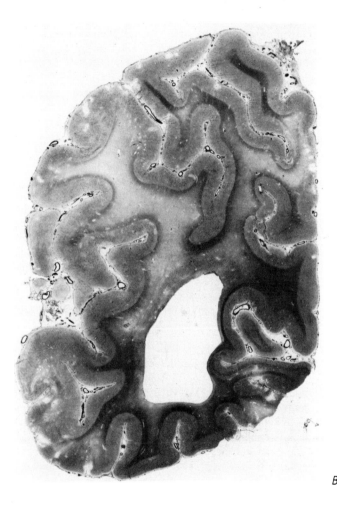

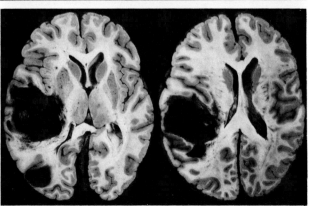

Figure 5–3. Primary cerebral amyloid angiopathy. *A*, Lower-power view of leptomeningeal and parenchymal arteries with neural amyloid deposition as demonstrated in thioflavin S-stained section viewed under ultraviolet light. *B*, Bodian-stained posterior section of cerebral hemisphere with multiple small critical infarcts (light-staining areas) and diffuse secondary degeneration of dorsal white matter. *C*, Horizontal sections of cerebral hemispheres with large and small hemorrhages in anterior temporal and posterior temporo-occipital regions, respectively.

Multiple infarcts, mostly cortical, can result from this change. Segmental hyalin-fibrinoid degeneration is often superimposed on affected medium-sized vessels, leading to microaneurysm formation. Recent and old extravasations from these microaneurysms are encountered, mainly in the cerebral cortex. Small or large, at times fatal, hemorrhages can also result. These hemorrhages are characteristically in the cerebral white matter, with partial involvement of the overlying cortex. The basal gray matter appears to be exempt from these vascular changes and resultant hemorrhages. Therefore, primary amyloid angiopathy is an infrequent but important cause of "multi-infarct dementia" (often preceded by episodes resembling transient ischemic attacks) and small or large fatal cerebral hemorrhage in elderly persons.

5.2 CONDITIONS WITH PREDOMINANT INVOLVEMENT OF THE EXTRAPYRAMIDAL SYSTEM

A. Huntington's chorea (Fig. 5–4)

There is diffuse loss of small ganglion cells in the caudate nucleus and putamen, with atrophic, lipochrome-laden surviving neurons, accompanied by pronounced reactive astrocytosis. This results in macroscopic atrophy of these nuclei and dilatation of the frontal horns of the lateral ventricles. The cerebral cortex, particularly in the frontal lobe, shows variable degrees of simple atrophy. Similar but much less conspicuous atrophic changes are found more widespread in the brain, particularly in the substantia nigra and the thalamus.

B. Dystonia musculorum deformans

Despite the grotesque clinical movement disorder in this condition, the anatomic substrate has not been clearly elucidated. Neuronal degeneration involving the cortex and various brainstem nuclei has been described, but its significance is doubtful. The infantile form in which status marmoratus and status dysmyelinisatus are described in the basal ganglia most likely represents the end result of perinatal hypoxia (see section 8.7).

C. Parkinson's disease (paralysis agitans) (Fig. 5–5)

The main lesion lies in the substantia nigra (the zona compacta in particular) and locus ceruleus, in which pigment-bearing neurons have broken down and have left pigment granules behind, free in the tissue or within the cytoplasm of phagocytic cells. This results in grossly discernible depigmentation of these nuclei. There is reactive astrocytosis. One or more chracteristic hyaline eosinophilic intracytoplasmic inclusion bodies (Lewy bodies) are seen in some of the remaining neurons (Fig. 0–6 G). Simple atrophic neurons or ghost cells may also be found. Some other nuclei including the nucleus basalis and the dorsal vagal nucleus, neurons of the reticular formation, and sympathetic ganglia are known to show similar changes.

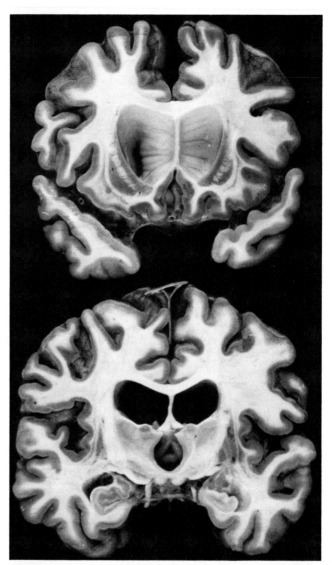

A

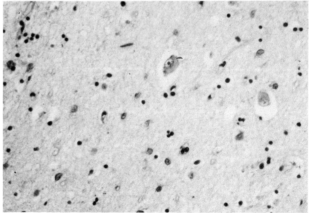

B

Figure 5–4. Huntington's chorea. A, Coronal sections of anterior cerebral hemispheres, showing pronounced atrophy of caudate nucleus and milder atrophy of putamen, bilaterally. Ventricles are correspondingly enlarged. B, Photomicrograph of caudate nucleus with near-total disappearance of small neurons and reactive astrocytosis in their place. Two preserved large neurons are also seen (H&E).

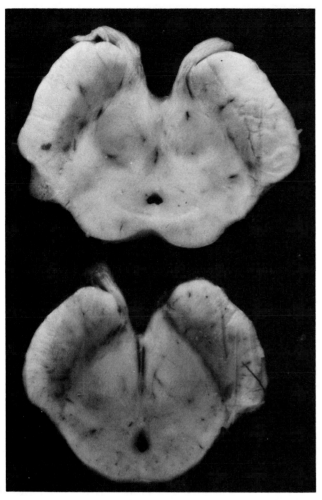

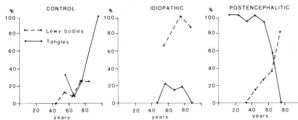

Figure 5-5. Parkinson's disease. *A,* Midbrain sections from a patient with Parkinson's disease and from an age-matched control, the former *(above)* showing pronounced nigral depigmentation. *B,* Diagrams illustrating relative frequencies of Lewy bodies and Alzheimer's tangles. (*B* modified from Alvord EC Jr: The pathology of parkinsonism. In *Pathology of the Nervous System.* Vol 1. Edited by J Minckler. New York, McGraw-Hill Book Company, 1968, pp 1152–1161.)

For a long time the basal ganglia were thought to be the seat of a primary lesion (état criblé, "perivascular degeneration"). However, this change is now known to be indistinguishable from that seen among otherwise healthy elderly persons. Aside from some loss of nerve fibers (of nigral neurons) in the globus pallidus, no distinctive morphologic features have been authenticated in the basal ganglia.

D. Postencephalitic parkinsonism

The gross appearance is nearly identical to that in Parkinson's disease, with destruction of melanin-bearing neurons and reactive gliosis, primarily in the substantia nigra. Here characteristic changes include Alzheimer's neurofibrillary tangles, saccules of lipochrome granules, and rare binucleated neurons.

Note: The "specificity" of these inclusions is only relative; Lewy bodies are age dependent and are found, although relatively few in number, in otherwise normal elderly persons (up to 20% at age 80). They show increased prevalence even among the elderly postencephalitic parkinsonian patients. Alzheimer's tangles in contrast show a drastic reduction in number in the postencephalitic group beyond age 60, whereas they become very frequent beyond age 80 in the control group (Fig. 5-5 *B*).

E. Parkinsonism-dementia complex of Guam

This disease of unknown cause which affects natives of the island of Guam in the Pacific Ocean is characterized by the widespread presence of Alzheimer's tangles associated with neuronal loss throughout the brain, in the absence of senile plaques, Lewy bodies, or inflammatory reactions. The sites of predilection are the hippocampus, amygdaloid nucleus, and adjacent temporal cortex and frontal cortex. The basal ganglia, substantia nigra, periaqueductal gray matter, midline raphe, and reticular nuclei and dorsal vagal nucleus are also preferentially involved. The anterior horn of the spinal cord is also affected in some patients, and this explains a clinical picture resembling that of amyotrophic lateral sclerosis.

F. Progressive supranuclear palsy (Steele-Richardson-Olszewski syndrome); heterogeneous system degeneration (Fig. 5–6)

In this condition, neuronal loss associated with Alzheimer's neurofibrillary tangles is the main feature, involving the various regions of the basal ganglia (especially the pallidum), the brainstem (the substantia nigra, subthalamic nucleus, superior colliculi, periaqueductal gray matter, pontine tegmentum, and some of the cranial nerve nuclei), and the cerebellum (especially the dentate nuclei). Fibrillary gliosis marks the sites of the involved gray matter and their tracts. Only rarely are neuronophagia, microglial nodules, and inflammatory reaction reported.

G. Hallervorden-Spatz disease (Fig. 5–7)

The essential lesion consists of rust-brown discoloration of the globus pallidus and substantia nigra (especially the reticular zone) due to accumulation of abnormal pigment (with shades of yellow, green, and blue in a Nissl stain) in these areas. Pigment granules are free in the tissue, perivascular, or intracellular in nerve cells, astrocytes, and microglial cells. Mineralization (mainly iron incrustation) of vascular walls and in free concretion forms adds to the discoloration. Various degrees of neuronal loss, the presence of focal axonal swelling (spheroids, neuroaxonal dystrophy), demyelination, and reactive astrocytosis are additional important findings.

Other areas, including the cerebral cortex and Purkinje

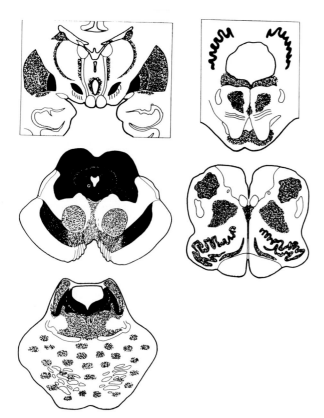

Figure 5–6. Heterogeneous system degeneration. In this diagrammatic demonstration of the distribution of lesions, the intensity of shading corresponds to the severity of involvement. (From Steel JC, Richardson JC, Olszewski J: Progressive supranuclear palsy: a heterogeneous degeneration involving the brain stem, basal ganglia, and cerebellum with vertical gaze and pseudobulbar palsy, nuchal dystonia and dementia. *Arch Neurol* 10:333–359, 1964. By permission of the American Medical Association.)

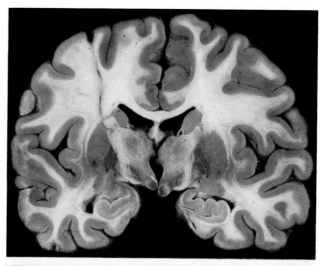

A

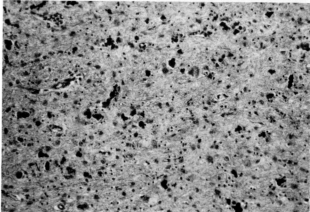

B

Figure 5–7. Hallervorden-Spatz disease. *A,* Bilateral atrophy and light-brownish discoloration of globus pallidus, subthalamic nucleus, and substantia nigra (only anterior portion is shown). *B,* Photomicrograph of affected globus pallidus with swollen neurites (neuraxonal dystrophy) and iron pigment granules (iron and H&E).

cell layer of the cerebellum, are also reported to show some neuronal loss. Some consider this to be a locally restricted form of generalized neuraxonal dystrophy, which is a rare autosomal recessively transmitted disease that usually manifests itself in the second year of life (infantile or late infantile neuraxonal dystrophy) and has a progressive course (3 to 8 years) of motor and mental deterioration leading to a decorticate state and death. In either of these conditions, there is no known biochemical test that would help to establish the diagnosis during life.

5.3 SPINOCEREBELLAR DEGENERATION (FIG. 5–8)

A fully satisfactory and universally acceptable classification of spinocerebellar degeneration has not been achieved. Clinically, numerous different combinations of signs and symptoms have been recorded, and similarly, numerous variations of neuronal and tract involvement have been described

pathologically. The problem is compounded by frequent lack of correlation between clinical findings and anatomic lesions. The following classification, given here for reference, is based largely on that of Greenfield. It is to be remembered that intermediate forms are numerous.

Figure 5–8. Spinocerebellar degeneration. *A,* Friedreich's ataxia. Myelin-stained cross section of thoracic spinal cord is shown. *B,* Pontocerebellar atrophy as a component of multiple system atrophy (LFB/C), showing pronounced pallor of pontocerebellar fibers. Note the preservation of dentatofugal fibers. *C,* Cerebellar cortical atrophy, primarily associated with dropping out of Purkinje cells and proliferation of Bergmann's astrocytes in their place, in a case of olivopontocerebellar atrophy (H&E). *D,* Diagrammatic demonstration of affected areas in multiple system atrophy. *E,* Atrophy of intermediolateral nucleus (*circle*) of lower thoracic cord as a partial anatomic substrate of Shy-Drager syndrome.

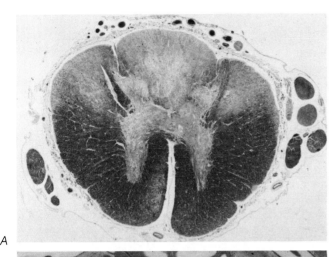

A

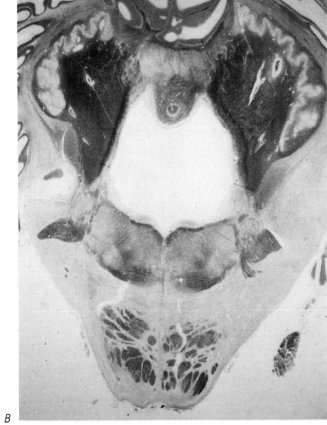

B

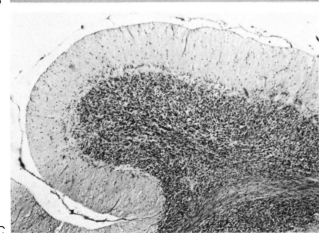

C

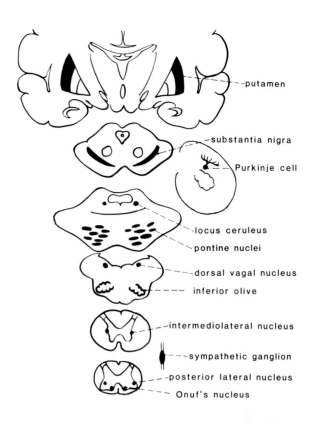

putamen

substantia nigra

Purkinje cell

locus ceruleus

pontine nuclei

dorsal vagal nucleus

inferior olive

intermediolateral nucleus

sympathetic ganglion

posterior lateral nucleus

Onuf's nucleus

D

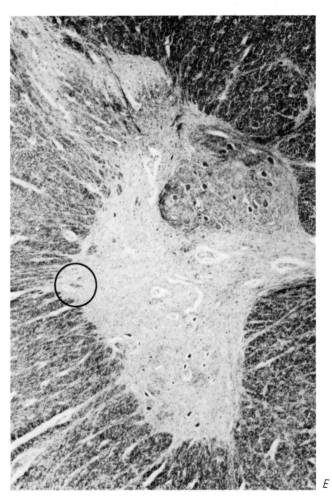

E

161

Histologically, these diseases (or syndromes) are characterized by nonspecific degeneration and eventual loss of neurons and myelinated nerve fibers. It is assumed that the pathogenesis for all is primary neuronal degeneration (atrophy). When the process is very slow, the cell body and proximal part of the nerve fibers may survive, but often the whole neuron atrophies and disappears. In some, however, it is not conclusively established whether the disorders begin in the neurons or in the myelin sheaths.

This group of diseases is also associated, in varying degree, with hereditary degeneration of the retina and inner ear and with dementia.

Designation	*Degenerated Areas*
A. Predominantly spinal forms	
1. Friedreich's ataxia	Dorsal root ganglia, dorsal roots, dorsal columns
	Clarke's columns, spinocerebellar tracts
	Pyramidal tracts
	(Nuclei gracilis and cuneatus)
	(Other brainstem nuclei and tracts)
2. Variant and related forms	
a. Familial spastic paraplegia	Lateral (and dorsal) columns
b. Posterior-column ataxia of Biemond	Dorsal roots, dorsal columns
3. Friedreich's ataxia associated with peroneal muscular atrophy (hereditary areflexic dystasia of Roussy-Levy)	(See section 5.5)
B. Predominantly cerebellar forms	
1. Cerebello-olivary degeneration (Holmes type of hereditary ataxia), including late cortical cerebellar atrophy (Marie-Foix-Alajouánine) and subacute familial type (Akelaitis)	Purkinje cells and granular cells
	Olivary nuclei
C. Predominantly cerebellar and spinal forms	
1. Olivopontocerebellar atrophy (Menzel type of hereditary ataxia)	Pontine nuclei, pontocerebellar tract
	Olivary nucleus, olivocerebellar tract
	Purkinje cells and granular cells
	Pyramidal tract
	Spinocerebellar tracts
	Dorsal columns
	Lower motor neuron
	Substantia nigra, corpus striatum, etc.

D. Multiple system atrophy (Fig. 5–8)

As described above, many reported cases of olivopontocerebellar atrophy show concomitant involvement of the striatum (especially the putamen) and substantia nigra (without Lewy bodies). The latter combination of lesions alone has been previously reported as striatonigral degeneration with a clinical picture indistinguishable from that of Parkinson's disease. Some other cases of pontocerebellar atrophy include degeneration of the long tracts of the spinal cord similar to but less extensive than that seen in Friedreich's ataxia, with or without additional loss of motor neurons of the anterior horns, preganglionic spinal sympathetic nuclei, intermediolateral nucleus of the thoracolumbar segments (and the nucleus of Onuf), and other nuclei of the midsacral segments.

The distribution and relative intensity of these lesions vary considerably from case to case even within a single family, as in the large family reported by Schut and Haymaker. The term "multiple system atrophy" has been coined to encompass cases exhibiting combined degeneration of these loci.

Its clinical counterpart, Shy-Drager syndrome, represents a clinical combination of autonomic symptoms of orthostatic hypotension, urinary incontinence, sexual impotence, and parkinsonian or spinocerebellar ataxic symptoms.

E. Cerebellar ataxias associated with systemic metabolic disorders

These naturally are not "degenerative disorders" but must be kept in mind for differential diagnosis and are therefore briefly mentioned here.

1. Ataxia-telangiectasia (Louis-Bar disease)

This autosomal recessive disorder with deficiency of immunoglobulin (IgA) is associated with progressive oculocutaneous telangiectasia and severe degeneration of the cerebellar cortex involving both Purkinje and granular cells. Irregular dendritic expansions and eosinophilic cytoplasmic inclusions in some of the remaining Purkinje cells have also been described. Other lesions include degeneration of the posterior column, spinocerebellar tracts, anterior horn cells, peripheral nerves, and cells of the sympathetic ganglion. The sympathetic ganglion often contains abnormally large cells with a bizarrely shaped nucleus, as seen in various visceral organs, including the anterior lobe of the pituitary.

2. Other, rarer, conditions include
Bassen-Kornzweig syndrome (abetalipoproteinemia)
Refsum's disease
Lipidoses
Hartnup disease
Maple syrup urine disease
Pyruvate decarboxylase deficiency

F. Myoclonus epilepsy

Myoclonus, as a phenomenon, is seen in many disorders of diverse cause and with varied anatomic lesions. Even the familial form of myoclonus epilepsy originally described (without pathologic accounts) by Unverricht (1891) and

Lundborg (1903) now appears to be a mixture of different degenerative diseases.

1. Lafora's disease (or Lafora-body polymyoclonus)

This disease is characterized by the presence of large basophilic intracytoplasmic inclusion bodies (Fig. 0–6 *H*) with staining reaction of amyloid in neurons, varying degrees of neuronal loss, and gliosis. These changes are rather diffuse but are most extensive in the dentate nucleus, substantia nigra, thalamus and globus pallidus, and anterior frontal and central gyri. These bodies are chemically composed of unusual polymers of glucose (polyglucosans) and are also found in the heart, liver, and other visceral tissues.

The disease is autosomal recessive in hereditary pattern and begins in late childhood and adolescence with epilepsy and progressive myoclonic jerks and dementia. Death usually occurs within 5 to 6 years.

2. Myoclonus epilepsy of degenerative type

In this form of myoclonus epilepsy, Lafora bodies are absent, and only nonspecific neuronal atrophy and loss accompanied by reactive astrocytosis has been reported in various regions of the brain, most consistently including the cerebellar cortex (Purkinje cells), dentate nucleus, inferior olive, and substantia nigra.

This form takes a much more benign course with longer survival and only mild or absent dementia. Whether this form represents a single disease entity or a syndrome has not been established.

3. Myoclonus is a major feature of late childhood and adolescent forms of cerebral lipidoses such as Jansky-Bielschowsky, Spielmeyer-Vogt, and Kufs types (see section 6.1, *A*).

4. Familial myoclonus and ataxia

This is an uncommon condition inherited as an autosomal dominant trait. Ramsay Hunt coined the term "dyssynergia cerebellaris myoclonica" to describe a syndrome of myoclonus (with or without seizures) and cerebellar signs and attributed it to lesions of the dentatofugal pathway. Its nosologic position is still uncertain. It is regarded as either a form of spinocerebellar degeneration (dentato-ruberal atrophy) or a variant of myoclonus epilepsy.

5. Other conditions

Other conditions in which myoclonus is a feature are mentioned here for comparison. It is often observed in association with epilepsy, and this association is commonly designated "myoclonic epilepsy." In some of the viral encephalitides, especially subacute sclerosing panencephalitis and Creutzfeldt-Jakob disease (presumed viral), myoclonus is a major symptom. Anoxic encephalopathy is another relatively common condition with myoclonus. It is also seen in Alzheimer's disease, somatic neuroblastoma (often occult), and bronchogenic carcinoma, among other disorders.

5.4 RETINAL AND OPTIC DEGENERATION IN ASSOCIATION WITH HEREDOFAMILIAL NEUROLOGIC DISORDERS

A. Pigmentary retinal degeneration ("retinitis pigmentosa")

This is the most frequently encountered form of chorioretinal degeneration in patients with or without other systemic abnormalities. The vast majority occur as autosomal recessive traits. Pathologically, it is characterized by degeneration and loss of photoreceptors (rods and cones) accompanied by both degenerative and proliferative changes in the retinal pigment epithelium. Liberated pigment granules are phagocytosed by macrophages, which along with proliferating retinal pigment epithelial cells migrate into the retina and lie adjacent to blood vessels in upper retinal layers. The optic nerves show relatively inconsistent changes.

Various forms of spinocerebellar degeneration, motor neuron disease, and muscle dystrophy are known to be associated with this disorder.

Similar combined degeneration of the photoreceptors and pigment epithelium is seen in many other known or suspected inborn errors of metabolism, including juvenile (Batten-Mayou; Spielmeyer-Vogt) and late infantile (Jansky-Bielschowsky) familial amaurotic idiocies, Refsum's disease, Gaucher's disease, mucopolysaccharidoses, and abetalipoproteinemia (Bassen-Kornzweig syndrome), among others.

B. Optic atrophies

This disorder is characterized primarily by degeneration and loss of ganglion cells of the retina and secondary optic atrophy. Leber's disease (? sex-linked recessive), which usually appears as an isolated optic nerve disorder, is likely to show minor neurologic abnormalities, usually pyramidal and cerebellar symptoms and those of the peripheral nerves. Degeneration of the lateral geniculate bodies and geniculocalcarine fibers is described in the brain. Behr's (complicated) optic atrophy (autosomal recessive) is associated with corticospinal and cerebellar signs and mental retardation and, at times, epilepsy. Ophthalmoscopically indistinguishable optic atrophy is also often reported in hereditary spinocerebellar ataxias (up to 20%) and motor neuron disorders.

5.5 CONDITIONS WITH PREDOMINANT INVOLVEMENT OF THE MOTOR SYSTEM (PROGRESSIVE NUCLEAR MYELOPATHIES, NUCLEAR AMYOTROPHIES, OR MOTOR NEURON DISEASE)

This group is characterized by degeneration primarily of either lower or lower and upper motor neurons. Three main subgroups representing different combinations are diagrammatically illustrated in Figure 5–9.

A. Amyotrophic lateral sclerosis (ALS; Charcot's disease) (Fig. 5–10)

1. Sporadic variety

There is loss of large motor neurons, leading to astrocytosis, which is most easily seen in the anterior horns of

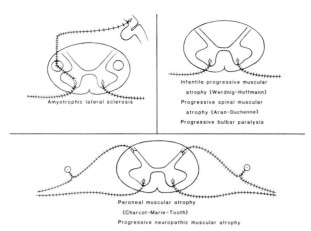

Figure 5–9. Component disorders of motor neuron disease.

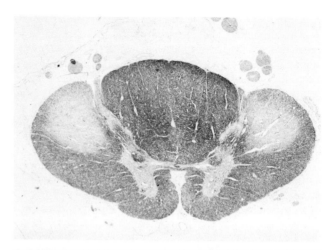

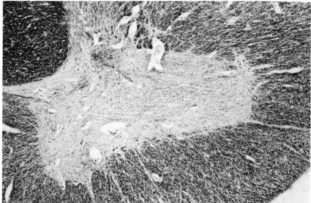

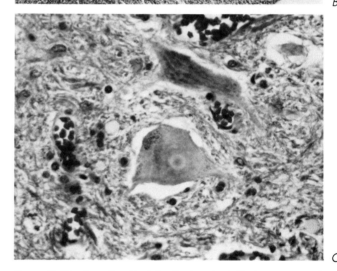

the cervical and lumbar enlargements and in the hypoglossal nuclei (and other motor nuclei of the brainstem, for example, nuclei V and VII). Nuclei III, IV, and VI are rarely, if ever, involved. Surviving motor neurons are often shrunken and pyknotic. Neuronophagia may be seen in some rapidly progressive cases.

There is a variable degeneration of the pyramidal tracts, crossed and uncrossed, in the spinal cord; it may be traced upward into various levels, including the cerebral white matter. This is attributed to the loss of large pyramidal cells of the precentral gyrus. There may be diffuse reduction of stainable myelin in the lateral and anterior columns, with intact posterior columns. The significance and pathogenesis of these changes are undetermined.

Progressive spinal muscular atrophy (Aran-Duchenne) and progressive bulbar palsy (Duchenne) are generally considered one and the same condition as ALS with variations in the distribution and severity of the lesions, involvement of the spinal lower motor neurons and of the bulbar lower motor neurons being in the foreground, respectively. These three conditions are often collectively referred to as "motor neuron disease."

2. Familial ALS

An estimated 10 to 15% of motor neuron diseases in the United States occur on a familial basis (Kurland & Mulder, 1954). Special histologic features reported in these cases include (1) eosinophilic hyaline intracytoplasmic inclusions in anterior horn cells and (2) degeneration of Clarke's columns and spinocerebellar tracts and of the posterior columns.

3. Guamanian ALS

This appears to represent part of the spectrum of a single disease entity, which includes parkinsonism-dementia complex (see section 5.2, E) and is characterized by the presence of Alzheimer's neurofibrillary tangles in the involved areas. The disease takes a much more protracted course than classic ALS.

B. Infantile spinal muscular atrophy (Werdnig-Hoffmann disease)

There is loss of motor neurons of the spinal anterior horns and the brainstem (nucleus XII and VII, nucleus am-

Figure 5–10. Amyotrophic lateral sclerosis. *A,* Photomacrograph of cervical segment with pronounced degeneration of pyramidal tracts (LFB/CV). *B,* Closer-up view of anterior horn, showing depopulation of motor neurons. *C,* Familial amyotrophic lateral sclerosis. Eosinophilic intracytoplasmic inclusions are present in anterior horn cell (H&E).

biguus). Among the remaining cells, pale swollen neurons and neuronophagia may be seen. Long tracts in the brainstem and spinal cord are not involved.

The disease is transmitted by simple autosomal recessive inheritance. It is manifest at birth or becomes so within the first few months of life, and the affected children are dead by 12 to 24 months. There are cases with later onset and these merge with the juvenile proximal spinal muscular atrophy or the Kugelberg-Welander syndrome, which is often seen sporadically. Generally, the later the onset, the slower is the progression of the disease (with a more favorable prognosis).

C. Peroneal muscular atrophy (Charcot-Marie-Tooth disease)

In this inherited disorder, distal portions of the peripheral nerves show degeneration of myelin sheaths and axons (segmental demyelination and remyelination and some wallerian degeneration with onion-bulb type proliferation of Schwann cells). This is thought by some to represent a degenerative neuropathy with dying back of axons, distinct from a primary neuronal disease.

However, there is a combined degeneration of the spinal *motor* neurons, indistinguishable from that of motor neuron disease described above, and of spinal *sensory* ganglion cells and their processes, resembling that of Friedreich's ataxia. For this reason, this disorder is sometimes included among spinocerebellar degenerations (see section 5.3). When associated with evident spinocerebellar degeneration, it is known as the Roussy-Lévy syndrome.

D. Hypertrophic interstitial neuritis (or neuropathy) (Dejerine-Sottas disease)

This was for a long time thought to be a specific disease entity, consisting grossly of swelling of peripheral nerves and histologically of widely separated and poorly myelinated axons surrounded by concentric onion-bulb proliferation of Schwann cells (Fig. 0–8 *B*). It is usually familial (autosomal dominant) but occasionally reported to be sporadic.

More recently, identical histologic changes have been recognized in Refsum's disease (heredopathia atactica polyneuritiformis, see Chapter 6), in acromegaly, and in post-infectious polyneuropathy (as a rare sequela). It is now realized that this histologic feature can occur in any disease that is associated with segmental demyelination and remyelination, albeit to a limited degree.

REFERENCES

Fischer O: Miliare Nekrosen mit drusigen Wucherungen der Neurofibrillen, eine regelmässige Veränderung der Hirnrinde bei seniler Demenz. *Monatsschr Psychiatr Neurol* (Berlin) 22:361–372, 1907

Greenfield JG: *The Spino-cerebellar Degenerations.* Springfield, Illinois, Charles C Thomas, Publisher, 1954.

Kurland LT, Mulder DW: Epidemiologic investigations of amyotrophic lateral sclerosis. 1. Preliminary report on geographic distribution, with special reference to the Mariana Islands, including clinical and pathologic observations. *Neurology* (Minneap) 4:355–378; 438–448, 1954.

McMenemey WH: Present concepts of Alzheimer's disease. *Monogr Pathol Int Acad Pathol,* 1968, No. 9, pp 201–208.

Schut JW: The hereditary ataxias. *Res Publ Assoc Res Nerv Ment Dis* 33:293–324, 1954.

6. Metabolic and Toxic Diseases

Every known disease of the nervous system, even those due to vascular pathology, trauma, or infection, ultimately requires the presence of a chemical, and therefore metabolic, abnormality. It is apparent that the term "metabolic" by itself is almost meaningless for the purpose of differentiating one class of neuropathologic state from another. Therefore, the term "metabolic" has been more meaningfully restricted to two classes of nervous system disorders:

1. Those commonly referred to as "inborn errors of metabolism," particularly those with prominent, if not exclusive, nervous system involvement. Before the discovery of their true nature, many of these diseases had been classified among "degenerative disorders" of the nervous system. The majority of them were also called "storage" diseases because of accumulation of abnormal substances in the cytoplasm of neurons or other cellular components of the nervous system.

2. A group of conditions in which the disorder of the nervous system is secondary to a metabolic disturbance created by a disease of another viscus.

This aforementioned metabolic category contrasts with a *toxic* state of the nervous system, in which the abnormality of nervous function or structure is due to the presence of an exogenous poison or a demonstrable metabolite. Naturally, if the disorder is due to an offending metabolite that results from a visceral metabolic abnormality, as in uremia, the condition may be considered both metabolic and toxic. Only some of the more common or significant conditions in neurologic practice will be discussed here.

6.1 STORAGE DISEASES

A. Disorders of lipid metabolism

A simplified overview of the relationship between the chemical compounds and the enzymatic defects which exists in various "lipid storage" diseases is presented in Table 6–1.

Gangliosidoses may be subclassified according to their specific enzyme defect(s) as in Table 6–2.

1. Classic Tay-Sachs disease (infantile G_{M2} gangliosidosis, type I) (Fig. 6–1)

This is the morphologic prototype of lipidoses. There is a ubiquitous neuronal storage phenomenon with displacement of the nuclei, often toward the apical dendrite, which prevents expansion of the dendrite. Ultrastructurally, the stored lipid material is composed of membranous cytoplasmic bodies, probably of lysosomal origin.

Affected neurons disintegrate, rarely attended by neuronophagia, and lipid is phagocytosed and degraded by macrophages, which migrate toward perivascular spaces and to the leptomeninges. Neuronal loss elicits a reactive astrocytosis. Astrocytes also contain degraded lipid in their cytoplasm.

There is massive destruction of the white matter, which shows wallerian degeneration and also evidence of arrested myelination. The brain grossly shows generalized atrophy with thickened meninges and thin optic nerves. The cerebellum is particularly sclerotic and contrasts sharply, in protracted cases, with the cerebral hemispheres, which are enlarged (megalencephaly) as a result of a massive increase of extracellular space.

Note: For a group of neuronal storage disorders without identification of enzymatic defect(s) or chemical nature of the stored material, designations based on the time of onset or by eponym have been traditionally applied: for example, the late infantile type or Jansky-Bielschowsky form, the juvenile type or Batten-Mayou or Spielmeyer-Vogt disease, and the adult type or Kufs' disease.

Generally, the later the onset of the disease, the less prominent is the storage phenomenon in neurons. Also, the involvement becomes more selective, and the brainstem and cerebellum are more favored. The traditional collective name for these disorders, "familial amaurotic idiocy," is inaccurate, for some patients are not amaurotic or mentally deteriorated. Alternatively, the term "atypical juvenile neurolipidosis" was proposed to encompass all of these cases.

Many of these disorders are characterized by the presence of pigment that ultrastructurally resembles lipofuscin pigment or shows a configuration described as curvilinear bodies or a fingerprint pattern. The term "neuronal ceroid-lipofuscinoses" was proposed for this group of disorders. The pigment accumulation is also noted in endothelial cells and pericytes of the vascular wall of the somatic tissue, and this feature provides easy access to a biopsy diagnosis. Nosologic identity of these cases is not universally accepted.

2. Cerebrosidoses

    a. Gaucher's disease (Fig. 6–2) (glucocerebroside lipidosis), infantile form

TABLE 6–1. Interrelationship of Disorders of Lipid Metabolism

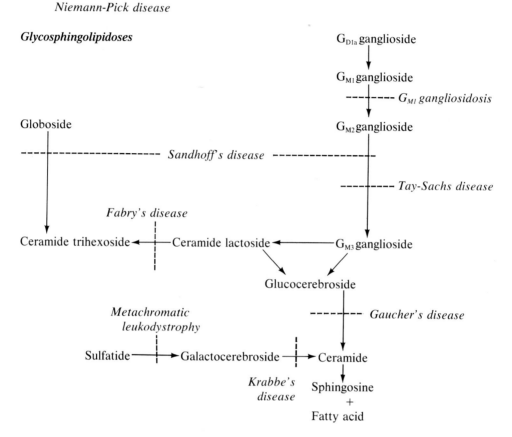

TABLE 6–2. Classification of Gangliosidoses

	Eponyms	Defective Enzyme(s)	Storage Material	Tissue Affected
1.a. G_{M2} gangliosidosis, type I (or variant B)	Classic infantile Tay-Sachs disease	Hexosaminidase A	G_{M2} gangliosides and asialo derivative of G_{M2} ganglioside	Neurons
b. G_{M2} gangliosidosis, type II	Late infantile and juvenile amaurotic idiocy	Hexosaminidase A (partial)	As above (to a lesser degree)	Neurons
c. G_{M2} gangliosidosis, type III (variant O)	Sandhoff's disease	Hexosaminidase A and B	Asialo-G_{M2} gangliosides G_{M2} ganglioside Ceramide tetrahexoside + globosides, especially in viscera	Neurons Viscera
2.a. G_{M1} gangliosidosis, type I (variant O)	Pseudo-Hurler's syndrome	β-galactosidase A, B, and C	G_{M1} gangliosides	Neurons
b. G_{M1} gangliosidosis, type II (variant A)	Derry's disease	β-galactosidase B and C	Glycosaminoglycan and mucopolysaccharides	Visceral reticulohistiocytic cells (especially pericytes)

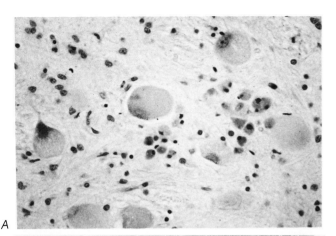

A

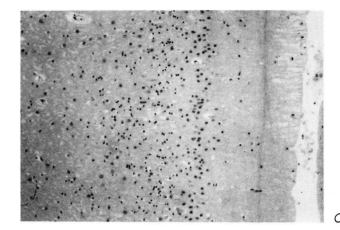

C

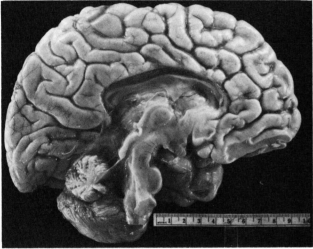

B

Figure 6-1. Tay-Sachs disease. *A*, Neuronal storage phenomenon and phagocytotic intracellular "digestion" (degradation) of ganglioside by macrophage (LFB/PAS/H). *B*, Mesial surface of left cerebral hemisphere with pronounced atrophy of cerebellum in contrast to fullness of cerebral hemisphere. *C*, Microscopic appearance of devastated cerebellar cortex, with no Purkinje cells and few granular cells remaining (H&E). (*B* courtesy of Dr. Bruno Volk.)

In Gaucher's disease there is glucocerebroside storage as a result of a deficiency of glucocerebroside-β-galactosidase. Typical Gaucher cells are found in perivascular spaces of the brain (the gray and white matter). Ultrastructurally, they contain elongated rod-shaped

Figure 6-2. Gaucher's disease. Perivascular collection of elongated "Gaucher cells" is seen in the cerebral white matter.

structures with smooth-walled tubules. Obvious neuronal storage is absent, but neuronal degeneration and neuronophagia may be found in the deep gray matter and brainstem. Only very occasionally are Gaucher bodies seen in some neurons (under the electron microscope).

b. Krabbe's disease (galactocerebrosidosis)

Krabbe's disease is associated with galactocerebroside storage due to deficiency of galactocerebroside-β-galactosidase. This disease is discussed under leukodystrophies as globoid cell leukodystrophy (see section 4.2, B). Fine tubules are demonstrated by electron microscopy in globoid cells and in Schwann cells.

3. Sulfatidoses
a. Metachromatic leukodystrophy (cerebroside sulfatidosis)

Sulfatide storage occurs in this disorder as a result of deficiency of sulfatidase A. The main manifestation of the disease is diffuse "dysmyelination" and metachromatic inclusions in macrophages and glial cells. Electron microscopy shows structures with periodic striation and transverse partitions and fragments of degenerated myelin. This disease is discussed in Section 4.2, A.

b. Austin's disease (mucosulfatidosis or variant O)

In Austin's disease there is accumulation of sulfatide and mucopolysaccharide due to a total deficiency of arylsulfatases A, B, and C. The disease shows the typical features of sulfatidosis and the neuronal and visceral lesions of mucopolysaccharidosis reminiscent of those in Hurler's disease.

c. Fabry's disease (ceramide trihexosidosis)

This sex-linked recessive disorder is due to a deficiency of ceramide trihexoside α-galactosidase, resulting in accumulation of trihexosylceramide (ceramide glucose-galactose-glucose). The disease is characterized by the presence of foamy cells in the reticuloendothelial tissues of the somatic tissues, particularly the liver, spleen, and lymph nodes, and also in the epithelia of the kidney and skin. This pathologic change underlies the development of characteristic cutaneous and mucous angiokeratomas.

The nervous system involvement is for the most part limited to infiltration of the abnormal material in neurons of the autonomic nervous system, including those of the hypothalamus, brainstem, thoracolumbar and sacral spinal cord segments, spinal dorsal root, ganglia, sympathetic ganglia, and myenteric plexuses. The peripheral nerves are also involved, and the result is painful polyneuropathy clinically.

Slowly progressive lipid accumulation in the vessel walls will eventually lead to the late manifestations of the disease which include chronic renal insufficiency, cardiovascular disorders, and cerebrovascular disease (cerebral infarcts).

4. Sphingolipidoses
   a. Niemann-Pick disease (sphingomyelinosis)

Of several genetic and clinical forms of Niemann-Pick disease, the nervous system is primarily involved in the acute infantile form (type A). The basic neuronal storage phenomenon is similar to that seen in Tay-Sachs disease. Lipid storage is also seen in endothelial cells of blood vessels and arachnoid cells of the leptomeninges. The underlying enzymatic deficit is that of sphingomyelinase, and there is accumulation of sphingomyelin. Cholesterol also accumulates. Under the electron microscope, the stored lipid appears as membrane-bound inclusions containing a few loosely arranged membranes (vacuole-like lipid bodies).

The juvenile form (type C), a less common and more slowly evolving form, may involve the nervous system, but its manifestations appear later in the course of the disease.

b. Refsum's disease (heredopathia atactica polyneuritiformis)

There is in Refsum's disease an absence of phytanic oxidase, which oxidizes phytanic acid to pristanic acid, leading to excessive accumulation of phytanic acid (either free or in association with triglycerides and phospholipids). The principal nervous system lesion is a demyelinating neuropathy, which is associated with onion-bulb Schwann cell hyperplasia in the later stages. Considerable axonal loss may also be noted. Clinically, there is a distal sensorimotor polyneuropathy associated with neurogenic deafness and ataxia. Centrally, variable demyelination of the posterior columns, cerebellar peduncles, and rubrospinal and olivocerebellar tracts has been reported. Schwann cells may contain osmophilic lipid (heterogeneous or crystalline) inclusions.

B. Disorders of mucopolysaccharide (glycosaminoglycan) metabolism (Table 6–3)

In these disorders, there is a lipid neuronal storage phenomenon, primarily involving gangliosides, as a secondary disturbance. Swollen neurons contain, ultrastructurally, "zebra bodies" and structures that are intermediary to the membranous cytoplasmic bodies of Tay-Sachs disease. Capillary pericytes may show pronounced vacuolation due to

TABLE 6–3. Disorders of Mucopolysaccharide Metabolism

Type	Name	Defective Enzyme(s)	Storage Material	Systemic Changes
Type I	Hurler's disease (recessive)	L-Iduronidase	Mucopolysaccharide with excessive chondroitin sulfate B and heparan sulfate	Facial and skeletal deformities (gargoylism) (more conspicuous)
Type II	Hunter's disease (sex-linked)	Sulfoiduronate sulfatase	Biochemically identical with Hurler's disease	Similar to Hurler's disease but no corneal opacities
Type III	Sanfilippo's disease (recessive)	Heparan N-sulfatase (type I or A) N-Acetylglucosaminidase (type II or B)	Heparan sulfate	Facial and skeletal deformities (discrete)

excessive accumulation of glycosaminoglycans. Vacuolation is noted in the CNS, in various visceral organs (liver, myocardium, and bone marrow), and in lymphocytes. In Hurler's disease, distention of perivascular spaces in the white matter is seen, with loose fibrous tissue and a few macrophages (Fig. 6–3). The leptomeninges also show fibrous thickening and macrophages.

The CNS involvement is often conspicuous in Sanfilippo's disease but is limited in Hurler's and Hunter's disease.

C. Disorders of carbohydrate metabolism

1. Glycogen storage disease (glycogenoses)

Pompe's disease, McArdle's disease, and Forbes' disease are the principal examples, but they chiefly affect the skeletal muscles. Pompe's disease (or type II glycogenosis) shows an excess storage of type α glycogen in selected groups of neurons, including the spinal anterior horn, some of the brainstem nuclei, the cerebellum, and, to a lesser extent, the cerebral cortex. The involved neurons appear swollen and vacuolated. The glial cells also store glycogen. The disease is caused by acid maltase deficiency.

2. Galactosemia

In this disorder, there is a deficit of galactose-1-phosphate-N-uridyl transferase, resulting in accumulation of galactose-1-phosphate. When the CNS is involved (in some slowly progressive cases), there is no excessive neuronal storage. Neurons are indirectly affected, and the result is neuronal loss and astrocytosis in the cerebral cortex and cerebellum. Pallidonigral degeneration may also be seen.

3. Subacute necrotizing encephalopathy (Leigh's disease) (Fig. 6–4)

This disorder results in a spongy degeneration of neuropil with relative sparing of neurons, capillary hypertrophy and hyperplasia, and, later, astrocytosis, which closely resembles the lesion of Wernicke's encephalopathy (see section 6.2). The lesions are distributed characteristically in the basal ganglia and thalamus, brainstem tegmentum, corpora quadrigemina, and inferior olive. The cerebral white matter may be involved. However, the absence of involvement of the mamillary bodies contrasts sharply with Wernicke's disease. The precise biochemical nature of the disease has not been identified, but a disturbance of the Krebs cycle is suspected.

4. Lafora's disease

This disorder is considered in Chapter 5 (section 5.3).

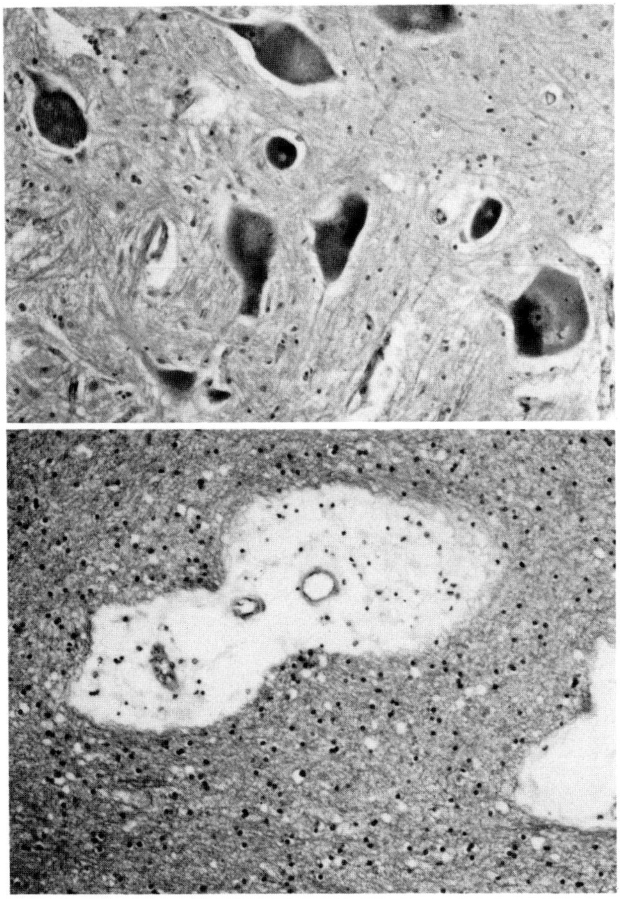

A

B

Figure 6–3. Hurler's disease (gargoylism). *A*, Distended neurons with displaced Nissl bodies (darker areas) in large motor neurons. *B*, Photomicrograph of distended perivascular spaces in low power.

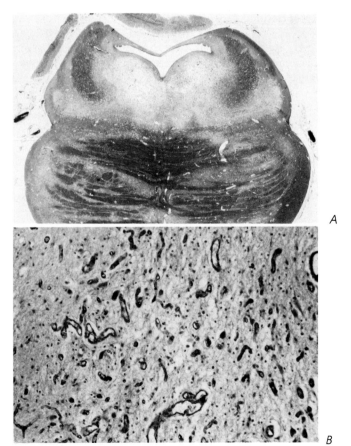

A

B

Figure 6–4. Subacute necrotizing encephalopathy (Leigh's disease). *A*, Bilateral spongy degeneration in tegmentum of pons (Weil). *B*, Capillary proliferation and mild sponginess of neuropil in affected area.

D. Disorders of amino acid metabolism

In most aminoacidopathies, the structural alterations are quite nonspecific and often consist of fatty infiltration of liver and foci of necrosis in liver, kidney, brain, myocardium, and, to a lesser extent, other organs. Thus, the morphologic studies of tissues in patients with aminoacidopathies have not been fundamental in gaining insight into the nature of these disorders, contrary to the findings in most errors in lipid and carbohydrate metabolism. The various disorders are listed in Table 6–4.

E. Disorders of metal metabolism

1. Hepatolenticular degeneration (Wilson's disease)

In this disorder there is increased absorption of copper from the intestinal tract and failure of albumin-bound copper to become converted to ceruloplasmin (copper-globulin complex). The copper-albumin complex is deposited in the tissue and causes tissue damage. The brain and liver are most severely affected. The cerebral change is most obvious in the basal ganglia (the striatum mainly), which shows a brownish to brick-red discoloration. Microscopically, there is spongy degeneration of the involved area, leading to gross cavitation with macrophages. Neurons are reduced in number. There is little evidence of reactive scarring by either neuroglial or collagen fibers. Instead, Alzheimer's type II astrocytes with large, vesicular nuclei and little visible cytoplasm ("naked nuclei") contribute to an increased cellularity. They are also diffusely scattered in the brain. Larger, sometimes multinucleated, Alzheimer's type I astrocytes are rarer and are not present in every case (Fig. 0–10 C and D).

Milder changes may be seen, among others, in the globus pallidus, subthalamic nuclei, and the cerebral cortex, especially in the frontal lobes.

Opalski cells, which are large cells with relatively small nuclei and without processes, are occasionally present in the thalamus, globus pallidus, and substantia nigra but very rarely in the striatum. Their origin is uncertain. They have been variously considered to be degenerating neurons, derivatives of astrocytes, or phagocytes.

Note: Kayser-Fleischer rings are produced by rows of brown pigment granules (containing copper) in Descemet's membrane near the limbus of the cornea.

2. Disorders of iron and calcium metabolism (Fig. 6–5)

The conditions described in this section are not due to inborn errors of metabolism but are discussed for convenience here.

a. The commonest form of "calcification," and for the most part an asymptomatic change, occurs in and around blood vessels of the globus pallidus in middle-aged or elderly persons, without any discernible cause. It is preceded by deposition of colloid hyaline material (matrix or pseudo calcium), which has the histochemical staining characteristics of acid mucopolysaccharides. The deposited minerals are mainly iron and calcium with some mixture of magnesium and aluminum; therefore, this process is more appropriately referred to as mineralization rather than calcification. The mineralization takes the form of small droplets in and about capillaries and mural impregnation of larger arteries. Microscopic pallidal mineralization is found as often as in 30 to 40% of the autopsy population. It is detected clinically in about 1% of persons examined by computed tomography for a variety of reasons. The hippocampus and cerebellar white matter in the vicinity of the dentate nucleus are less often affected.

b. In hypoparathyroidism and pseudohypoparathyroidism, calcification (reported in 40 to 80% of cases) is not limited to the putamen but is seen in more widespread areas, including the putamen, thalamus, caudate and dentate nuclei, and white matter. Extrapyramidal signs and symptoms reported in isolated cases do not appear to have any relationship to the calcification of the basal ganglia.

TABLE 6–4. Disorders of Amino Acid Metabolism

Disorder	Enzyme Deficit	Neuropathology
Phenylketonuria	Absence of phenylalanine hydroxylase	Microcephaly, status spongiosus, and white matter change resembling leukodystrophy
Tyrosinosis	Deficiency of parahydroxy-phenylpyruvic acid oxidation	
Leucinosis (maple syrup urine disease)	Decrease in decarboxylase activity (hydroxybutyric acid in urine)	Spongy white matter degeneration resembling that of spongy degeneration of Bertrand-van Bogaert (see Chapter 4)
Homocystinuria	Deficit in cystathionine synthesis	Foci of necrosis, suspected of being of vascular origin in the brain
Hartnup's disease	Disorder of tryptophan absorption	Pellagra-like cerebral lesion

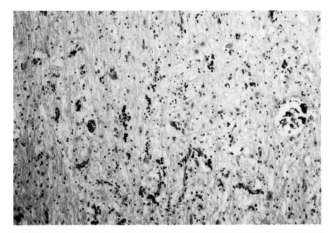

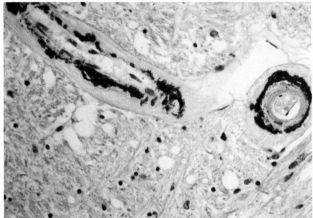

Figure 6–5. Abnormal deposition of iron and calcium. *A,* Droplets of pericapillary mineralization in globus pallidus. *B,* Vascular mural mineralization of globus pallidus.

c. Similarly, extensive calcification may be found in the absence of demonstrable metabolic disorders, and this phenomenon was often in the past referred to as "Fahr's disease" or "idiopathic nonarteriosclerotic cerebral calcification." The term appears to have been applied to many different conditions almost indiscriminately, and the condition had been known for many years before this eponymic designation, and so there is little justification for the continued use of the term "Fahr's disease."

A sporadic form is now recognized as being unassociated with signs and symptoms of basal ganglia involvement. A familial form of idiopathic bilateral calcification of the basal ganglia, on the other hand, tends to show extrapyramidal and cerebellar signs, convulsions, and dementia in the third or fourth decades. The deposited material is reported to be hydroxyapatite, which occurs also in renal calculi, teeth, and bones. The process of idiopathic cerebral calcification is thought to be similar to physiologic calcification elsewhere and is not thought to originate from the blood vessels. The original matrix appears to consist mainly of proteins.

d. It is well known that calcification of the choroid plexus, pineal body, falx cerebri, and adjacent dura (often with ossification) occurs often in older persons without clinical significance. Varieties of intracranial lesions show the tendency to become calcified, including vascular malformations, toxoplasmosis, cytomegalovirus, encephalitis, and phakomatoses, among others. These will not be discussed further here.

F. Disorders of pigment metabolism

1. Porphyria

In the acute intermittent form of porphyria, a dominantly inherited disorder, there is polyneuropathy characterized by the wallerian type of degeneration, with a greater involvement of motor axons than sensory fibers. The CNS may reflect these changes in the form of central chromatolysis of spinal motor neurons. In some of the cases with cerebral signs and symptoms, focal loss of cells in association with ischemic neuronal alteration in the gray matter or of focal myelin pallor in the white matter (or both) is described. Focal ischemia, possibly due to vasospasm, is thought to account for these changes.

The disease is due to deficiency of porphobilinogen deaminase (uroporphyrinogen I synthetase), with accumulation of both δ-aminolevulinic acid and porphobilinogen. The precise mechanism of the peripheral nerve lesion is unknown.

6.2 CHRONIC ALCOHOLISM AND THIAMINE- AND OTHER VITAMIN-DEFICIENCY STATES

A. Nutritional polyneuropathy (Fig. 6–6)

This condition consists of degeneration of peripheral nerves, more intense in the distal segments, which is man-

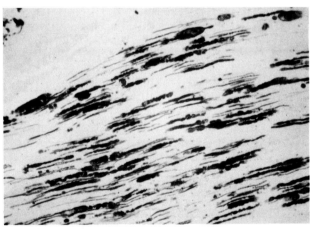

Figure 6–6. Nutritional (alcoholic) polyneuropathy. Frozen section-myelin stain demonstrates multiple focal swelling with eventual disappearance of myelin sheaths, one of the more readily discernible features of this condition. Axonal degeneration is not seen in this section.

ifested clinically as distal sensorimotor neuropathy. A wallerian type of degeneration (and segmental degeneration in some proximal portions) with variable loss of posterior root ganglion cells and axonal reaction of spinal motor neurons is the basic histologic finding.

B.1. Wernicke's encephalopathy (Fig. 6–7)

Characteristic histologic changes are distributed in a characteristic pattern. The basic changes consist of destruction of myelinated fibers with relative preservation of nerve cell bodies and hypertrophy and hyperplasia of capillary and small blood vessels, with or without fresh petechiae, macrophage formation, and astrocytosis at the periphery. The lesions are distributed symmetrically along the ventricular walls of the brainstem, involving the mamillary bodies and other regions of the hypothalamus and the thalami (especially the dorsal and anterior medial nuclei and the pulvinar), the periaqueductal gray matter, and the floor of the fourth ventricle, particularly the dorsal vagal and the vestibular nuclei. Grossly, the affected areas appear somewhat granulated and soft, with varying extent of petechial hemorrhages, which are not invariably present. Occasionally, more extensive hemorrhages occur and the course is rapidly fatal.

The mechanism of and the reason for this particular pattern of the lesions are not known, other than that vitamin B_1 deficiency is the cause of the disease.

B.2. Korsakoff's disease (Fig. 6–8)

This disease is now recognized to be a chronic stage of Wernicke's encephalopathy and is seen in patients who have survived it, presumably because they experienced a relatively less fulminant course. The consistent lesion is atrophy of the mamillary bodies, which show neuronal loss and fibrous astrocytosis but no vascular proliferation. The dorsomedial nucleus of the thalamus is reported to be regularly involved in the same series. Other changes are also reported, but they are less consistent and their relationship remains controversial.

C. Alcoholic cerebral atrophy

The presence of cerebral atrophy in persons with chronic alcoholism as compared with age-matched neurologic controls has been documented in clinical roentgenographic and neuropathologic studies. No data are available in regard to the amount or duration of alcohol abuse which is necessary to cause cerebral atrophy, and degrees of atrophy demonstrable by computed tomography (CT) do not correlate well with functional impairment. Histologic changes ("aging-like cortical neuronal loss") are nonspecific, and variable degrees of reversal of CT-recognized atrophy after abstinence have been reported. Better understanding of the neurobiologic substrates of alcoholism-induced cerebral dysfunction will be necessary before the actual relevance of this form of cerebral atrophy can be assessed.

D. Alcoholic cerebellar degeneration (or atrophy) (Fig. 6–9)

There is loss of Purkinje cells and, to a lesser extent, of granular cells accompanied by astrocytosis. The lesion is largely confined to the superior vermis and the adjacent anterior lobe, which appears grossly shrunken with wider sub-

arachnoid spaces. This particular distribution accounts for the predominantly truncal type of ataxia seen clinically. Gross cerebellar atrophy may be present, however, without clinical cerebellar dysfunction.

E. Marchiafava-Bignami disease

This disease is reported to occur mainly but by no means exclusively among Italians who drink cheap red wine.

The lesion consists of degeneration of the central fibers of the corpus callosum. Demyelination is a consistent feature, and axonal damage is variable. Myelin breakdown products are generally sparse, and astrocytosis is not pronounced. Proliferation and fibrous sclerosis of blood vessels within the lesion are also prominent features. The callosal lesion may be accompanied by degeneration of other symmetric fiber tracts such as the anterior commissure, middle cerebellar peduncles, optic chiasm, and centrum semiovale.

This rare condition is seldom recognized clinically, and its pathogenesis and cause are unknown.

F. Central pontine myelinolysis (Fig. 6–10)

The lesion is situated in the center of the pontine base and is characterized by demyelination, with relative preservation of axons and neural bodies. Additional areas in which similar demyelination is described include the striatum, thalamus, lateral geniculate body, internal and external capsules, and white matter of the cerebellar folia. Although originally described in alcoholics with severe nutritional deficiency, other patients with uremia, electrolyte disturbances, and related disorders are also known to be affected. The cause is unknown but a rapid overcorrection of hyponatremia has recently been recognized to be associated with this condition in many instances. Clinically, a syndrome consisting of progressive upper motor neuron quadriparesis, lower cranial nerve paresis, and preserved mental responsiveness in the setting of severe metabolic derangement is now recognized.

G. Pellagra

Nicotinic acid deficiency is regarded as the etiologic factor, but involvement of multiple factors is considered probable. The main histologic change is central chromatolysis of neurons with inconsistent axonal damage to account for it. More prominently involved are the cerebral cortex (particularly Betz cells), basal ganglia, pontine nuclei, dorsal vagal nuclei, and cuneate nucleus and nucleus gracilis.

Peripheral neuropathy, with demyelination alone when it is mild and axonal degeneration when it is severe, and degeneration of the dorsal and lateral columns of the spinal cord (without the spongy appearance characteristic of vitamin B_{12} deficiency) have also been reported in pellagra. These are likely to be an admixture rather than an integral part of pellagra.

H. Subacute combined degeneration of the spinal cord (Fig. 6–11)

This disorder is seen in pernicious anemia due to vitamin B_{12} deficiency, but many other conditions, including folic acid deficiency and other malabsorptive and malnutritive states, have been listed as a cause of this pathologic state. The main feature is rapid fragmentation of myelinated fibers,

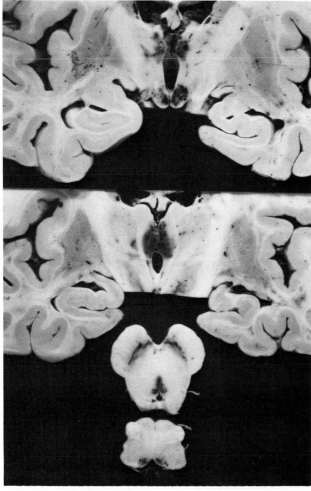

A

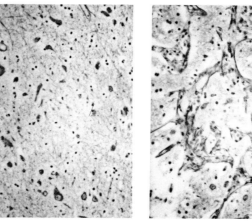

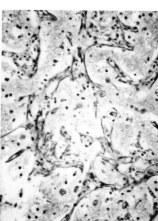

C

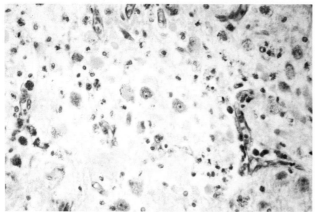

B

Figure 6–7. Wernicke's encephalopathy. *A,* Gross appearance characterized by petechial hemorrhages in typical locations, including mamillary bodies, hypothalamus and thalamus, periaqueductal gray matter, and floor of the fourth ventricle. *B,* Photomicrograph of affected mamillary body, showing breakdown of neuropil, a few macrophages, capillary prominence, and relative preservation of neurons (LFB/PAS/H). *C,* Capillary prominence and proliferation in affected mamillary body (*right*) in contrast to normal control (*left*) (reticulin). (*A* courtesy of Dr. Emmanuel Stadlan.)

with conspicuous absence of glial reactions. Both myelin sheaths and axons are affected, the former being damaged earlier and more severely. This leads to the characteristic spongy change of the white matter, particularly in the dorsal and lateral columns. The change may extend into the brainstem, optic nerves, and cerebrum in a few cases. Fibrous astrocytosis will follow successful treatment. Peripheral nerve lesions consisting of demyelination have been described by some.

6.3 SOMATIC METABOLIC DISEASES AFFECTING THE NERVOUS SYSTEM

A. Hepatic encephalopathy (Fig. 6–12)

There is a diffuse proliferation of Alzheimer's type II astrocytes (with prominent glycogen granules in their vesicular nuclei), particularly in the gray matter. This is more conspicuous in the cerebral cortex, basal ganglia, and cer-

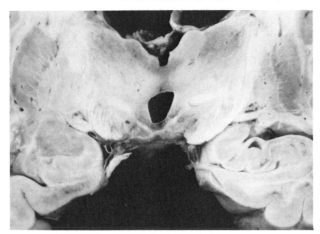

Figure 6-8. Korsakoff's disease. Atrophic mamillary bodies.

ebellar cortex (particularly along the layer of Bergmann's astrocytes).

Less commonly, pseudolaminar necrosis of the cerebral cortex, reminiscent of that caused by diffuse cerebral hypoxia, is seen. In fact, it is possible that at least one of the etiologic factors in this condition is hypoxia. Rarely, necrosis and microcavitation of the lenticular nuclei are present, but less conspicuously than is seen in Wilson's disease.

Hepatic cirrhosis is found to be associated with an increased incidence of intracerebral hemorrhage, presumably related to a coagulation abnormality due to vitamin K deficiency.

B. Uremia

Peripheral neuropathy, more pronounced distally and characterized by segmental demyelination and remyelination, is the main feature. Loss of all populations of nerve fibers (myelinated and unmyelinated), which is greatest distally, is also observed.

Specific alterations underlying clinical uremic encephalopathy have not been clearly defined and are debatable.

Some patients who receive long-term hemodialysis acquire a clinical syndrome, "progressive dialysis encephalop-

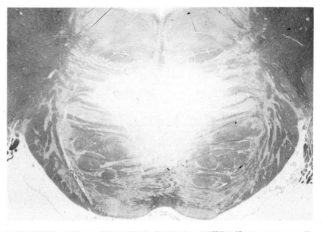

A

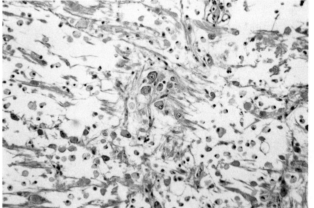

B

Figure 6-10. Central pontine myelinolysis. A, Moderate-sized area of demyelination in central portion of pontine base (LFB/PAS/H). B, Photomicrograph of more severely affected central portion of lesion with complete demyelination and some axonal loss and phagocytosis by macrophages but with preserved neurons in the midst of it (H&E).

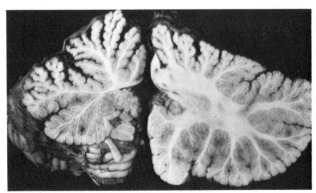

Figure 6-9. Alcoholic cerebellar degeneration (atrophy). Atrophy of folia of dorsal vermis and adjacent anterior lobe is evidenced by wide separation of sulci. (Courtesy of Kings County Hospital, Brooklyn, New York.)

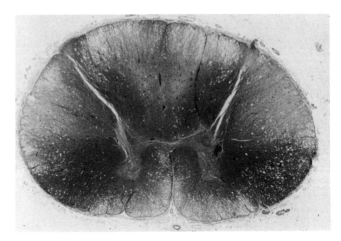

Figure 6-11. Subacute combined degeneration of spinal cord. Photomacrograph of thoracic cord segment shows spongy degeneration of white matter as demonstrable by myelin stain (Weil).

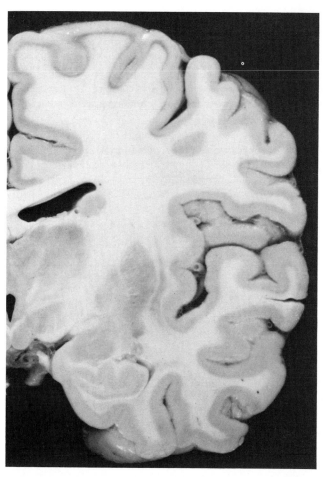

Figure 6–12. Hepatic encephalopathy. Pseudolaminar cortical necrosis (and sclerosis) predominantly in dorsal arterial border zone is seen in a patient with repeated episodes of hepatic coma.

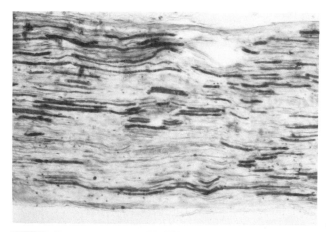

A

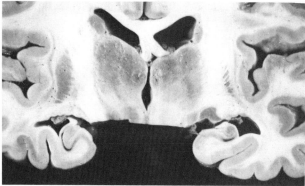

B

Figure 6–13. Diabetes mellitus. *A,* Diabetic neuropathy as evidenced by pronounced reduction of myelinated fibers in peripheral nerve (Weil). *B,* Hypoglycemic encephalopathy with hippocampal sclerosis (bilateral) in a patient who remained in coma for 8 months after hypoglycemic shock.

athy.'' Sudden onset of hesitant, nonfluent speech is usually the earliest sign. This is followed by difficulty in gait, myoclonus, dementia, and seizures, among other changes, in association with a markedly abnormal electroencephalogram. A rapidly fatal outcome may be seen if hemodialysis is continued. Neuropathologic changes are mild and nonspecific. Aluminum toxicity due to a high concentration of aluminum in the dialysate is generally regarded as the pathogenetic mechanism.

C. Diabetes mellitus (Fig. 6–13)

Peripheral polyneuropathy with predominant distal (''stocking and glove'') sensory symptoms occurs most commonly in the fifth or sixth decade in mild, chronic cases. An increased frequency of segmental demyelination and remyelination is seen in the nerves of untreated patients who are free of symptoms of neuropathy. In symptomatic cases, a mixture of abnormal fibers with segmental demyelination and remyelination and fibers undergoing axonal degeneration is seen. The axonal degeneration predominates in longstanding treated neuropathic cases. The precise pathogenetic mechanism has not yet been clarified, but the role of ischemia and metabolic damage to Schwann cells received

the greatest interest in the past. More recently, primary atrophic and then degenerative changes of axons has also been offered as a likely mechanism.

CNS lesions are parenchymal consequences of accelerated atherosclerosis, which often involves, in addition to large arteries at the base of the brain, smaller arterial branches that are usually spared in the absence of diabetes. No specific diabetic vascular disease is known.

In *hypoglycemic encephalopathy,* pathologic changes are seen that are closely similar to those of diffuse hypoxia, except for a greater predilection for the hippocampus and a lesser involvement of Purkinje cells of the cerebellar cortex. *Note:* Glucose is probably the only substrate that the brain can use for its oxidative process, but the extent of cortical injury does not correlate accurately with the circulating glucose concentration. In contrast to hypoxia, cerebral oxygen tension is not reduced and lactic acid content is not increased. Energy-rich phosphate bonds such as ATP decrease in the brain tissue, and glucose and glycogen stores are depleted. The precise biochemical mechanism of hypoglycemic encephalopathy has not been elucidated.

Rough clinical correlates of hypoglycemia are as follows:

Blood glucose <30 mg/dl—drowsiness, confusion, and delirium
<20 mg/dl—coma after seizures
lower concentrations—neuronal loss

D. Somatic malignancies (Fig. 6–14)

Indirect or remote effects of a malignant growth elsewhere in the body on the nervous system are discussed here,
excluding those due to direct or metastatic invasion. Several
forms are recognized, but they sometimes occur together.
These are known as paraneoplastic syndromes.

1. Cerebellar cortical degeneration, subacute or acute

There is widespread degeneration and loss of Purkinje
cells, with lesser involvement of granular cells. The spinocerebellar and other spinal tracts may also be affected. Meningeal and perivascular infiltration is infrequently reported
in this condition.

The association between this condition and ovarian and
lung carcinomas is particularly high. Lymphomas are also
known to be associated with this condition.

2. Peripheral neuropathy

This occurs primarily as sensory neuropathy, with degeneration and loss of neurons of the posterior ganglion
associated with wallerian degeneration of fibers in the peripheral nerves, posterior roots, and posterior columns. Inflammatory reaction is occasionally observed. Bronchogenic
carcinoma is the most frequent carcinoma associated with
this condition.

3. Necrotizing myelopathy; subacute necrotic myelopathy

This change is an infrequent but relatively acute complication of a malignant tumor, usually a bronchogenic carcinoma. The spinal cord, usually the thoracic segment, shows
a fairly symmetric necrosis of myelin sheaths and axons with
a mild inflammatory reaction, over several segments (radiation necrosis should be excluded). A similar, if not identical,
condition occurs sometimes in the absence of a somatic malignancy, often after a mild febrile disease of presumed viral
origin. A close relationship of this condition to postinfectious, perivenous encephalomyelopathy (see section 4.1) is
suspected.

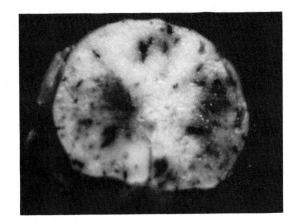

A

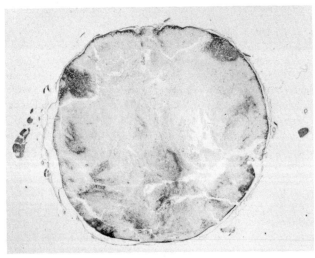

B

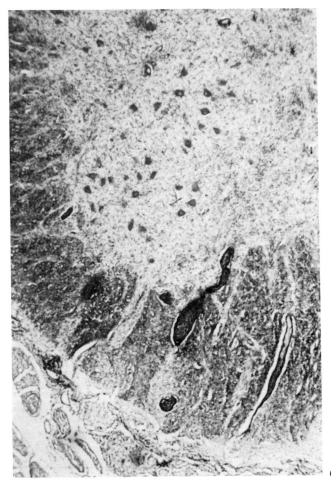

C

Figure 6–14. Remote effects of somatic malignancy on nervous
system. *A* and *B,* Necrotizing myelopathy. Gross cross sections (*A*)
and photomicrograph (LFB/CV) (*B*) of affected thoracic segments
of thoracic cord. *C,* Low-power photomicrograph of lumbar anterior horn with perivascular lymphocytic cuffing, neuronophagia,
and microglial nodules.

4. Encephalomyeloradiculitis

This condition is characterized by changes reminiscent of a viral infection and consisting of neuronal destruction, microglial proliferation, either diffuse or focal (forming "glial nodules"), and perivascular lymphocytic infiltration associated with reactive astrocytosis of the affected areas. Depending on the areas of preferential involvement, the following subtypes are recognized, although the lesions are often distributed in more than one of these sites.

    a. Limbic encephalitis, affecting mainly the hippocampus, amygdaloid nucleus, and cingulate and orbital cortex

    b. Bulbar or brainstem encephalitis, involving mainly the lower brainstem

    c. Myelitis, damaging primarily anterior horn cells at varying levels, but also affecting other cell groups and tracts in some instances

    d. Ganglio-radiculo-neuritis, affecting the posterior ganglia with wallerian degeneration in the peripheral nerves, posterior roots, and columns

        The disease process is generally subacute and may burn out after several months, but it may continue longer.

5. Carcinomatous myopathy

This disorder may show the typical findings of polymyositis in some cases; in others, atrophy of type II muscle fibers occurs without inflammatory reaction. Progressive proximal muscle weakness is the clinical feature. Carcinomas of the lung, breast, stomach, or ovary are usually associated with this myopathy.

6. Abnormal coagulability in somatic malignancy is also an important factor in secondary central nervous system involvement. This is usually mediated through cerebral embolism from nonbacterial thrombotic endocarditis, but less frequently it is due to local cerebral vascular thrombosis. Tumor embolism is also a rare complication. These conditions have already been discussed in Chapter 1.

E. Amyloidosis (Fig. 6–15)

Amyloid deposition in peripheral nerves occurs frequently in the hereditary systemic amyloidosis and less often in other forms. Deposits are seen mainly in the endoneurium and to a lesser extent in the interfascicular epineurium, and they are often related to blood vessels, where amyloid material is present both in the media and in the adventitia. Both wallerian degeneration (with predominant but not exclusive involvement of small myelinated and unmyelinated fibers) and segmental demyelination have been described. Clinically, a painful distal symmetric sensory neuropathy with prominent autonomic features is commonly seen.

The pathogenesis of these lesions has not been clearly elucidated. An ischemic or a mechanical compressive basis is open to doubt, and some authors believe that nerve fiber degeneration is independent of amyloid deposition. The clinical picture is that of a sensorimotor neuropathy of insidious onset and slow progression.

F. Reye's syndrome

In this condition, children, after upper respiratory tract infection (approximately 90%, often by influenza virus), gas-

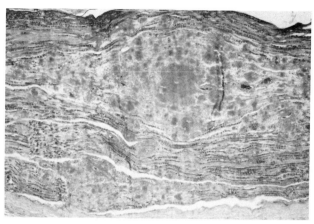

Figure 6–15. Primary amyloidosis with peripheral nerve infiltration. Large amount of amorphous amyloid material apparently originating from blood vessels is seen between nerve bundles, associated with reduced numbers of myelinated fibers (LFB/PAS/H).

trointestinal illness, or varicella, suddenly experience a toxic encephalopathic syndrome including vomiting, convulsions, and coma along with signs of hepatic failure (very high blood ammonia levels, high serum glutamic-oxalacetic transaminase, mild hypoglycemia). Delirium may also be seen. The liver and other viscera are fatty. The brain at autopsy shows cerebral edema. The conditions of "respirator brain" (see section 1.2) usually exist and this makes research for the initial and essential alteration(s) difficult with autopsy material. Cerebral edema is said to be primarily cytotoxic, associated with swollen, myelin blebs and intact cerebral microvasculature. Mitochondrial injury in all tissue, including the brain, is considered to be the primary morphologic change, but its origin is obscure.

6.4 ANOXIC POISONS

A. Anesthetics and hypnotics

CNS changes found in cases of overdosage of these agents are secondary to the respiratory and cardiac failure induced by them; therefore, the pattern of CNS damage is essentially similar to that of hypoxia.

B. Carbon monoxide poisoning (Fig. 6–16)

In cases in which death occurs immediately after acute intoxication, there is general visceral pink discoloration (due to carboxyhemoglobin), but no other morphologic changes are present.

Several, though not mutually exclusive, patterns of tissue damage are found in patients who survive for some time.

Factors determining which type of CNS lesions any given patient will experience are not clearly understood at present.

1. Cerebral cortical (pseudolaminar type) and pallidal necrosis essentially similar to that seen in hypoxia or ischemia.

2. Widespread petechiae and thrombosis leading to focal infarcts predominantly involving the white matter. These changes are attributed to anoxic damage to capillary vessels. The basal ganglia, especially the globus pallidus, may show similar changes.

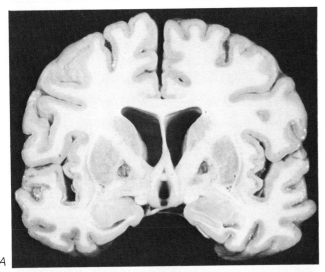

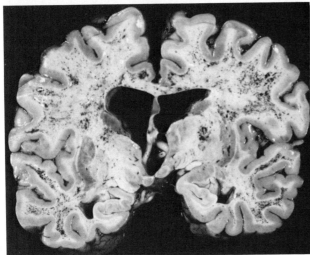

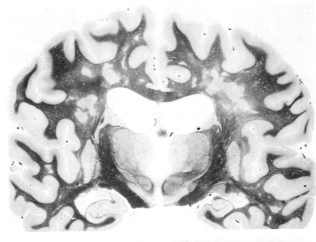

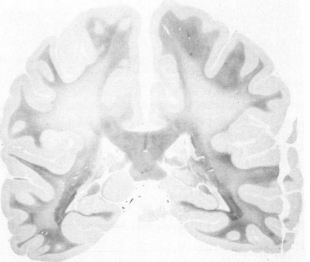

Figure 6–16. Carbon monoxide poisoning. *A,* Pseudolaminar cortical and cystic globus pallidus necrosis 16 days after a suicide attempt by means of carbon monoxide. *B* and *C,* Gross (*B*) and celloidin sections (LFB/CV) (*C*) of cerebral hemispheres with multiple petechiae and infarcts, predominantly in white matter. *D,* Delayed diffuse leukoencephalopathy of Grinker (LFB/CV).

3. Leukoencephalopathy (of Grinker), which consists of patchy or confluent areas of demyelination with preservation of axons. The change may advance to scattered spongy and necrotic lesions accompanied by phagocytosis by macrophages. This type of lesion is often associated with a relapsing clinical course after an initial recovery from the acute phase. Experimental studies suggest that the size of the white matter lesion correlates with the degree of metabolic acidosis and systemic hypotension sustained during the original exposure to carbon monoxide but not with the extent of hypoxia per se.

6.5 OTHER POISONS

A. Lead poisoning (Fig. 6–17)

The childhood disorder takes the form of acute encephalopathy characterized histologically by diffuse cerebral edema. There is seepage of plasma fluid into the white matter with little if any morphologic changes in the blood vessels. In the gray matter, particularly in the cerebral cortex and the molecular layer of the cerebellar folia, droplets with the same staining characteristics as plasma are conspicuous about capillaries, which appear prominent and have probably undergone proliferation. Subpial accumulation of plasma fluid is also characteristic. The neuronal degeneration and Purkinje cell loss (often attended by glial shrubs) that are often found are probably related to anoxia incident to seizures.

The adult form manifests itself as a chronic neuropathy with predominant motor paralysis. Segmental demyelination of the affected nerve fibers is the anatomic substrate.

B. Organic mercury poisoning

Industrial contamination by methyl mercury has resulted in large-scale poisoning of the populace (through ingestion of fish caught in the poisoned bay) in Japan (Min-

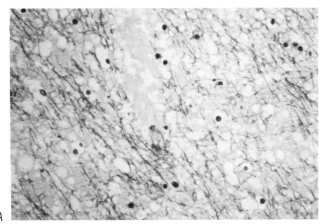

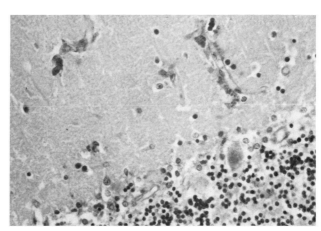

Figure 6–17. Acute lead encephalopathy. *A*, Photomicrograph of edematous cerebral white matter (LFB/PAS/H). *B*, Droplets of plasma exudate along prominent capillaries in molecular layer of cerebellar cortex.

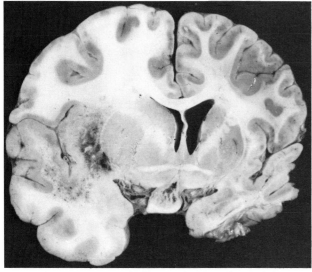

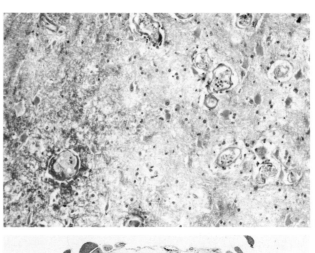

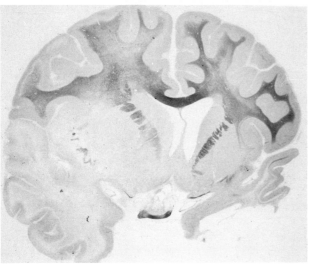

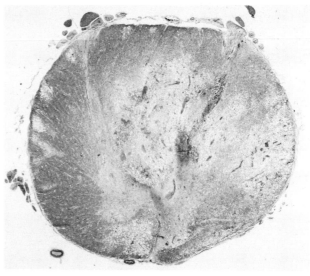

eration in left insular region and extensive white matter edema (right temporal lobe had been partially resected). *C*, Vascular and parenchymal necrosis of fibrinoid type associated with proliferation of dilated blood vessel and astrocytosis. *D*, Radiation myelopathy with asymmetrically placed vascular lesions (dark appearing) and parenchymal lesions (spongy areas).

Figure 6–18. Radiation necrosis of CNS. *A* and *B*, Gross (*A*) and celloidin sections (LFB/CV) (*B*) of cerebral hemispheres of child irradiated for medulloblastoma. Note gray-yellowish area of degen-

181

amata disease), with devastating clinical consequences. There is diffuse neuronal degeneration and loss of the granular layer of the cerebellum and patchy loss of neurons in the cerebral cortex which is most pronounced in the calcarine cortex. Degenerative changes may also occur in the peripheral nerves, posterior nerve roots, and posterior columns of the spinal cord.

6.6 NERVOUS SYSTEM DAMAGE BY PHYSICAL AGENTS: RADIATION NECROSIS OF THE CNS (FIG. 6–18)

Coagulative necrosis of the affected tissue associated with fibrinoid necrosis of local blood vessels is the principal lesion, which favors the white matter over the gray and is bordered by a wide zone of edema and astrocytosis. Petechial hemorrhages occur not infrequently from the involved vessels. Foci of microscopic calcification are occasionally seen.

The pathogenesis of this necrosis, which characteristically develops insidiously and progressively after a period of latency (usually 6 months or more) after a course of radiation therapy, has not been clearly established. Because it occurs within a standard "safe" dosage in some patients, individual susceptibility must be involved. Primary vascular damage has been favored as the primary etiologic factor, but other evidence suggests that the direct effects of radiation in the neuronal elements are of primary importance. Wide areas of demyelination (and subsequent axonal damage) without vascular necrosis are known to occur.

7. *Neoplastic and Related Lesions*

7.0 GENERAL DISCUSSION

In this series, neoplasms of the central and peripheral nervous systems and adjacent structures which are of clinical neurologic importance are considered. Some nonneoplastic mass lesions ("tumors" and "cysts") are also discussed, for convenience. The classification adopted here and outlined below corresponds, with minor variations, to those that are popular with most modern pathologists and clinicians. The first two categories (7.1 and 7.2) correspond to what is generally known as "glioma."

It must be realized that a certain number of tumors of the brain (and the spinal cord) are currently unclassifiable or at least create considerable disagreement among recognized authorities. These tend to occur in younger age groups and to be highly malignant.

7.1 Tumors of neuroglial cells	A. Astrocytoma B. Oligodendroglioma C. Ependymoma D. Papilloma of choroid plexus E. Colloid cyst of the third ventricle
7.2 Tumors of primitive bipotential precursors and nerve cells	A. Medulloblastoma B. Ganglioneuroma and ganglioglioma C. Other, rare, primitive central neuroectodermal tumors D. Tumors of pineal parenchyma
7.3 Nerve sheath tumors	A. Schwannoma B. Neurofibroma C. Malignancy in nerve sheath tumors
7.4 Tumors of mesenchymal tissue	A. Meningioma B. Xanthomatous tumors C. (Capillary) hemangioblastoma D. Sarcomas (primary and secondary)
7.5 Tumors of the lymphoreticular system and leukemia	
7.6 Tumors of maldevelopmental origin	A. Primary germ cell tumor B. Dermoid and epidermoid C. Lipoma D. Neuroepithelial ectopic tumors and hamartoma, craniopharyngioma, and others
7.7 Phakomatoses	A. Tuberous sclerosis B. Multiple neurofibromatosis C. Sturge-Weber disease D. Von Hippel-Lindau disease E. Neurocutaneous melanoma and primary meningeal melanoma
7.8 Tumors of adjacent structures compromising the CNS	A. Pituitary adenoma B. Paraganglioma C. Chordoma D. Other bone tumors of skull and spine
7.9 Metastatic neoplasms	

The relative frequencies of major lesions are shown in tabular form below. Because of their different clinical manifestations, they are considered in two topographic forms: A, intracranial tumors, and B, spinal tumors.

A. Intracranial tumors

The crude incidence rate of brain tumors in the United States is estimated to be 4.5 persons per 100,000 population. Brain tumors are found in approximately 2% of autopsy examinations and most clinical series. They account for 1% of admissions. The relative frequency of different kinds of primary brain tumors is fairly constant, within certain ranges, in all large series. The figures given here should be considered only as rough measures of their relative incidence.

Note: The term "brain tumors" encompasses neoplasms and related mass lesions of the brain parenchyma and those arising from the meninges. Also conventionally included are such tumors as pituitary adenomas and chordomas, which arise from structures adjacent to the brain and indirectly affect the brain tissue. In this regard, the term "brain tumors" also implies tumors that affect the brain, either primarily or secondarily, but do not arise in the brain. The term "intracranial" may be anatomically more correct for such tumors and is often used interchangeably with brain tumors. Here again, the tumor might arise in the bone or adjacent soft tissue and project into the intracranial space. Similar considerations apply to "spinal tumors."

There is a topographic difference between brain tumors of adults and those of children which is in part determined by the types of tumors encountered. In adults, roughly 70% of brain tumors are located in the supratentorial compartment, whereas in children, 70% are infratentorial.

1. Primary neoplasms (see chart below)

2. Secondary neoplasms

Metastatic tumors (to CNS)—15 to 30% of all intracranial tumors in pathologic series. There is considerable variability in reported incidence of metastatic CNS tumors, depending on sources—surgical versus autopsy, general hospital versus specialty clinic, and so on. They are rare in childhood.

B. Spinal tumors

Included under spinal tumors are neoplasms and related mass lesions of the spinal cord parenchyma and its coverings. The term does not apply to tumors of the spinal column (vertebrae), although some of these become our concern if the cord parenchyma is secondarily affected.

Primary neoplasms (see chart on next page)

Primary Intracranial Tumors

Found in All Ages			Found in Children (less than 15 years old)	
Glioma 45 to 50%	Malignant astrocytoma—50 to 60% (predominantly cerebral)		Astrocytoma—>50% Cerebellar—30% Brainstem—10%	Glioma >75%
	Benign astrocytoma—25 to 30%			
	Oligodendroglioma	5%	Oligodendroglioma <1 to 2%	
	Ependymoma	5%	Ependymoma 8%	
	Medulloblastoma	6%	Medulloblastoma 20 to 25%	
Schwannoma		6%		
Meningioma		15%		
Hemangioblastoma		1 to 2%		
Lymphoma		<1%		
Sarcoma		1 to 2%	Schwannoma, meningioma, hemangioblastoma, sarcoma Rare	
Germ cell tumor		1 to 2%	Germ cell tumor 2 to 4%	
Dermoid, epidermoid		<1%	Dermoid, epidermoid 1 to 2%	
Craniopharyngioma		3%	Craniopharyngioma 5 to 10%	
Pituitary adenoma		5%	Pituitary adenoma Rare	
Others			Others	

100%

15 to 20% of all intracranial tumors occur in childhood. CNS tumors are the second commonest form of cancer—second only to leukemia—in children under the age of 15.

Primary Spinal Tumors

Found in All Ages				Found in Children (less than 15 years old)	
Glioma 20 to 25%	Astrocytoma	30%		Glioma 20% (15 to 30%)	
	Oligodendro-glioma	3%			
	Ependymoma	65%			
Schwannoma		30%		Schwannoma	10%
				Meningioma	3 to 5%
Meningioma		25%		Congenital tumors	20 to 40%
				Sarcoma (including extension from spinal metastasis)	15 to 25%
Others					

These are 1/10 as frequent as intracranial tumors. Roughly 70% are extramedullary and 30% are intramedullary.

Spinal tumors are rare (constituting 5 to 10% of intracranial tumors). Wide disagreement exists as to the true incidence of these lesions in infancy and childhood, primarily because of the lack of uniformity in the reported studies.

Intramedullary types are mainly gliomas. Vascular malformations also present as clinical problems in this age group.

An *intradural-extramedullary* type is infrequent (10 to 15%) and is made up of schwannomas and meningiomas.

An *extradural-intradural* type is the largest group and includes teratoma, dermoid, and lipoma, often associated with local bony abnormalities. The extradural type, roughly one-fourth of spinal tumors, is composed largely of sarcomas arising from the vertebrae.

7.1 TUMORS OF NEUROGLIAL CELLS (GLIOMAS)

Corresponding to three types of glial cells are three major types of gliomas: astrocytoma, oligodendroglioma, and ependymoma. Although they often occur in relatively "pure" forms, some degree of mixture is probably the rule. The term "mixed glioma" may be appropriate when there is a high degree of mixture, either as separate areas of different cell types (compact type—more frequent) or as equal mixtures of different cells (diffuse type—less frequent). The incidence of these types is probably less than 5% of all gliomas.

A. Astrocytomas

This type of glioma is composed of neoplastically transformed astrocytes, which vary in degree of histologic resemblance to normal astrocytes; some can be readily identified as astrocytes (well differentiated or benign), and others show a great deal of anaplasia (undifferentiated or malignant), in which case identification of individual cells with respect to astrocytic derivation is only presumptive. The transition from one end of the spectrum to the other is gradual.

Kernohan and Sayre simplified previously complicated nomenclatures of astrocytic neoplasms by dividing them into four numerical grades on a benignancy-malignancy scale, with the intent of gaining a better tool for prognostication from biopsy specimens. The system is shown in Table 1.

It must be realized that in this classification an attempt is being made to separate a biologic continuum into somewhat arbitrary classes and that the scale itself lacks morphometric precision. As is readily apparent from the imprecise qualifying adverbs or adjectives used for quantitation, other, equally arbitrary, systems of grading of three or four stages—for example, benign through malignant or differentiated through undifferentiated (or anaplastic)—could be used instead of the grade 1 through 4 scale. The scale as displayed contains possible internal contradictions between different parameters. For instance, degrees of cellularity and anaplasia do not necessarily go hand in hand. Also, in certain areas of an astrocytoma, the cellularity may appear to be reduced from what is expected for that anatomic region.

The designations "benign" and "malignant" are used here in the histologic sense (i.e., differentiated or anaplastic) by convention and for brevity and do not necessarily reflect the biologic behavior patterns of the neoplasms, which must also take into account invasiveness, size, location, and so on. Compounding the clinical problem, many astrocytic tumors contain areas of different degrees of anaplasia, and there is no assurance that what one sees in a biopsy specimen is representative of the whole tumor. But the histologic features do serve as a guide, an informed estimate of malignant potential. In practice, a given tumor is often assigned to a category by a more or less impressionistic (although experienced) appraisal.

Astrocytomas of grades 3 and 4 correspond to the age-honored term "glioblastoma multiforme." The term was coined to represent a glioma that is presumed to be derived from and composed of primitive embryonal glial cells. Even those who are reluctant to equate glioblastomas with high-grade astrocytomas describe the former as being "now widely accepted as an extreme manifestation of anaplasia and dedifferentiation on the part of mature glial tumor cells, mostly astrocytic" (Rubinstein).

It is quite possible that, in smaller numbers of cases, the picture of glioblastoma multiforme arises from anaplasia of oligodendroglial or, more rarely, ependymal cells, and thus that some of the glioblastomas are possibly examples of anaplastic oligodendroglioma or ependymoma. Placing glioblastomas among astrocytomas is a matter of practical convenience, for this type of transformation appears to be rather rare.

Examination of autopsy cases makes it quite reasonable to assume that most, if not all, malignant (anaplastic) forms of astrocytomas have arisen within more benign (well differentiated, mature) tumors, with all shades of transition being noted in a given tumor. Generally, the central portions of the tumor show a higher grade of anaplasia and the peripheral portions show a better differentiation.

Some authors favor dividing glioblastomas into two categories: (1) anaplastic astrocytomas or secondary glioblastomas, those demonstrably derived from the preexisting (benign) astrocytomas; and (2) primary glioblastomas, with absence of any definitive evidence of the above type or a form of astrocytoma with evident anaplastic features de novo.

Also to be discussed here is a "malignant astrocytoma" (in apparent contrast to an "anaplastic" one), which is said to be a form of astrocytoma which shows evident

Table 1. Classification of Astrocytomas

Histologic Features	Grades of Malignancy			
	1	2	3	4
Constituent cells				
Cellularity	Normal to slightly increased	As in grade 1	Increased (by 50% or more)	Markedly increased (up to three times as many cells)
Degree and frequency of anaplasia	None to early in a small number of cells	Early in roughly half of cells	Moderate in roughly half of cells	Pronounced in most cells
Mitotic figures	None	None	One in every high-power field on average	Numerous—four to five per high-power field on average
Giant cells	None	None	Occasional	Frequent
Necrosis	None	None	Frequent	Frequent
Blood vessels				
Numbers	Normal or near normal	As in grade 1	Increased	Markedly increased
Endothelial and adventitial proliferation	None	Minimal	Quite prominent	Markedly increased

anaplastic features de novo but which, histologically, falls short of the classic picture of glioblastoma multiforme and shows evident astrocytic lineage. This form is equated with grade 3 astrocytoma. This distinction is somewhat contrived and confusing, for these two terms, anaplastic and malignant, are used interchangeably on a histologic level.

After all this, some authors readily concede that most examples are probably derived by anaplasia from a preexisting astrocytoma of relatively restricted size which has undergone rapid progression of anaplastic changes spreading throughout the entire neoplastic area. Despite its theoretic importance in understanding CNS neoplasia, the above scheme is of limited practical value. In fact, glioblastomas that are totally devoid of recognizable astrocytic components cannot be conclusively separated from sarcomas (see section 7.4, D, 5).

Malignant astrocytomas are not always larger than their benign counterparts. Rarely, at autopsy, relatively small astrocytomas composed largely of anaplastic cells are also encountered.

It is not an uncommon experience to see previously benign astrocytomas, as diagnosed by biopsy, turn up some time later—either at second operation or at autopsy—as essentially malignant astrocytomas. This may be regarded as temporal or longitudinal evidence of transformation from benign to malignant, as opposed to the topographic, cross-sectional, or static manifestation discussed above. However, sampling bias must also be taken into account as an explanation, at least in some of these cases, before one accepts the possibility of malignant transformation.

With respect to general histologic features, in better-differentiated astrocytomas the following subtypes of component cells are commonly recognized:

Fibrillary. Elongated cells with little visible cytoplasm and long glial fibers. This is the predominant cell type. When these fibers form parallel rows or trabeculae, the term "piloid" or "pilocytic" ("hairlike") is applied.

Protoplasmic. Stellate cells with delicate processes that have few or no stainable neuroglial fibrils, forming a fine cobweb matrix

Gemistocytic. Plump cells with abundant eosinophilic cytoplasm, one or more eccentric nuclei, and short glial fibers (from the German word "gemästet," meaning bloated or swollen)

It must again be stressed that these descriptive distinctions are relative. Also, although one type of cell may predominate over the others, astrocytomas are rarely pure in their cytologic component cells. Finally, as stated above, there is a continuum of transition from mature, benign types to anaplastic forms within a given tumor and also between different individual cases.

In more malignant (i.e., anaplastic) forms (glioblastoma multiforme), the bulk of the tumor consists of (1) small, round, (2) spindle or fusiform, or (3) giant, pleomorphic cells, alone or in varying combinations. There is a greater departure from a recognizably astrocytic appearance as anaplasia progresses.

Commonly, bizarre multinucleated giant cells are considered a symbol or embodiment of malignant growth potentials of astrocytomas. More recent cytokinetic investigations of dying human patients by means of a tritiated-thimidine autoradiography technique indicate that these cells, and even gemistocytic cells, are more like dead wood and that active cellular multiplication is carried out by more innocuous-looking smaller cells.

Note: The term "astroblastoma" was coined originally to describe tumors that are presumably composed of developing astrocytes, or "astroblasts." The term refers to the histologic feature of a perivascular arrangement of astrocytic cells with thick processes radiating toward a central blood vessel. This feature, however, is seen both in relatively benign and in malignant astrocytomas, rarely in pure or totally dominant forms. The need to create a self-standing entity bearing this name is questionable at best.

It is feasible and practicable to separate astrocytomas into fairly well defined clinicopathologic entities in which a particular localization in the brain is generally associated with a prevalent age incidence, a readily recognizable microscopic feature, and a fairly predictable biologic behavior. Therefore, astrocytomas will be discussed under the following topographic categories:

1. Cerebral
2. Third ventricle and optic
3. Brainstem
4. Cerebellar
5. Spinal

1. Cerebral astrocytomas

Although, for contrast, benign and malignant types will be described separately, it must be remembered that all degrees of transition are seen in reality (Fig. 7–1 to Fig. 7–10).

a. Benign varieties

These types tend to occur in young age groups. They can be found in every portion of the cerebrum, except for relative sparing of the occipital lobe. They produce an ill-defined, infiltrating growth that obscures the normal structural boundaries and has no obvious demarcation from the adjacent tissue. Preexisting normal neurons or myelinated axons are often easily demonstrable among tumor cells.

The consistency of these tumors depends on the density of fibrillary processes of astrocytes; some are firm (when predominantly fibrillary) and others are soft and gelatinous (when predominantly protoplastic). Calcification occurs in roughly 15% of cases; this feature is helpful in diagnosis because it is rare in reactive gliosis.

Some of the special secondary features are (1) subpial and subependymal tumor cell aggregates, (2) perivascular accumulations, (3) perineuronal accumulations, (4) more distant infiltration along major nerve fiber tracts, and (5) occasional invasion of the subarachnoid space, despite their cytologic benignancy.

Note: Rare examples of diffuse leptomeningeal astrocytoma with no apparent primary parenchymal focus have been reported and are thought to take origin in ectopic glial nodules in the leptomeninges. However, the presence of an associ-

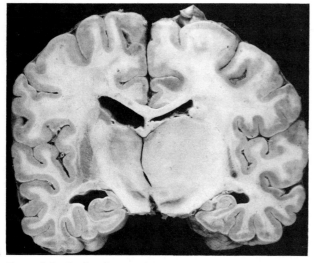

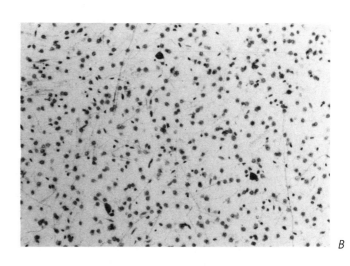

Figure 7–1. Benign (low-grade) astrocytoma of the right thalamus in an adult. *A*, Gross appearance of the involved right thalamus and caudate nucleus, which are enlarged diffusely and are indistinct. *B*, Photomicrograph of tumor cells and local neurons (LFB/CV).

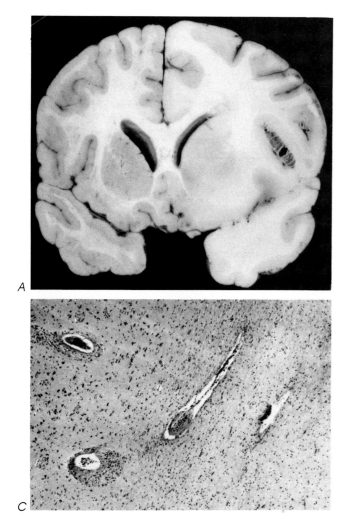

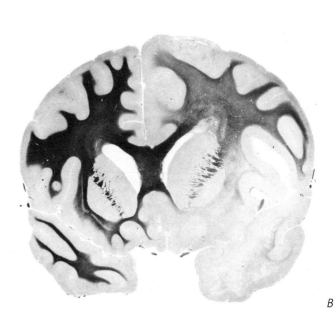

Figure 7–2. Benign (low-grade) astrocytoma of the right frontal and temporal lobes in an adult. *A*, Gross appearance of diffuse infiltration. *B*, Pattern of involvement as demonstrated by LFB/CV stain, which shows myelin pallor of infiltrated areas. *C*, Low-power photomicrograph of corticomedullary junction, showing concentration of fibrous astrocytes around blood vessels.

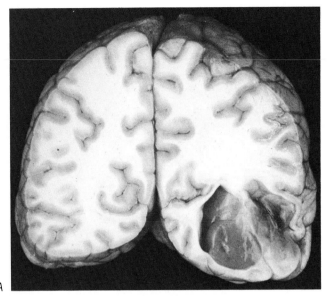

A

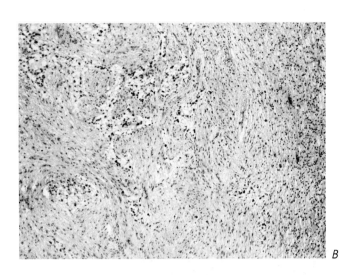

B

Figure 7–3. Benign circumscribed and cystic astrocytoma of right temporal lobe in teenage girl (so-called cerebellar type). *A,* Gross appearance. Cystic space on left side of tumor mass is the occip- ital horn of the lateral ventricle; and cyst on right is produced by tumor. *B,* Low-power photomicrograph of tumor shows fibrillar area.

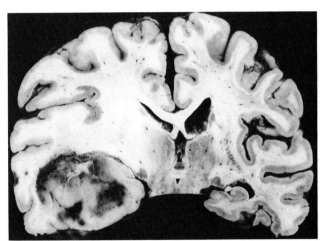

A

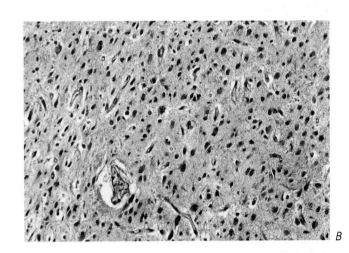

B

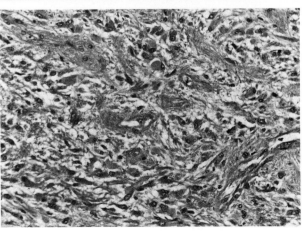

C

Figure 7–4. Astrocytoma of left temporal lobe with intermediate grade of malignancy (grade 2 to 3) in an adult. *A,* Grossly more circumscribed tumor with areas of necrosis and hemorrhage. Note edematous swelling of adjacent white matter. *B* and *C,* Variable histologic features within tumor (H&E).

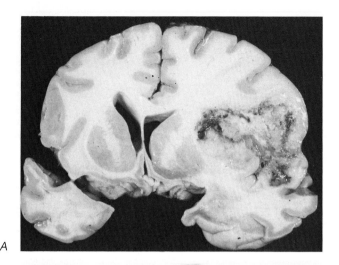

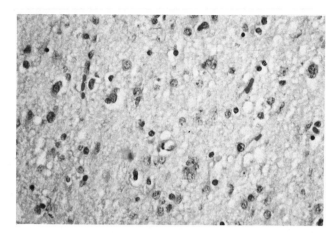

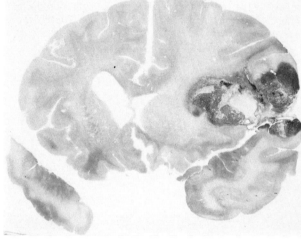

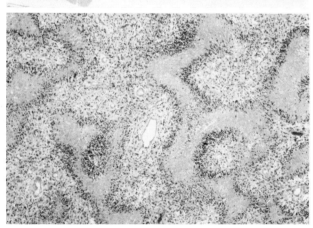

Figure 7–5. Malignant astrocytoma, fairly well circumscribed, mainly involving right insula, inferior frontal gyrus, and adjacent portion of superior temporal gyrus. *A*, Gross appearance showing areas of necrosis and hemorrhage. *B*, CV preparation not only delineates main tumor site but also demonstrates, by virtue of dark staining (increased nuclear counts), diffuse, mainly cortical infiltration of adjacent right temporal lobe and distant and separate left temporal lobe. *C*, Low-power (H&E) view of main tumor with a pseudopalisading pattern due to irregular necrosis. *D*, Histologic features of left involved temporal cortex (H&E).

ated ill-defined low-grade astrocytoma in the parenchyma is not infrequently missed by casual inspection.

An infrequent variety is the tumor closely resembling the cystic astrocytoma of the cerebellum in childhood (see below).

Rare, small, well-circumscribed, slow-growing astro-

cytomas are also recognized. They may represent hamartomas rather than neoplasms.

b. Malignant varieties

Some degree of anaplasia is found in nearly 80% of all patients with cerebral astrocytoma who come to autopsy. Frankly malignant tumors tend to occur in older

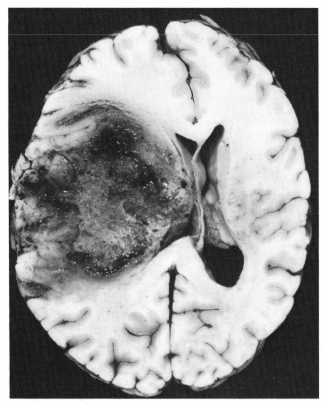

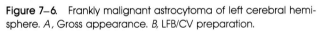

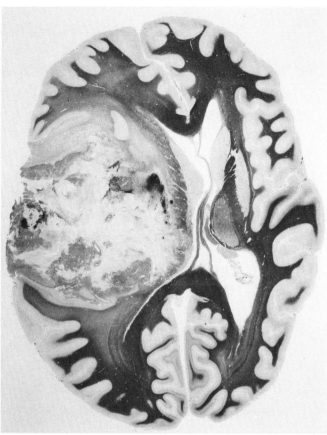

Figure 7–6. Frankly malignant astrocytoma of left cerebral hemisphere. *A*, Gross appearance. *B*, LFB/CV preparation.

patients. Their peak incidence is in the age group 45 to 55 years; however, they can be seen at any age, including the neonatal period ("congenital").

Any part of the cerebral hemispheres may be involved. The frontal and temporal lobes are most often affected. Involvement of the central portion, especially the corpus callosum, with a "butterfly" type of distribution is not uncommon. Others apparently arise in one hemisphere and spread to the opposite side by way of the corpus callosum.

Frankly malignant tumors are, on gross inspection, relatively well circumscribed and are surrounded by a zone of edematous white matter of varying extent, where reactive gliosis is present. Hemorrhages (red) and necrosis (yellow) are common and give rise to a variegated appearance. Better-differentiated cells are usually found at the more peripheral portions of the tumor. Thrombosis (causing tissue necrosis) and hyperplasia of small blood vessels are often present. The hyperplasia may become frankly neoplastic (see below).

These malignant tumors exhibit a considerable tendency to invade the leptomeninges and dura and to spread through the subarachnoid spaces, particularly after surgical exploration.

Apparent multiplicity has been reported in 5 to 15% of cases. This may be due to multifocal anaplasia in a

diffusely infiltrating benign tumor or clearly separate foci of neoplasia.

Sudden, massive hemorrhage into the tumor may reveal its presence after an otherwise clinically silent period.

c. Special forms

• Gliomatosis cerebri (Fig. 7–11)

This is a very rare type of widespread glial (astrocytic) neoplasia in which no grossly discernible focal masses form; the process may be more concentrated in certain areas than in others. Some degree of enlargement of the involved tissue is inevitable, however subtle it may be. The tumor is usually found in patients in the second and third decades.

The cerebral hemispheres are primarily affected, but the brainstem, cerebellum, and even spinal cord may be involved. Tumor cells are primarily elongated, dark-staining bipolar cells; one or more areas of focal anaplasia may occur. The grading depends on the degree of anaplasia of the component cells, which can be variable even within a given case.

• Giant cell fibrosarcoma or monstrocellular sarcoma

The majority, if not all, of the tumors so designated appear to be examples of malignant astrocytoma made up largely of large, bizarre, often multinucleated cells. Some also appear to belong to the

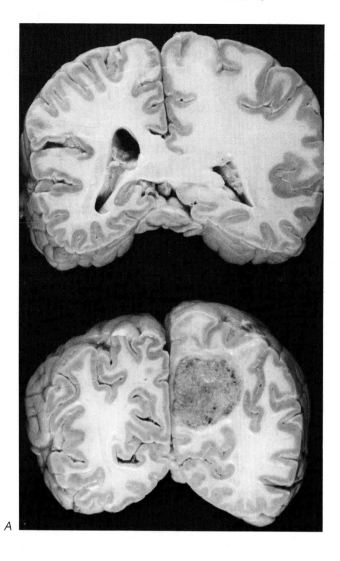

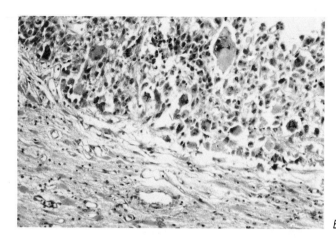

Figure 7–7. Medium-sized, well-circumscribed malignant astrocytoma of right parietal lobe, simulating metastatic carcinoma. *A,* Gross appearance. Note rather sharp border of tumor and extensive edema of the white matter, extending well into the right frontal lobe. *B,* Histologic picture at the border of tumor, which shows features of "giant cell glioblastoma."

group of mixed glioblastoma and fibrosarcoma (see under sarcoma, section 7.4, D).

2. Astrocytoma of the third ventricular region, including the optic pathway (Fig. 7–12 to 7–14).

These tumors represent 1 to 2% of intracranial gliomas of all ages and a slightly higher percentage (3%) of childhood gliomas. In regard to the optic pathway, only 10 to 20% are confined to the intraorbital portion (below); the rest involve the intracranial portions or both. Nearly 50% of all "optic" astrocytomas appear to be hypothalamic in origin.

The tumors are seen predominantly in childhood and adolescence and are slow-growing, relatively well-circumscribed (but microscopically infiltrating) tumors on the floor or in the wall of the third ventricle. The chiasmatic region may be invaded. Some grow primarily within the third ventricle and fill it, causing obstructive hydrocephalus of the lateral ventricles.

They are composed mainly of elongated astrocytes with unipolar or bipolar processes ("pilocytic") arranged in bundles; some areas exhibit looser, microcystic foci containing stellate cells. Rosenthal fibers may be abundant in more solid fibrillated areas (known as "pilocytic astrocytomas of the juvenile type"). Some authors (e.g., Zülch) call this type of tumor (along with astrocytoma of the cerebellum) "polar spongioblastoma," a term vigorously objected to by others (e.g., Rubinstein).

A more anaplastic variety as seen elsewhere in adults is occasionally found in this region. Examples of involvement of this region by adjacent astrocytomas are also seen, particularly in adults.

A variant of this tumor is the astrocytoma of the optic nerve. It is found predominantly in children (about 75% in patients less than 12 years old) and is a slow-growing tumor. An association with Recklinghausen's disease is known. Up to 30 to 50% of children with optic nerve glioma are reported to have stigmata of Recklinghausen's disease (see below).

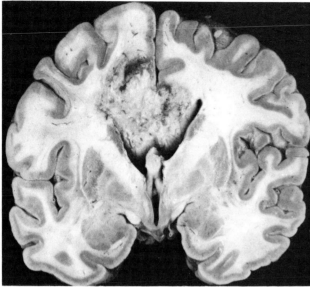

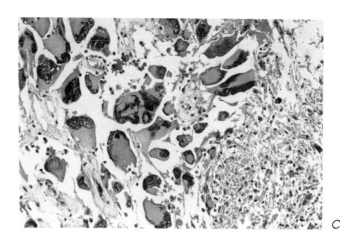

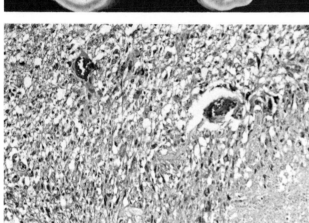

Figure 7–8. Malignant astrocytoma involving anterior corpus callosum and adjacent tissue, more on the left. *A*, Gross appearance. *B* and *C*, Two different histologic views of tumor (H&E).

These tumors most often arise as fusiform enlargements in the intraorbital division and frequently extend posteriorly toward the chiasm. A small number extend anteriorly toward the globe. (They may arise within the retina itself.) Some originate in the osseous intracranial portion or in the chiasm.

The tumors are largely composed of highly fibrillated piloid astrocytes; some areas are composed of loosely packed cells of reduced polarity with mucoid matrix, and this has given rise to the view that oligodendroglial cells are involved. Some authors therefore prefer a noncommittal term, "optic gliomas," for these tumors.

The leptomeninges are regularly invaded. This causes a vigorous fibroblastic proliferation and results in an intimate intermingling of astrocytic and fibroblastic cells.

3. Astrocytoma of the brainstem (Fig. 7–15 and 7–16)

These lesions occur most often in children but are not uncommon in adults. The tumors are generally diffusely infiltrating and of uniform texture; most often they involve one or both sides of the pons, which becomes enlarged ("pontine hypertrophy"), and they extend rostrally into the midbrain and thalamus or caudally into the medulla and cervical cord. Extension into the cerebellar peduncle(s) may occur. Some are more or less limited to the medulla or midbrain.

These tumors closely resemble histologically the diffuse cerebral astrocytomas of adults; they have a greater tendency to be pilocytic, most likely as a result of the alignment of infiltrating tumor cells along preexisting nerve fibers. The tumor mass may not be continuous but have many separate "masses" connected by rather indistinct bands of inconspicuous cells. The tumors often extend by a fungate growth into the subarachnoid space, even enclosing the basilar artery and occasionally seeding the subarachnoid space. An equivalent of diffuse cerebral gliomatosis is also known to occur, primarily involving the brainstem.

Anaplastic features in these diffuse forms, with gross hemorrhage and necrosis, are not infrequently seen (about

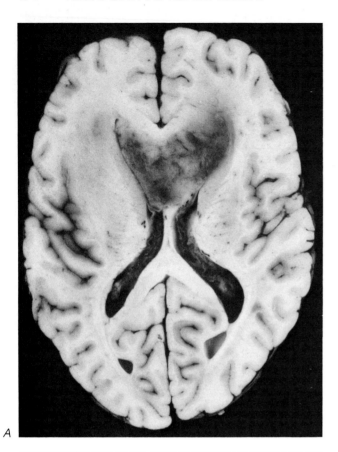

A

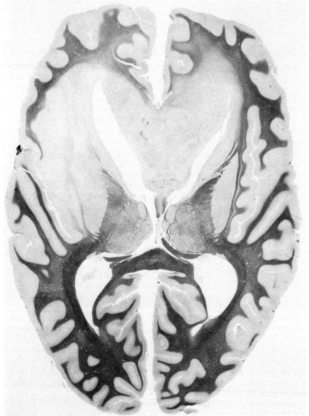

B

Figure 7–9. "Butterfly" pattern of involvement by malignant astrocytoma. A and B, Gross appearance (A) and LFB/CV preparation (B) of bifrontal tumor.

60%). Much more circumscribed tumors are occasionally found in the tegmental and tectal regions. The tumor cells are usually stellate and have a varying amount of fibrillary background. Some grow almost exclusively within the ventricular space.

Nodular, extruding tumors of the tectal region composed of piloid astrocytes are also known, with or without involvement of the aqueduct.

Rarely, relatively localized but infiltrating periaqueductal astrocytomas cause serious consequences despite their small size.

4. Astrocytoma of the cerebellum (Fig. 7–17)

This type of astrocytoma occurs predominantly in childhood and adolescence. Although it constitutes less than 5% of all brain tumors, it represents 16% of brain tumors in this age group.

These tumors are well-circumscribed masses of homogeneous texture, with microcysts and a few hemorrhagic areas. They may occur as largely solid masses or, more often (60 to 80%), they appear as large cysts that contain a small, solid tumor in one portion of the wall (mural tumor nodule). The protein-rich, xanthochromic cyst fluid coagulates on standing in room temperature. Although the tumor lies largely in one hemisphere, the midline structure and opposite hemisphere may be involved.

Histologically, the tumors show a varying mixture of (1) compact areas composed of strongly fibrillated cells, which are often fusiform or polar, and (2) loosely microcytic (containing protein-rich eosinophilic fluid) areas composed mostly of nonfibrillated stellate astrocytes. Both areas are of a low (1 or 2) grade of malignancy. Vascular proliferation, often with mural fibrosis, is common (at times simulating a vascular tumor or malformation).

A small proportion (10 to 15%), usually in the older age group, are more diffuse (with a greater tendency toward anaplasia) and resemble the infiltrating cerebral astrocytoma of adults. These may simultaneously involve the cerebellum and portions of the brainstem.

5. Astrocytoma of the spinal cord (Fig. 7–18)

These tumors are relatively uncommon, accounting for less than 1% of all central nervous system tumors. Among the spinal tumors, they are less frequent than schwannomas and meningiomas. The ratio of astrocytomas in the spinal cord to those in the brain is 1:20, reflecting the ratio of the weight of these two anatomic components of the CNS. Adults are much more commonly affected than children.

The lesion is most often found in the thoracic and cervical segments as a fairly circumscribed fusiform enlargement over several segments. The incidence is roughly proportional to the length of those divisions.

Histologically, these tumors resemble the fibrillary astrocytomas of the cerebral hemispheres, with a pronounced tendency to be more pilocytic, usually because of infiltration of the preexisting fiber tracts; anaplastic features are relatively infrequent. More than 75% of tumors are grade 1 or 2. Some infiltrate the leptomeninges or grow primarily in exophytic fashion. Spinal astrocytomas may be associated with syringomyelia (up to 40% in some series).

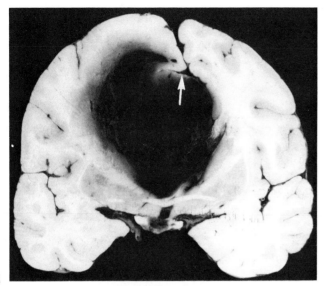

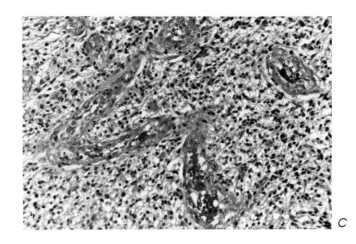

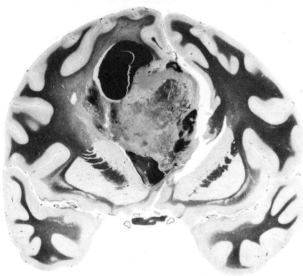

Figure 7–10. Sudden massive hemorrhage into left mesial frontal astrocytoma (grade 2 to 3). *A*, Gross appearance. Infiltration of left cingulate gyrus (*arrow*) is the only grossly discernible feature of the underlying neoplasia. *B*, LFB/CV preparation of same area as in *A*. *C*, Histologic appearance of tumor.

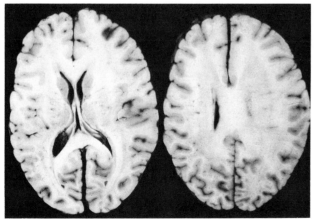

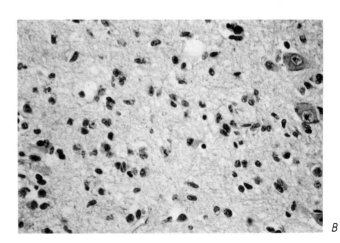

Figure 7–11. Diffuse gliomatosis. *A*, Slight enlargement of right frontal white matter with no discernible tumor mass. *B*, Histologic appearance of right frontal white matter (H&E).

195

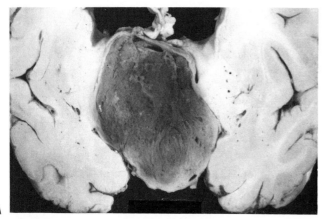

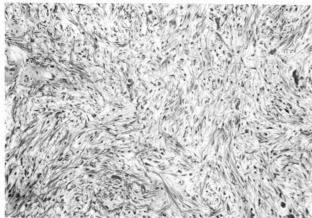

Figure 7–12. "Benign" astrocytoma of optic chiasm (in a child). *A,* Large tumor extending into and completely filling the third ventricle. *B,* Typical "pilocytic" appearance of tumor (H&E). (*A* from Gomez MR, Okazaki H: Intracranial neoplasms in infants and children. In *Brennemann-Kelley Practice of Pediatrics.* Vol 4, Part 1, Chap 12. Edited by VC Kelley. New York, Harper & Row, Publishers, 1974, pp 1–24. By permission.)

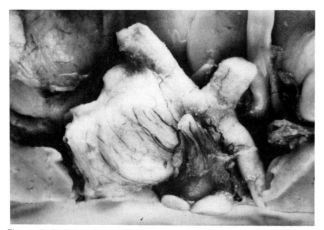

Figure 7–13. Astrocytoma of right optic tract in an adult, ventral view.

B. Oligodendroglioma (Figs. 7–19 and 7–20)

These tumors occur mainly in adults, with a peak incidence in the age group 35 to 40 years. They are usually well-defined, circumscribed, globular, slow-growing masses with little tendency to hemorrhage or cyst formation; they arise almost exclusively in the cerebral hemispheres, mostly in the frontal lobes. Often the bulk of the tumor is in the white matter, with extension into the cortex and leptomeninges. Thalamic examples tend to occur in younger age groups. Some occur as intraventricular tumors.

Histologically, the tumor is composed of patternless sheets of uniform cells with regular spherical central nuclei and a small amount of clear cytoplasm, which often appears ruptured, giving rise to a honeycombed appearance. These diagnostically useful pericellular halos are by-products of the histologic tissue preparation and are exaggerated in paraffin sections. Most of these tumors correspond to grade 2. The stroma consists of capillary-size vessels, which may show varying degrees of endothelial proliferation.

Calcification is seen in more than 70% on histologic study and in 40% on plain x-ray films.

Additional cellular elements, mostly astrocytes and what are considered by some to be transitional cells between the two, are often present. Nearly 50% of the tumors are regarded as mixed oligodendroglioma and astrocytoma.

Larger, somewhat irregular cells and mitotic figures are variable, but frank anaplasia is rarely seen. Occasional glioblastomatous features are regarded by many as a result of malignant changes in the astrocytomatous component; others maintain that the oligodendroglial cells are capable of pleomorphism and pronounced anaplasia ("polymorphous oligodendroglioma").

C. Ependymoma (Figs. 7–21 to 7–24)

These are slow-growing, circumscribed, usually homogeneous, but often lobulated neoplasms; typically intraventricular in location, they seldom spread far or display cytologic characteristics of malignancy. They are usually quite large when discovered clinically; some contain fine foci of calcification and cysts.

1. Several topographic subtypes are noted:
   a. Cerebral tumors (40% of intracranial ependymomas) occur and are evenly distributed throughout all age groups. They have a greater tendency to expand into the surrounding parenchyma of the brain. Calcification is seen on x-ray films in 20%.
   b. Infratentorial tumors (60 to 70% of intracranial ependymomas) occur mainly in childhood and adolescence. They usually arise in the floor of the lower portion of the fourth ventricle, fill it, and protrude into the subarachnoid space of the cisterna magna to form a tongue-like projection; others are more laterally located and extend through the foramen of Luschka into the cerebellopontine angle. Calcification is found in 10%.
   c. Spinal tumors occur with fairly even distribution from the second to the sixth decade (with a peak at the fourth). They constitute the majority of intramedullary masses

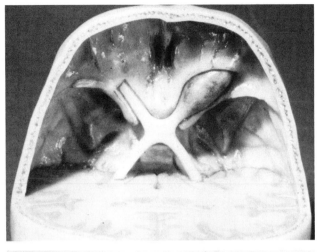

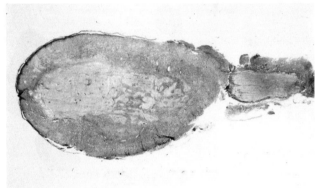

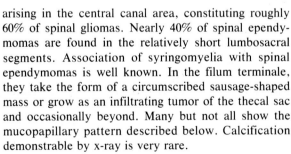

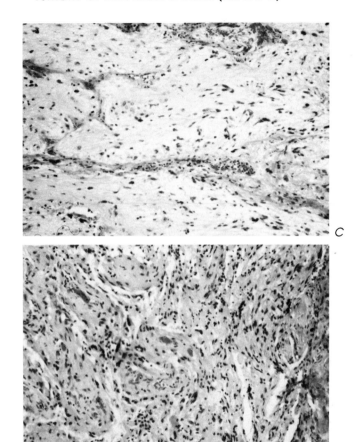

Figure 7–14. Astrocytomas of optic nerve, chiasm, and tract. *A,* Wax model of astrocytoma of intraorbital right optic nerve (roof of orbit has been partially removed). *B,* Longitudinal section of surgical specimen, showing extensive infiltration of leptomeninges. *C* and *D,* Histologic appearance of tumor within substance of optic nerve (*C*) and leptomeninges (*D*).

arising in the central canal area, constituting roughly 60% of spinal gliomas. Nearly 40% of spinal ependymomas are found in the relatively short lumbosacral segments. Association of syringomyelia with spinal ependymomas is well known. In the filum terminale, they take the form of a circumscribed sausage-shaped mass or grow as an infiltrating tumor of the thecal sac and occasionally beyond. Many but not all show the mucopapillary pattern described below. Calcification demonstrable by x-ray is very rare.

2. Histologically, several types of cellular arrangements are recognized. The pure forms are rare and mixtures of varying degree are the rule. They correspond for the most part to grade 1 or 2 in malignancy.

a. A cellular type (the most frequent) is composed of fusiform cells with a tapering fibrillary process arranged equidistantly about thin-walled small blood vessels (''perivascular pseudorosette'') and cell masses with a relatively compact mosaic arrangement between them, giving rise to a leopard-skin pattern on low-power magnification. Blood vessels may become sclerotic and have a more fibrillary background between them and the tumor nuclei.

b. An epithelial type shows tumor cells (some ciliated) aligned to reproduce in miniature the lining of the normal ependymal cavity (as in the central canal of the spinal cord)—that is, rosette formation. Some assume a more elongated canal configuration. This is diagnostic but is infrequently seen. Rod-shaped blepharoblasts in the cytoplasm along the free borders (identified as basal bodies or rudimentary ciliary bodies by electron microscopy) may be demonstrable at high-power magnification by special stain (e.g., PTAH). Although their presence in ependymoma is characteristic, they cannot be relied on for diagnosis.

c. A papillary type (uncommon) is made up of single or multiple layers of tumor cells, which are arranged to cover papillae composed of glial tissue (not collagenous tissue as in a choroid plexus papilloma).

d. A myxopapillary type is seen exclusively in the conus medullaris or filum terminale, although not all ependymomas here show this feature. Cuboidal or low-columnar cells are arranged in a papillary fashion around a vascular core, which shows increasing amounts of hyaline acellular connective tissue and stains positively with mucicarmine and PAS.

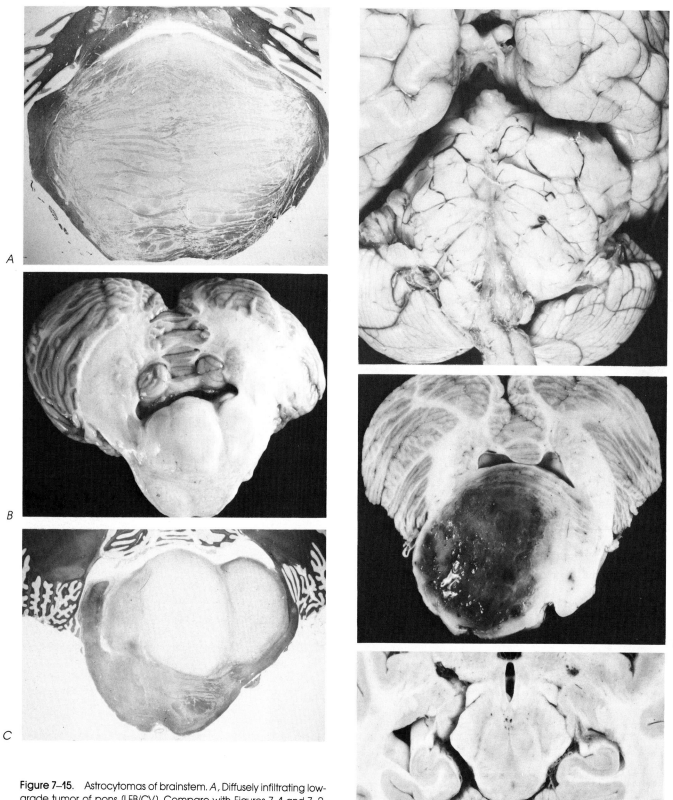

Figure 7–15. Astrocytomas of brainstem. *A*, Diffusely infiltrating low-grade tumor of pons (LFB/CV). Compare with Figures 7–1 and 7–2. *B* and *C*, Gross appearance (*B*) and LFB/CV preparation (*C*) of nodular (tegmentum) and diffusely infiltrating (base) low-grade astrocytoma of mid pons. *D* and *E*, External (*D*) and cross-sectional (*E*) views of diffuse but locally malignant astrocytoma of the pons in a child. *F* and *G*, Gross appearance (*F*) and LFB/CV preparation

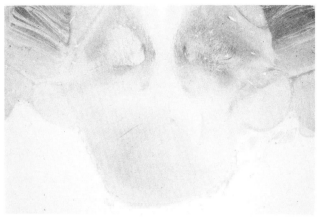

G

(*G*) of a diffuse low-grade astrocytoma of midbrain, tegmentum, and tectum, obliterating aqueduct and extending into subarachnoid space. (*D* courtesy of Kings County Hospital, Brooklyn, New York; previously published in Rosai J: *Ackerman's Surgical Pathology.* Vol 2. Sixth edition. St Louis, CV Mosby Company, 1981, pp 1555–1628, reproduced with permission. *E* from Gomez MR, Okazaki H: Intracranial neoplasms in infants and children. In *Brennemann-Kelley Practice of Pediatrics.* Vol 4, Part 1, Chap 12. Edited by VC Kelley. New York, Harper & Row, Publishers, 1974, pp 1–24. By permission.)

Malignancy is rare, unlike the case with astrocytomas. However, with progressive anaplasia, an ultimate histologic picture reminiscent of glioblastoma multiforme may be reached. This is usually seen in the cerebral hemispheres of adults. Some reported cases of grade 3 or 4 fourth ventricular ependymomas in children with dissemination appear to be in reality medulloblastomas. The term ''ependymoblastoma,'' previously applied to an anaplastic form of ependymoma, has now by and large been abandoned by most neuropathologists and applied to a different tumor type (see section 7.2, C, 4).

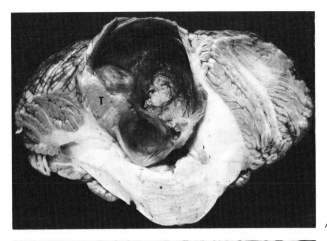

A

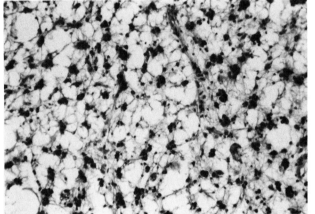

B

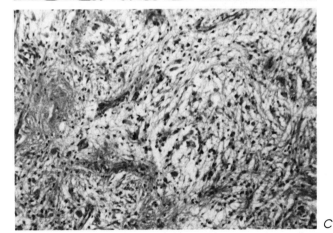

C

Figure 7–17. Astrocytoma of cerebellum. *A,* Typical cystic tumor with "mural tumor nodule" (*T*). *B* and *C,* Two different histologic appearances of tumor (H&E). (From Gomez MR, Okazaki H: Intracranial neoplasms in infants and children. In *Brennemann-Kelley Practice of Pediatrics.* Vol 4, Part 1, Chap 12. Edited by VC Kelley. New York, Harper & Row, Publishers, 1974, pp 1–24. By permission.)

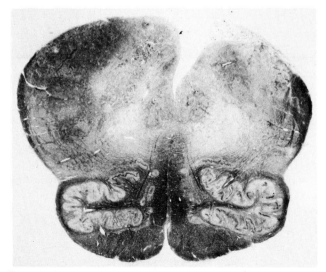

Figure 7–16. Diffuse gliomatosis of brainstem. LFB/CV preparation of medulla shows diffuse but focally accentuated pattern of tumor infiltration.

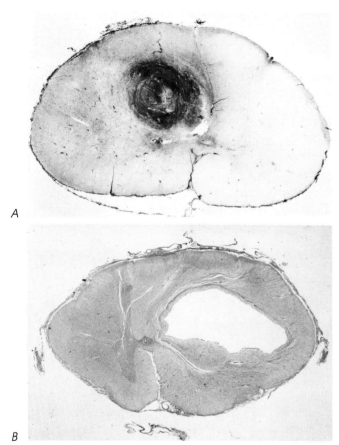

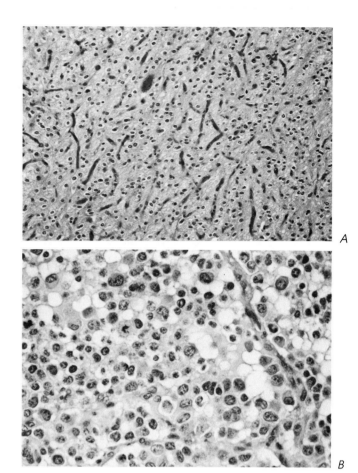

Figure 7–18. Astrocytomas of spinal cord. *A*, Relatively localized, low-grade fibrillary astrocytoma as demonstrated by PTAH stain. *B*, Low-grade astrocytoma at ventral border of syringomyelic cavity.

Figure 7–20. Oligodendroglioma (histologic features). *A* and *B*, Typically benign and more pleomorphic appearance (H&E).

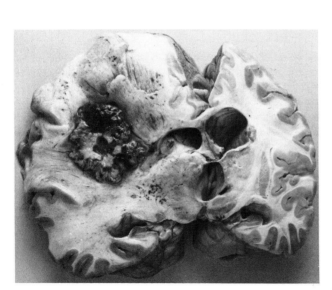

Figure 7–19. Oligodendroglioma (gross appearance). Medium-sized tumor is located in the deep periventricular parietal white matter in a young adult.

A variant—subependymoma (subependymal astrocytoma)—occurs mostly as small, lobulated nodules attached to the lower medulla and projecting into the caudal fourth ventricle; these tumors are most often found incidentally at autopsy among middle-aged or elderly persons. Rarely, they are symptomatic and cause obstructive hydrocephalus. Some are reported in the lateral ventricle and in the spinal cord. Histologically, they are composed of small cells forming small cell nests scattered in a poorly cellular, fibrillated matrix, which often shows microcystic changes. The cells of origin have been controversial, but they are most often considered to be a variant of ependymomas. Some appear to be more clearly of astrocytic origin. Many believe that they are derived from subependymal astrocytes and that they represent a transitional form between ependymomas and astrocytomas.

D. Papilloma of the choroid plexus (Fig. 7–25)

These are rare tumors, most of them (50%) occurring in the lateral recess of the fourth ventricle, often as cerebellopontine angle tumors. Those in the lateral ventricles (more often on the left) are second in frequency; they are seldom found in the third ventricle.

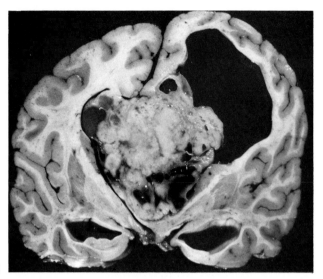
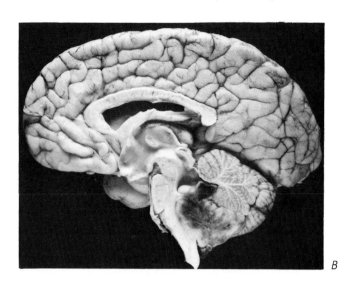

Figure 7–21. Ependymoma of brain. *A*, Large right para-midline tumor (arising from the septum?). *B*, Caudal fourth ventricular tumor. (*A* courtesy of Dr. Juan Olvera-Rabiela; previously published in Rosai J: *Ackerman's Surgical Pathology*. Vol 2. Sixth edition. St Louis, CV Mosby Company, 1981, pp 1555–1628. Reproduced with permission.

B, from Gomez MR, Okazaki H: Intracranial neoplasms in infants and children. In *Brennemann-Kelley Practice of Pediatrics*. Vol 4, Part 1, Chap 12. Edited by VC Kelley. New York, Harper & Row, Publishers, 1974, pp 1–24. By permission.)

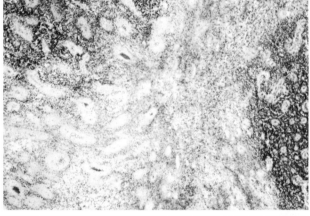
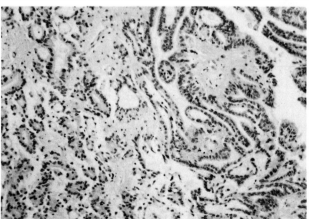

Figure 7–22. Histologic features of ependymoma. *A*, Cellular type with varying degrees of cellularity and fibrillary components. *B*, Epithelial and papillary types in adjacent areas.

Most commonly they affect children and young adults, especially in the first decade (50% occur in children less than 10 years old); in adults, the tumors are more likely to be infratentorial.

Grossly, they are reddish cauliflower-like masses, which may show cystic degeneration when large. Although not invasive, the tumor is often, at least in part, buried in the brain parenchyma.

Histologically, the tumor is composed of delicate papillary formations closely resembling the normal choroid plexus (grade 1) except that occasional piling up of the epithelial cells is present. Unlike the papillary type of ependymoma, the stromal tissue here is a vascular connective tissue. Cilia and blepharoblasts are reported in some infantile examples only. Exceptionally, mucus-producing cells are present. Significant calcification that is easily demonstrable by roentgenography may be seen, particularly in the infantile lateral ventricular variety. It is essential to exclude the possibility of a primary adenocarcinoma of another origin before the diagnosis can be established.

Malignancy (carcinoma of the choroid plexus) is very rarely seen in young children (age 2 to 4); it has a pronounced tendency to metastasize widely throughout the cerebrospinal fluid space.

E. Colloid cyst of the third ventricle (Fig. 7–26)

These are rare tumors (about 0.5% of brain tumors). Although they are considered to be developmental, and therefore congenital, in origin, they become symptomatic in late adolescence and young adulthood and are rarely seen before the age of 10 years.

The tumors are thin-walled, spherical cysts, commonly 1 to 3 cm in diameter when symptomatic, which may be

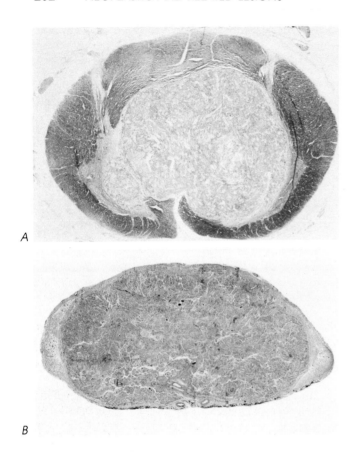

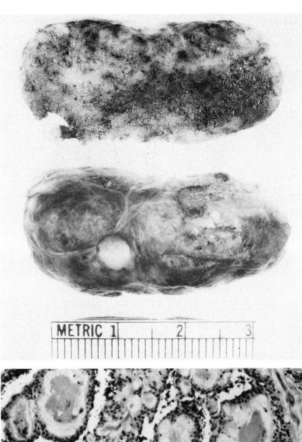

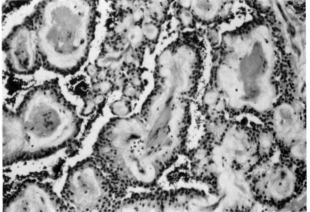

Figure 7–23. Spinal ependymoma. *A,* Cross section of centrally located tumor in LFB/CV preparation. *B,* Large tumor almost totally replaces a cross section of the cord. *C* and *D,* Surgical specimen (*C*) and histologic (H&E) features (*D*) of a myxopapillary ependymoma of the filum terminale.

attached to the anterior extremity of the velum interpositum or to the choroid plexus of the third ventricle in the region of the foramen of Monro. Here they often block passage of the cerebrospinal fluid and cause an acute obstructive hydrocephalus, which, if unrelieved, can rapidly cause death.

Histologically, the tumor is composed of an external thin collagenous capsule supporting cuboidal or low-columnar epithelial cells inside and encasing homogeneously gelatinous material, which is apparently secreted by these cells. Mucous goblet cells are often seen among the epithelial cells.

Considerable speculation exists concerning the origin of the tumor. No final resolution of the problem has been reached.

7.2 TUMORS OF PRIMITIVE BIPOTENTIAL PRECURSORS AND NERVE CELLS

A. Medulloblastoma (Fig. 7–27)

These tumors are now recognized as arising exclusively in the cerebellum. The majority occur in childhood—some 75% occur below the age of 15, 50% in the first decade. A male predominance (2 or 3 to 1) is noted. Considered a primitive tumor, it is thought to arise from the residual germinative cells that have persisted at some stage in the genesis of the external granular layer, which would normally disappear during the first year of life. Relatively numerous, small embryonal cell nests found in the posterior medullary

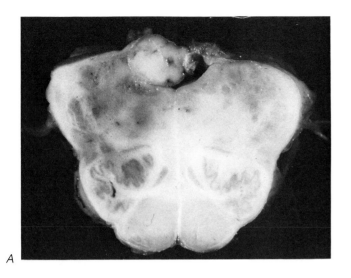

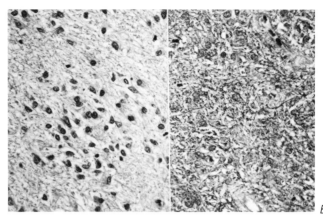

Figure 7–24. Subependymoma of fourth ventricle. *A*, Gross appearance of tumor attached to the medulla on one side. *B*, Histologic appearance (H&E on left; PTAH on right).

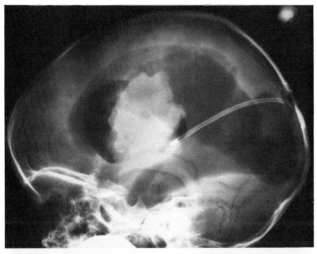

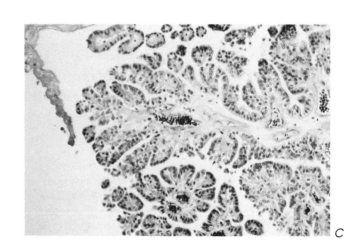

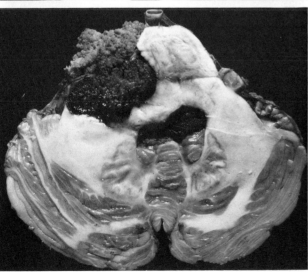

Figure 7–25. Papilloma of choroid plexus. *A*, Lateral view of a ventriculogram, demonstrating a large tumor in the left ventricle in a young child. *B* and *C*, Large fourth ventricular tumor largely projecting into right cerebellopontine angle in an adult, in its gross (*B*) and histologic (H&E) appearance (*C*). (*A* from Gomez MR, Okazaki H: Intracranial neoplasms in infants and children. In *Brennemann-Kelley Practice of Pediatrics*. Vol 4, Part 1, Chap 12. Edited by VC Kelley. New York, Harper & Row, Publishers, 1974, pp 1–24. By permission.)

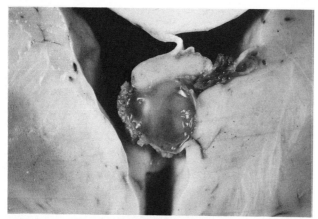

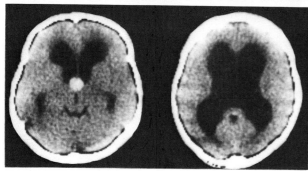

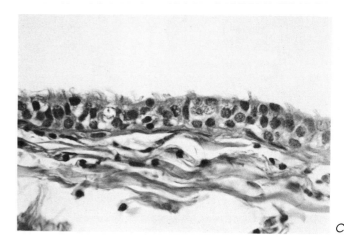

Figure 7–26. Colloid cyst of third ventricle. A, Small tumor inferior and posterior to crura of fornices partially obstructs foramen of Monro (frontal coronal section). B, Computed tomography image of obstructing tumor (left), which caused hydrocephalus of lateral ventricle (right). C, Typical histologic appearance of epithelial cell layer connective tissue capsule (H&E). (A courtesy of Kings County Hospital, Brooklyn, New York; previously published in Rosai J: Ackerman's Surgical Pathology. Vol 2. Sixth edition. St Louis, CV Mosby Company, 1981, pp 1555–1628, reproduced with permission.)

velum in infants and young children are thought to represent identical elements.

The name owes its origin to the presumed and hitherto unproved existence of a medulloblast during histogenesis. This cell was thought to represent a transitional stage of cellular differentiation from neuroepithelium and as such was presumed to possess the ability to differentiate into both neuronal and glial elements.

There are two subgroups:

1. Midline tumors (the most frequent type, about 75%, occurring mostly in children) are friable, homogeneous, pale-gray tumors that arise in the roof of the fourth ventricle, are relatively well circumscribed, and often completely fill the fourth ventricle. They frequently extend into the cisterna magna. Further spread over the cerebellar folia and beyond is a relatively early event.

2. Lateral tumors (the minority, mainly in adults) are smooth or lobulated masses on the surface of a cerebellar hemisphere (usually dorsal) with firm, homogeneous surfaces when cut; they occasionally spread en plaque on the surface of the hemisphere and are at times largely extracerebellar in location. Some of these are probably identical to the tumors described under the term "circumscribed sarcoma of the cerebellum" (see section 7.4, D, 5).

Histologically, the tumor is composed of dark-staining, spherical, oval, or polar cells, with hyperchromatic nuclei and ill-defined cytoplasm; the cells are densely crowded, usually without a definite architectural arrangement, against a finely fibrillated background. The vascular stroma is usually not prominent. Variable numbers of mitotic figures are seen. Although well circumscribed grossly, the tumor shows

a microscopic pattern of infiltration into the neighboring tissue, where individual tumor cells tend to assume a more elongated shape.

Tumor cells may show special patterns such as the following:

1. Pseudorosettes (of Bailey)—in which cells are arranged radially about an eosinophilic center containing a delicate tangle of fibrillary material, usually refractory to silver impregnation methods for axons or glial fibers. These formations were originally described in primitive tumors of the sympathetic nervous system (called "rosettes" by Homer Wright) and regarded as indicative of neuroblastic differentiation. They are highly characteristic of medulloblastoma when present (in less than one-third of cases).

2. Circular whorls—in some of which fine, delicately staining bipolar processes can be demonstrated with PTAH, suggesting possible spongioblastic (glial precursor) differentiation.

3. Palisades—showing a rhythmic pattern of cellular alignment, which may in places merge with a pattern of pseudorosettes.

Most medulloblastomas show little or no evidence of differentiation. Rare neuroblastic-ganglionic or spongioblastic-astrocytic differentiation is described; other authors consider these mature elements as resident neurons and astrocytes incorporated into the tumor mass.

Specifically important is the very frequent infiltration of the subarachnoid space seen in medulloblastomas; this usually happens early and often massively throughout the

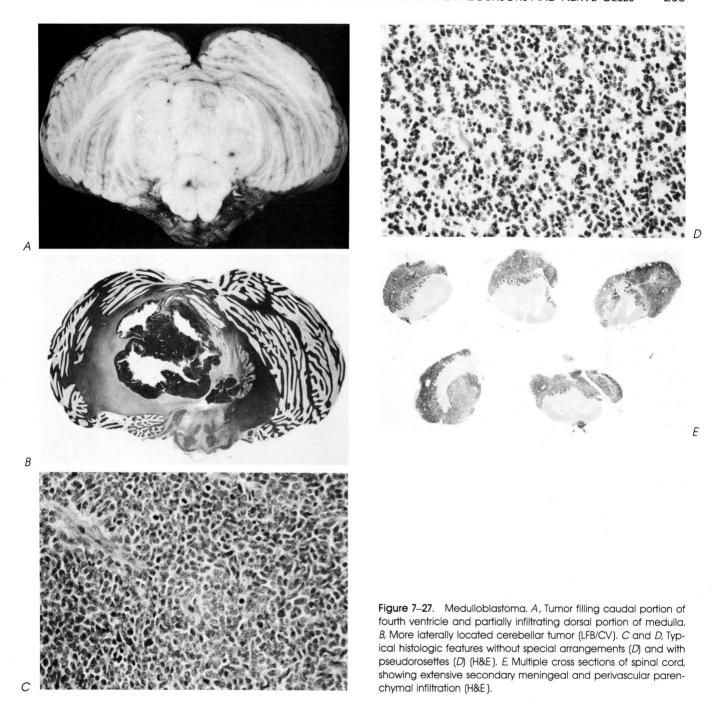

Figure 7–27. Medulloblastoma. *A*, Tumor filling caudal portion of fourth ventricle and partially infiltrating dorsal portion of medulla. *B*, More laterally located cerebellar tumor (LFB/CV). *C* and *D*, Typical histologic features without special arrangements (*D*) and with pseudorosettes (*D*) (H&E). *E*, Multiple cross sections of spinal cord, showing extensive secondary meningeal and perivascular parenchymal infiltration (H&E).

cerebrospinal fluid pathway. It evokes an intense proliferation of the connective tissue (desmoplastic reaction), which causes tumor cells to become aligned in long rows or reticulin-free islands and lobules. In many authors' views, the so-called circumscribed sarcoma of the cerebellum in fact represents the focal desmoplastic variant of laterally placed medulloblastomas.

Further dissemination of tumor cells throughout the entire cerebrospinal fluid pathways, including both the leptomeninges and the ventricular surfaces, either in diffuse or in nodular fashion, is notoriously frequent. This is said to be

present at the time of the first operation in 20 to 50% of the cases. The parenchymal tissue is secondarily invaded by extension of the tumor cells along the Virchow-Robin perivascular spaces.

The following variant rare tumors, although having a basic pattern identical to that of medulloblastoma, contain other elements.

1. Medullomyoblastoma contains smooth or striated muscle fibers and should probably be included in teratomatous tumors (see section 7.6A).

2. Pigmented papillary medulloblastoma includes melanin-containing cuboid or low-columnar epithelium in papillary and tubular formations. It is suggested that this tumor may be a variant of the pigmented neuroectodermal tumors of infancy, known variously as "retinal anlage" tumor, "melanotic progonoma," and other terms.

B. Ganglioneuroma and ganglioglioma (gangliocytoma, neuroastrocytoma)

These tumors are seen mostly in children and young adults (60% in those below the age of 30 years). They are composed of varying mixtures of differentiated but abnormal ganglion cells and glial stroma consisting of astrocytes and occasionally oligodendroglial cells, which may display evidence of concomitant neoplastic changes (almost always benign). They are therefore more often mixed tumors (ganglioglioma) rather than pure ganglionic tumors (ganglioneuromas). This is in contrast to ganglion cell tumors of the peripheral nervous system, which possess a stroma of capsular and Schwann cells. Considerable prominence of the fibrous connective tissue and vascular stroma may be seen in ganglionic areas (as in peripheral ganglioneuromas). Focal calcification and small cysts are common.

These are slow-growing, circumscribed lesions favoring the third ventricular region, the temporal lobes, and the frontal lobes. Focal forms are exceptional in the cerebellum (see variant below).

It is often postulated that these tumors are essentially hamartomatous, and some examples are heterotopic in location. They do, however, behave clinically and to some extent pathologically as expanding neoplastic lesions.

When, very rarely, malignant features are seen, they are invariably due to changes in the neuroglial elements.

A rare variant is dysplastic gangliocytoma of the cerebellum (gangliomatosis of the cerebellum, diffuse hypertrophy of the cerebellar cortex, Lhermitte-Duclos disease). This condition makes its clinical appearance in adult life as a gradually enlarging space-occupying lesion. The markedly thickened and enlarged cerebellar folia, locally or more diffusely, are thought to represent, essentially, hypertrophy of the internal granular layer neurons. The histologic appearance seems to combine the features of congenital malformation and neoplasia. Other malformations appearing elsewhere in the body have been reported in association with the CNS lesions.

C. Other, rare, primitive (embryonal) (and malignant) central neuroectodermal tumors occurring in early life

The following are other examples of "embryonal tumors," which, by inference, are thought to arise during embryonal, fetal, or early postnatal development from tissues that are still immature. These tissues may be said to contain dormant residual embryonal cells in which further multiplication and differentiation have been delayed until later in life. They are all reported almost exclusively in infants (even congenitally) and young children, and behave in a very malignant fashion.

1. Medulloepithelioma

These tumors are composed of papillary and tubular arrangements of medium or tall columnar cells reminiscent of the structure of the primitive neural or medullary epithelium. They rarely show differentiation into ganglion or glial (astrocytic and ependymal) cells. They are considered to be the most primitive and multipotential neoplasms in neuro-oncology.

The tumors occur in early life—from the neonatal period (congenital) to the age of 5 years—and grow very rapidly. They are sharply demarcated, highly necrotic, hemorrhagic masses, usually occurring in the cerebral hemispheres, often in or near the ventricles.

2. Cerebral neuroblastoma

These are very rare tumors about which there is still considerable uncertainty regarding incidence, clinical data, and pathologic features. Some consider these as examples of cerebral medulloblastoma.

They are very cellular, being composed of sheets of closely packed, poorly differentiated cells without special orientation or arranged in small clumps, short trabeculae, or irregular syncytial groups. Poorly defined Homer Wright "rosettes" (really pseudorosettes) may be seen. Rarely, more distinct maturation to ganglion cells is present (ganglioneuroblastoma). No spongioblastic differentiation has been demonstrated. The histologic features are similar to those of peripheral neuroblastomas but with rarer evidence of maturation toward mature ganglion cells. A remarkable degree of fibrous connective tissue stromal proliferation is not unusual.

These tumors are reported in infants and young children, and they present as well-defined, soft, granular, lobulated, grayish masses, often with areas of cystic degeneration. Dissemination through cerebrospinal fluid pathways is commonly reported.

Olfactory neuroblastoma or esthesioneuroblastoma is an uncommon tumor that presumably arises from the neural elements of the olfactory epithelium and usually grows as a friable reddish mass in the upper nasal cavity in adults or older children. The tumor is composed of small neuroblastic cells compacted into sheets or islands and separated by the often hyalinized stroma. The tumor may invade paranasal structures or extend intracranially to act as a brain tumor in the basal frontal region.

3. Polar spongioblastoma

These are thought to represent CNS tumors that show stages of differentiation along neuroglial cell lines. The polar tumor cells, with slender cytoplasmic processes, are aligned in parallel, forming compact bands or palisades separated by a delicate and regularly arranged vascular connective tissue stroma. There may be a limited or more extensive area of differentiation into astrocytes.

The tumors arise in the vicinity of the ventricular system (especially third and fourth) as well-demarcated masses with a propensity, however, to spread widely through the cerebrospinal fluid spaces. The highest incidence is in the first and second decades.

Note: This term is also applied by some authors (e.g., Zülch) to what have been described above as astrocytomas of the third ventricular region and of the cerebellum; this has added to the confusion in terminology.

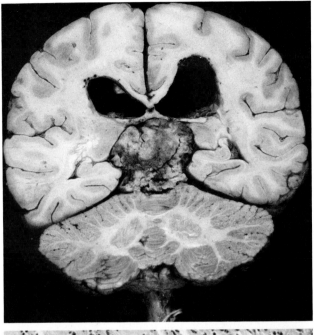

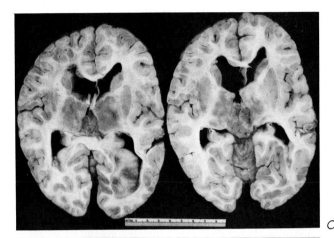

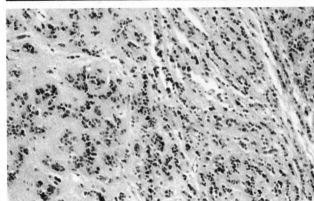

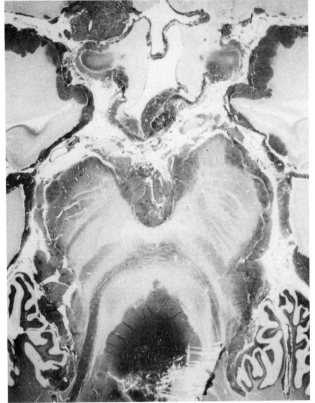

Figure 7–28. Pineal parenchymal tumors. *A* and *B,* Gross (*A*) and histologic (H&E) (*B*) appearance of pinealocytoma. *C* and *D,* Mixed pinealocytoma-pinealoblastoma with widespread dissemination through cerebrospinal fluid pathways, seen on horizontal sections of brain (*C*) and a histologic (LFB/CV) preparation through the lower midbrain level (*D*). (*A* from Baggenstoss AH, Love JG: Pinealomas. *Arch Neurol Psychiatry* 41:1187–1206, 1939. By permission of the American Medical Association.)

4. Ependymoblastoma

These tumors are composed mostly of undifferentiated embryonal cells, but in places they have distinct ependymal rosettes. They are seen in the cerebral hemisphere or within the ventricular system, exhibiting highly malignant characteristics, including rapid growth, local invasion, and diffuse spread.

Note: This term was originally used by Bailey and Cushing to describe the prominent perivascular pseudorosette pattern of ependymomas; these authors later discarded it. Subsequently, the term was applied by Kernohan to a rare malignant variant of ependymoma; he also subsequently discarded the usage in favor of the well-known grading system. A limited persistent use in the latter sense may be found in the modern literature.

D. Tumors of the pineal parenchyma (Fig. 7–28)

These rare tumors are thought to arise from pinealocytes, which are generally believed to represent modified nerve cells without long processes but rich in serotonin and other monoamines. The pineal gland contains no typical ganglion cells but has a rich network of nerve fibers, which are thought to arise in the superior cervical ganglion.

1. Pinealocytomas (preferred term) or pinealoma

These are circumscribed, noninvasive, slow-growing tumors (grade 1 or 2), which are seen at any age and in both sexes equally.

The histologic features are similar to those of the normal gland and include pseudorosettes, which, with appropriate silver stains, are found to contain delicate tangles of fine processes with small terminal clubs; also noted is the pattern of perivascular pseudorosette. Occasional larger cells may be found. Cases with ganglion cells, presumably differentiated from pineal parenchymal cells, have also been described.

Calcification may occur and can be detected roentgenologically. This is a useful sign because a normal gland rarely shows clinically detectable calcification before the age of 10. Premature pineal calcification should raise the suspicion of a pineal neoplasm, either this variety or those belonging to the germinal cell type (see section 7.6). Some examples of this tumor are known to disseminate widely along the cerebrospinal fluid spaces.

2. Pinealoblastoma

These tumors are composed of primitive cells closely resembling those of a medulloblastoma. Silver staining for pinealocytes is negative for the most part. They are highly malignant and behave like medulloblastomas, and they are found in both children and adults.

Note: 1. There are transitional or mixed forms containing the better-differentiated pinealocytoma cells and the more primitive pinealoblastoma cells.

2. The majority of the tumors formally included under the term "pinealoma" belong to the germinal tumor groups described below (section 7.6). Therefore, use of the term "pinealoma" should be discontinued.

3. Other neoplasms are found in the pineal region, if not in the pineal gland itself, although this distinction may be impossible when tumors are extensive. The list includes ganglioneuroma and ganglioglioma, chemodectoma, astrocytoma and glioblastoma, meningioma, and epidermoid and dermoid cysts (usually part of a well-differentiated teratoma).

7.3 NERVE SHEATH TUMORS

Two types of nerve sheath tumors derived from neoplasia of Schwann cells are distinguished on general morphologic grounds, especially in relation to the arrangement and form of the tumor cells and the character of the interstitial stroma and to the difference in their sites of predilection and their biologic behavior. The following three subtypes are recognized, and the two benign forms, A and B, are contrasted to emphasize their differences as well as their similarities:

A. Schwannoma
B. Neurofibroma
C. Malignant nerve sheath tumor

Note: 1. The term "schwannoma" is preferred over "neurinoma" and "neurilemoma." The last-named term is based on the now disproved belief that the neurilemma constituted an actual anatomic structure.

2. Schwann cells, best known for their role in the formation and maintenance of myelin sheaths in the peripheral nervous system, are apparently capable of synthesizing collagen, but they are also characterized by the presence of a basement membrane, in contrast to the better-known collagen-producing cells, the fibroblasts.

3. The term "neuroma," which has also been applied to these tumors, is now generally restricted to a nonneoplastic overgrowth of nerve fibers, Schwann cells, and scar tissue which occurs after traumatic transection of a peripheral nerve (traumatic neuroma) (see section 2.8).

A. Schwannoma (neurinoma, neurilemoma) (Fig. 7–29)	B. Neurofibroma (Fig. 7–30)

Gross Appearance

These tumors are encapsulated masses projecting from one side of the parent nerve. They have a relatively homogeneous surface when cut, with the frequent occurrence of yellow areas and cysts as they grow. Rarely, they are partially or completely hemorrhagic and are later converted to a fibrous-walled cyst filled with dark fluid with or without a recognizable nodule of viable tumor tissue (mostly seen in peripheral examples).	In the skin and subcutaneous fat, they are well circumscribed but not encapsulated, firm but rubbery, with pale-gray and translucent cut surfaces. The nerve of origin is almost never demonstrable. When the tumor is associated with a sizable nerve, the latter disappears into the substance of the tumor without being stretched over. Firm, rubbery cut surfaces show whirly patterns of fibrous strands but little, if any, tendency toward degeneration, cyst formation, or hemorrhage, even when large.

Histogenesis

Schwannomas apparently arise from a focal point and grow by expansion; they displace normal nerve fibers and produce round or lobulated, encapsulated masses over which the nerve of origin may be found stretched.	The tumors are initiated by diffuse proliferation of Schwann cells within a stretch of nerve, separating individual nerve fibers and causing fusiform enlargement of the involved nerve segment. The eventual gross shapes that are reached are fusiform (singly or more commonly at multiple points), in continuity with the nerve of origin.

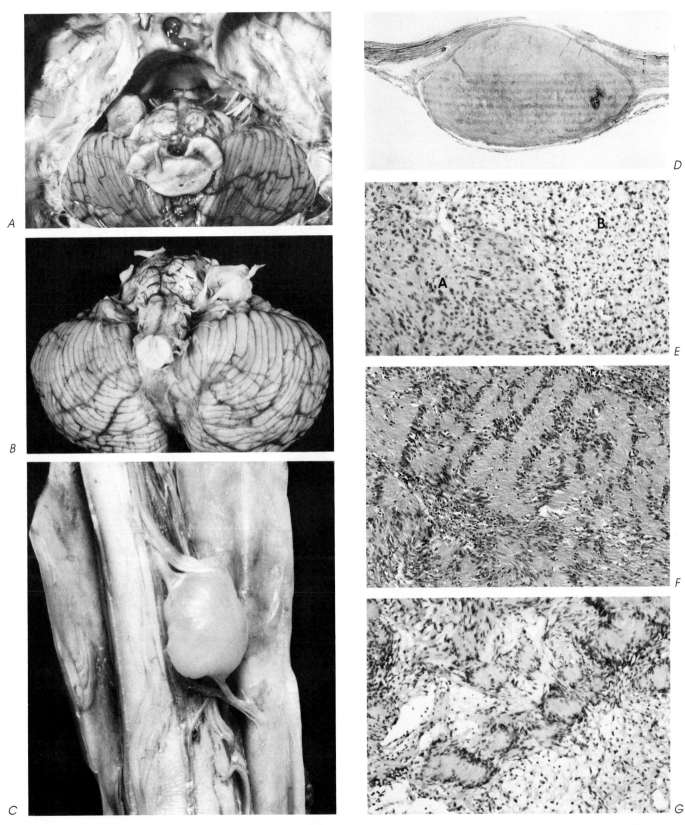

Figure 7–29. Schwannoma. *A* and *B,* Dorsal (in situ) (*A*) and ventral (*B*) views of schwannoma of left eighth cranial nerve. *C,* Schwannoma of left upper thoracic nerve root. *D,* Photomacrograph of similar tumor (H&E), demonstrating eccentric growth pattern and compressed parent nerve in brachial plexus. *E* to *G,* Histologic fea-

tures of schwannoma (H&E): typical Antoni A and B areas (*E*), palisading (*F*), and Verocay bodies (*G*). (*F* from Harlan WL, Okazaki H: Neurocutaneous diseases. In *Skin, Hereditary, and Malignant Neoplasms.* Edited by HT Lynch. Garden City, New York, Medical Examination Publishing Company, 1972, pp 104–148. By permission.)

209

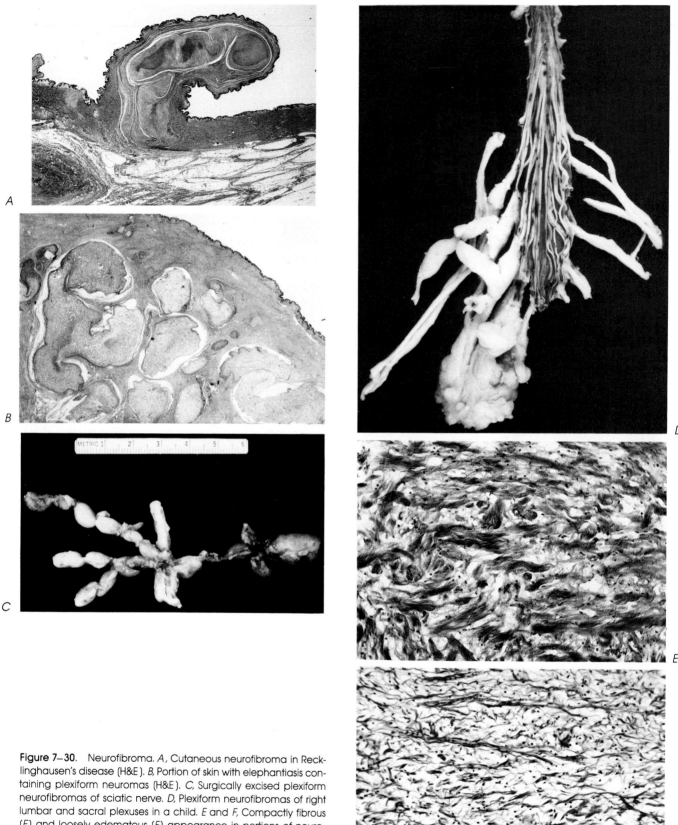

Figure 7–30. Neurofibroma. *A*, Cutaneous neurofibroma in Reck-linghausen's disease (H&E). *B*, Portion of skin with elephantiasis containing plexiform neuromas (H&E). *C*, Surgically excised plexiform neurofibromas of sciatic nerve. *D*, Plexiform neurofibromas of right lumbar and sacral plexuses in a child. *E* and *F*, Compactly fibrous (*E*) and loosely edematous (*F*) appearance in portions of neurofibromas (H&E). (*E* and *F* from Harlan WL, Okazaki H: Neurocutaneous diseases. In *Skin, Hereditary, and Malignant Neoplasms*. Edited by HT Lynch. Garden City, New York, Medical Examination Publishing Company, 1972, pp 104–148. By permission.)

Fusiform neoplastic Schwann cells form compact interlacing bundles accompanied by delicate fibers, which are positive for reticulin and collagen (Antoni type A pattern). Individual cytoplasmic bodies are indistinct. The pattern of palisading may be prominent in some of the spinal examples. Palisades with nuclei at either end of a bundle of parallel fibers result in Verocay bodies, which resemble Wagner-Meissner corpuscles. Other areas appear reticulated as a result of a loose mucinous matrix (rarely positive for mucin) and widely separated cells that are stellate in shape with long processes (Antoni type B pattern).

The lesion consists of a mixture of proliferated Schwann cells and fibroblasts between dispersed nerve fibers, accompanied by numerous fibrous strands of reticulin and collagen fibers and by a loose mucoid matrix. Eventually, axons disappear in the substance of the tumor. Decreased cellularity may be accompanied by a pronounced increase either in collagen fibers or in mucoid matrix.

Frequent secondary changes include the following:
1. Fatty degeneration with lipid-laden foam cells (xanthoma cells)
2. Cysts
3. Vascular changes consisting of hyalinization, sinusoid dilatation, and thrombosis
4. Hemorrhages, recent and old, with pigment-laden macrophages
5. Large atypical cells with irregular hyperchromatic nuclei, thought to be degenerative in nature without connoting malignancy

There is little tendency toward fatty degeneration, vascular change, or hemorrhage characteristic of schwannomas.

Note: Occasionally intermediate patterns occur: Schwannomas may have loose areas with abundant clear matrix as seen in neurofibromas.

Neurofibromas may show areas resembling the Antoni type A tissue of schwannomas.

The major problem is to determine whether a lesion is solitary or part of Recklinghausen's neurofibromatosis. Even though the pathologist can usually make the histologic distinction without difficulty in a given tumor, clinical information such as sites of lesions, presence or absence of associated lesions, and family history is very important in solving this problem.

The following characteristics apply to *solitary* forms (that is, those unrelated to multiple neurofibromatosis):

A. Schwannoma	Location	B. Neurofibroma
They are most commonly seen in the eighth nerve ("acoustic neurinomas"), mainly originating in the peripheral portion of the vestibular division; these constitute 5 to 10% of all intracranial tumors and occur predominantly in middle-aged or older patients. There is a female preponderance (2:1). Usually, these tumors are 1 to 4 cm in diameter when they are symptomatic. Compression and distortion of the brainstem and obstruction of the ventricular system cause symptoms other than those referrable to the eighth nerve impairment. Rarely, cranial nerve V, VII, or XII is involved as the origin of the tumor. More likely, these tumors are part of multiple neurofibromatosis.	Cranial nerve roots	Probably no true examples occur.
The tumors usually arise in the sensory roots and cause symptoms, mainly by compressing the spinal cord. Some grow through the spinal foramen and form a dumbbell shape. Surgical separation from the parent nerve is often impossible.	Spinal roots	They occur rarely. When found in these sites, neurofibromas, even solitary ones, are usually part of the phakomatosis of Recklinghausen's multiple neurofibromatosis.

	Peripheral nerve trunks	
They occur mainly on the flexor aspect of the elbow, wrist, knee, and so on. They often attain a very large size when located in the intercostal spaces, mediastinum, and retroperitoneal space.		
They are rarely, if ever, found.	Cutaneous nerves	The tumor is not infrequently found as a small circumscribed (nonplexiform) mass, the nerve origin of which is almost never demonstrable. The majority of neurofibromas in the skin are solitary, and occasionally several tumors occur in the absence of other features of neurofibromatosis.

The characteristics of *Recklinghausen's multiple neurofibromatosis* are as follows (for other associated neoplasms, see section 7.7, on phakomatosis):

A. Schwannoma	Location	B. Neurofibroma
Multiple involvement is characteristic, most often involving the eighth nerve, often bilaterally, and less often nerves V, IX, and X; even motor roots may become involved.	Cranial nerve roots	They occur in the region of the posterior ganglia as central extensions of peripheral tumors.
Multiple spinal (mainly sensory) roots are involved at multiple sites.	Spinal nerve roots	Same as above
Only exceptionally found	Peripheral nerve trunks	Exiting spinal nerves, nerve plexuses, and deep nerve trunks are involved in multiplicity.
Rarely, if ever, found	Cutaneous nerves	Plexiform neurofibromas occur which are collections of tortuously enlarged nerves under the skin and which are very characteristic of the disease. There is associated connective tissue proliferation resulting in a diffuse thickening of the skin known as "pachydermatocele" (the skin hangs down in folds) or as "elephantiasis neuromatosa" when it is more voluminous, particularly in the extremities. Nonplexiform (nodular fibromas) occur which are sessile or pedunculated projecting masses ("fibroma molluscum").
Multiple involvement occurs.	Visceral sympathetic plexuses	Multiple involvement occurs.

These relationships can also be expressed as follows:

Locations	Forms	
	In Solitary Forms	In Neurofibromatosis
Cranial Spinal	Schwannomas (almost exclusively)	Schwannomas Schwannomas > neurofibromas
Dumbbell tumor of spinal foramen	Schwannomas	Neurofibromas (often multiple)
Peripheral nervous system (trunks)	Schwannomas > neurofibromas	Neurofibromas > schwannomas (exceptional)
Cutaneous	Neurofibromas (almost exclusively)	Neurofibromas (almost exclusively)

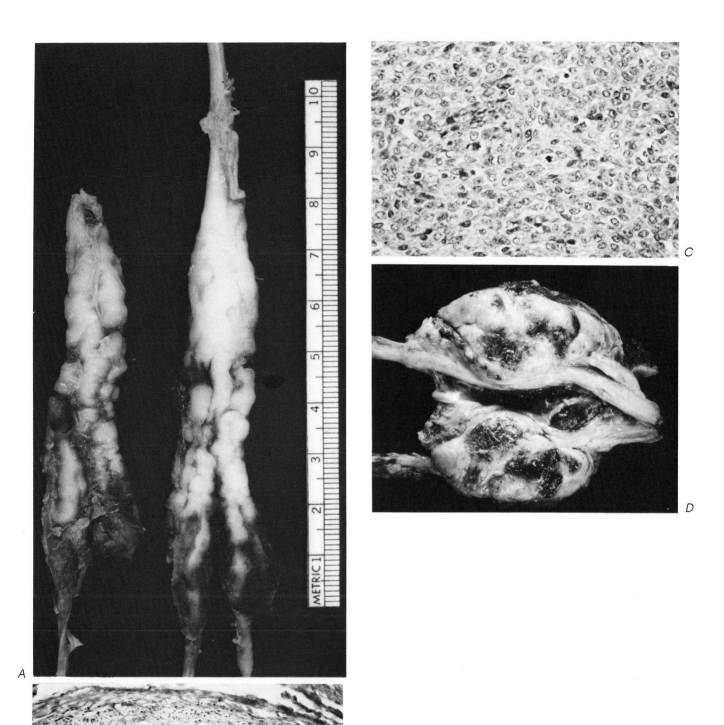

Figure 7–31. Malignant nerve sheath tumors. *A*, Gross appearance. *B* and *C*, Histologic features: excised nerve with progressive changes from benign neurofibromatosis to malignant neoplasm (H&E). *D*, Focal, frankly malignant tumor of sciatic nerve (longitudinally halved surgical specimen) in a child.

C. Malignancy in nerve sheath tumors (Fig. 7–31)

Malignant transformation occurs extremely rarely, if ever, in schwannomas. In Recklinghausen's disease, neurofibromas are known for their propensity to become malignant. The precise incidence is not known but was reported to be 13% in one series (which others believe was too selective). The problem lies in the difficulty of delineating the boundaries of the disease. There are obviously many mild cases that never come to medical attention. It is also difficult to be categorical about how many of the component lesions are necessary to constitute the disease.

Malignant nerve sheath tumors can arise de novo, independent of any preexisting neurofibroma.

In malignant primary tumors of the peripheral nervous system, the terminology is confusing, primarily because of the controversy concerning the cell or cells of origin for malignant growths arising in peripheral nerves. Representative terms include "malignant schwannoma" and "fibrosarcoma of the nerve (neurofibrosarcoma)," depending on whether Schwann cells or fibroblasts are considered the main cells of origin. Histologically, the distinction is usually not easily made. If distinctive features of Schwann cell differentiation are required for the designation of malignant schwannoma, this can seldom be satisfied; fibrosarcomas are therefore the most common type. The term "neurogenic sarcoma" is more noncommittal with regard to the problem of cell origin.

In tumors occurring in a preexisting neurofibroma, a gradual transition from a benign portion to cellular (spindle cell) sarcomatous areas can often be observed. The matrix may be more mucinous than collagenous; this morphologic feature makes the older terms "myxosarcoma" and "fibromyxosarcoma" justifiable. Chondroid, osseous, or rhabdomyoblastic metaplasia (differentiation) may be present in nerve sheath fibrosarcomas. These are indistinguishable from soft tissue tumors that are termed "malignant mesenchymomas" and they should perhaps be called such.

Compounding the problem is the occurrence of ordinary soft tissue sarcomas arising in the vicinity of the nerve trunks which can be confused with those arising in the nerve itself.

Other rare malignant primary neoplasms of the nerve whose nosologic position is not entirely clear include the following:

1. Malignant epithelioid schwannoma

Histologically, this tumor resembles malignant melanoma, but it usually fails to show melanin production. This pattern may be a focal feature of otherwise benign but cellular or frankly malignant nerve sheath tumors.

2. Malignant melanotic schwannoma

This tumor is composed of melanin-containing cells. The relationship of the tumor to Schwann cells and peripheral nerves is uncertain.

3. Neuroepithelioma and medulloepithelioma

About these tumors there is uncertainty whether they deserve a separate place or should be grouped with neuroblastomas (see below).

Note: Neuroectodermal neoplasms of the peripheral nervous system, which are of the primitive type and have the potential to develop into nerve cells, originate mainly in the ad-

renal medulla or in the sympathetic ganglia. They usually do not present as neurologic disorders and therefore are not discussed here. They include (1) neuroblastoma with or without ganglionic differentiation, (2) ganglioneuroma, and (3) pheochromocytoma.

7.4 TUMORS OF MESENCHYMAL TISSUE

The following tumors are included here:
A. Meningioma
B. Xanthomatous tumors
C. (Capillary) hemangioblastoma
D. Sarcoma

A. Meningioma (Fig. 7–32 to 7–37)

Adults are primarily affected, mostly between 20 and 60 years of age, with a peak incidence at about age 45.

The fundamental cells of origin are meningothelial arachnoid cells, in particular those packing the arachnoid (pacchionian) villi (or granulations), which project into the venous sinuses and tend to congregate in the region where the cerebral veins open into the sinuses. This accounts for the regularity with which meningiomas are attached to the dura and for their preferential sites of origin; other cells that may participate are dural fibroblasts and pial cells.

Characteristically, they are well-circumscribed, slow-growing, globular, or lobulated tumors of rubbery consistency, clearly demarcated from the brain. The size of the tumor at the time of discovery is largely dependent on its location and therefore its likelihood of producing clinical

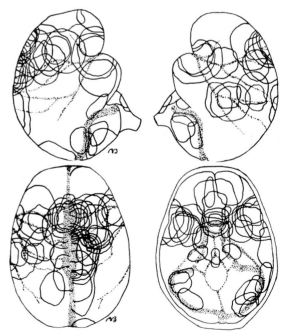

Figure 7–32. Meningioma. This diagrammatic presentation of the predilection sites of this meningioma is based on the distribution of a series of tumors studied by Cushing. (From Bailey P: *Intracranial Tumors.* Second edition. Springfield, Illinois, Charles C Thomas, Publisher, 1948. By permission.)

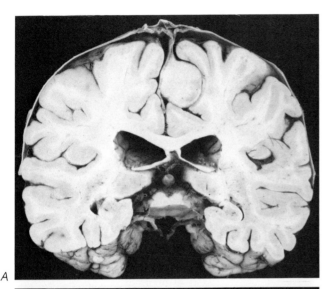

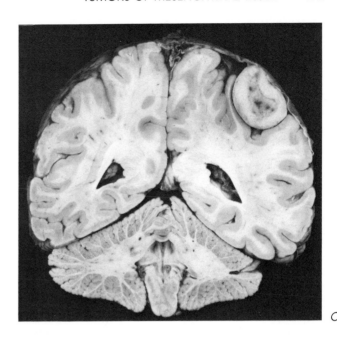

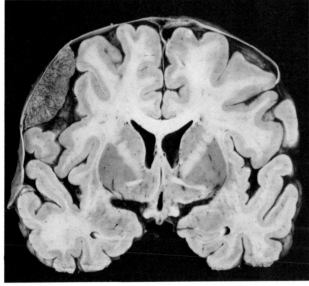

Figure 7–33. Convexity meningioma. *A,* Small globular tumor on right side of falx. *B,* Medium-sized, flat, dome-shaped left lateral convexity tumor. *C,* Medium-sized globular right lateral convexity tumor with central zone of necrosis. (*C* previously published in Kepes JJ: *Meningiomas: Biology, Pathology, and Differential Diagnosis.* New York, Masson Publishing USA, 1982.)

symptoms. Those in the "silent areas" of the brain tend to become quite large before being discovered.

Depending on the extent of dural attachment relative to the height of growth, meningiomas may be classified into (1) sessile (with a broad attachment), (2) pedunculated (with a narrow attachment), (3) flat ("meningioma en plaque"), and (4) tumor without dural attachment (often globular or sausage-shaped in the lateral ventricular cavities).

In the spinal canal a meningioma may form a collarlike mass around a spinal cord as a variant of the en plaque type. Rounded ovoid or globular tumors with considerable variability of the surface contour are much more common than flatly spreading carpets of tumor of the en plaque type. No fixed rules appear to exist in the size of the area of attachment in relation to the size of the tumor.

These tumors have firm, tough, yellowish or pinkish gray cut surfaces with a faintly lobular pattern of rather homogeneous tissue. When highly vascular, they are reddish in color. They may contain yellowish areas when xanthoma-

tous changes occur (see below). They derive their vascular supply mainly from the meningeal branches of the external carotid artery (in intracranial examples).

Meningiomas tend to occur in certain specific locations (as noted above). It has been pointed out that these locations correspond to regions in which arachnoid cell nests are commonly found in the dura. The knowledge of these sites is important, since certain stereotyped clinical signs and symptoms are expected from these patterns of tumor localization.

Roughly grouped together, the majority of meningiomas are found in the following sites—more than 90% are supratentorial and over two-thirds of those are in the anterior half of the skull:

Parasagittal	25%	
Convexity	20%	
Anterior basal	40%	
Sphenoid ridge		20%
Olfactory groove		10%
Suprasellar		10%

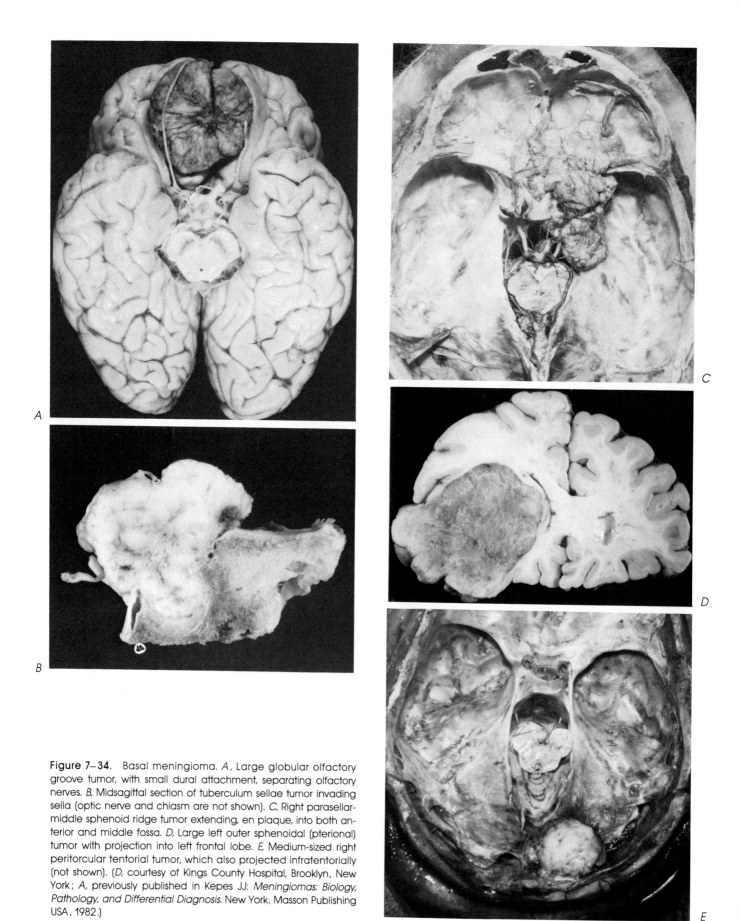

Figure 7-34. Basal meningioma. *A*, Large globular olfactory groove tumor, with small dural attachment, separating olfactory nerves. *B*, Midsagittal section of tuberculum sellae tumor invading sella (optic nerve and chiasm are not shown). *C*, Right parasellar-middle sphenoid ridge tumor extending, en plaque, into both anterior and middle fossa. *D*, Large left outer sphenoidal (pterional) tumor with projection into left frontal lobe. *E*, Medium-sized right peritorcular tentorial tumor, which also projected infratentorially (not shown). (*D*, courtesy of Kings County Hospital, Brooklyn, New York; *A*, previously published in Kepes JJ: *Meningiomas: Biology, Pathology, and Differential Diagnosis.* New York, Masson Publishing USA, 1982.)

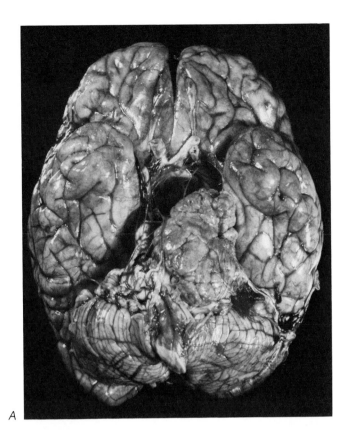

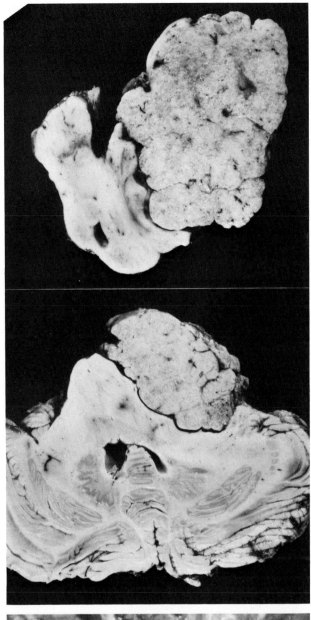

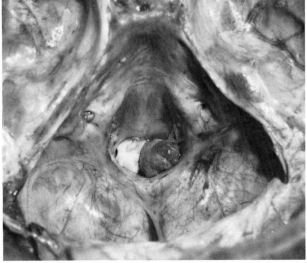

Figure 7–35. Infratentorial meningioma. *A* and *B*, Large Meckel cave (gassero-petrosal) tumor with smaller supratentorial and larger infratentorial (along right side of brainstem) components shown in situ (postoperative) (*A*) and on cross-sectional view (*B*). *C*, Small but compressive tumor arising on right side of foramen magnum. (*A* and *B* courtesy of Dr. Juan Olvera-Rabiela.)

217

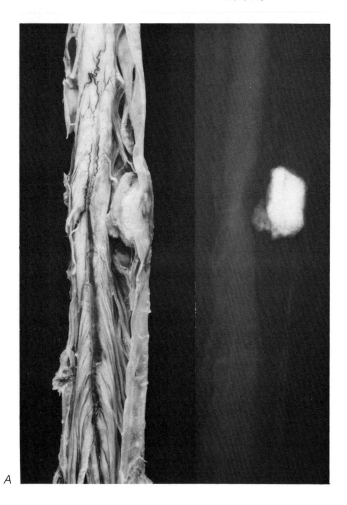

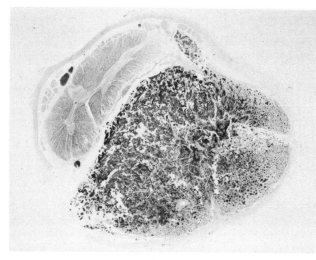

Figure 7–36. Spinal meningioma. *A*, Gross appearance and plain postmortem roentgenogram of heavily calcified low thoracic tumor on left with dura opened and tumor slightly reflected. *B*, Cross section of tumor and compressed spinal cord segment (LFB/CV). (See photomicrograph in Fig. 7–37 *F*.) (*A* previously published in Kepes JJ: *Meningiomas: Biology, Pathology, and Differential Diagnosis*. New York, Masson Publishing USA, 1982.)

An example of more detailed anatomic classifications (largely based on Cushing's scheme) is given below. It should be realized that a certain degree of overlap of location is possible in any given case (Fig. 7–32).

Convexity Meningiomas

Parasagittal—those arising in relation to the superior sagittal sinus, most often in its middle third, molding themselves in the angle between the falx and the convexity

Falcial—those relatively infrequent (2 to 3%) tumors arising primarily from the falx, usually with a broad attachment and not related to the superior sagittal sinus, favoring its anterior third and often growing bilaterally

Convexity—those arising from the lateral convexity dura away from the superior sagittal sinus. The majority (more than 50%) arise anterior to the central sulcus, and more than half arise along the coronal suture.

Meningiomas of the Base

Anterior fossa—those either in the olfactory groove (often becoming bilateral in location) or over the roof of the orbit. They project backward toward the sella and attain a large size before affecting vision by downward pressure on the optic nerves and chiasm. Extension of the sphenoid ridge meningiomas (see below) into the anterior fossa is also frequent.

Tuberculum sellae (suprasellar, prechiasmatic)—those apparently arising from arachnoid granulations of the anterior communicating branch of the cavernous sinuses and lying in the midline posterior to olfactory groove meningiomas. When large, they cause upward displacement of the optic chiasm and adjacent structures and may grow into the base of the frontal lobes and into the hypothalamus and over the sella. Closely related are tumors arising in the optic nerve sheath (of Schwalbe) which are located in the vicinity of the optic foramen, whence they may spread toward the orbit along the sheath.

Sphenoid ridge—those straddling the sphenoid ridge. They are rounded or flat and are capable of growing into either the anterior or the middle fossa to varying extents. Structures at the base of the brain can become surrounded by the carpetlike outgrowth of the tumor. Those in the inner (deep or clinoidal) or middle third may be termed "parasellar" and those in the extreme outer portion are called "pterional." The latter type is known for its tendency to be flat (en plaque), although some are global in shape and grow into the sylvian fissure. Rare deep sylvian tumors without dural attachment are presumed to have arisen from arachnoid cell nests deep in the fissure, perhaps from the carotid sheath.

Middle fossa—those primarily lying along the anterior floor of the fossa. Some are extensions of sphenoid ridge men-

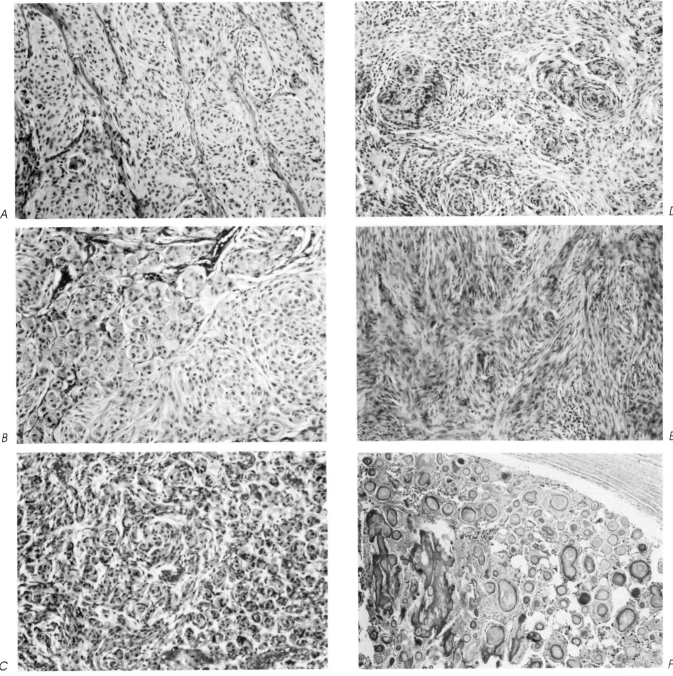

Figure 7–37. Histologic features of meningioma (H&E). *A* to *C,* Meningothelial nests of varying size, with psammoma in *C. D,* Mixture of whorls and streaming pattern (transitional type). *E,* Streaming pattern of fibrous meningioma. *F,* Spinal tumor (see Fig. 7–36) with numerous heavily calcified psammoma bodies.

ingiomas. Rare forms actually arise from the horizontal floor of the middle fossa and are surrounded everywhere by a margin of temporal lobe.

Meckel's cave (gassero-petrosal)—those initially lying en plaque at the petrous tip (which demarcates the middle fossa from the posterior fossa), where they are apparently contained for a long time by the superior envelope of the gasserian ganglion. Eventually, with enlargement, they become partially supratentorial and partially infratentorial, some of

them expanding more above and some more below. The major tissue damage tends to occur infratentorially.

Lateral ventricle—those principally arising in the glomus of the choroid plexus

Tentorial—those located on the upper surface of the tent and its sinusoid moorings, most frequently along the torcular Herophili, and expanding beneath the temporal or occipital lobe. They often have infratentorial components as well (see below).

Posterior Fossa Meningiomas

Tentorial (or cerebellar)—those located under the surface of the tent or arising from its flared marginal insertion along the transverse, sigmoid, and superior petrosal sinuses, either independently or as part of supratentorial tumor of the tent.

Clivus (basilar groove)—those that proceed from the lateral or medial clivus toward the temporal lobe, anterior surface of the cerebellum, or pontine region and may extend into the foramen magnum (craniospinal meningiomas).

Cerebellopontine angle—those growing along the medial portion of the petrous pyramid and growing more often toward the foramen magnum rather than toward the acoustic meatus. They constitute more than half the posterior fossa meningiomas and are often difficult to differentiate from acoustic schwannomas.

Foramen magnum—those arising at the rim of the foramen magnum or slightly below (actually upper cervical meningiomas), often causing symptoms early as a result of cord or lower medullary compression, despite their small size.

Spinal Meningioma

These tumors are most commonly found in the thoracic segment, although no pronounced predilection for any segmental level has been noted. They are firmly attached to the dura with a broad base and are often clearly related or at times attached to a nerve root and therefore mimick a nerve sheath tumor. Hyperostosis is generally lacking, but pronounced calcification of psammoma bodies is frequent.

Meningiomas are usually single, but multiplicity is the rule in Recklinghausen's disease. The overall incidence of multiplicity is 1 to 2%.

Meningiomas may stimulate new bone formation (hyperostosis) in the skull overlying the tumors. This may or may not be associated with actual invasion of the marrow spaces by meningioma cells. Sometimes, the tumors erode the adjacent bone. Invasion of the dura and major dural sinuses is also frequent; invasion of the orbit or paranasal sinuses occurs.

Although the tumors are, as a rule, easily separated from the adjacent brain tissue, the latter may, when the tumors are surgically removed, show total attenuation of the cortex, due to long and severe pressure and adherence to the surface of the tumors. The underlying brain may show either no or significant perifocal edema, which does not appear to be directly related to the size of the tumor. The rapid growth is considered to be one of the factors that favor the development of cerebral edema.

The morphologic diversity of meningiomas is generally regarded as an expression of the adaptive potential of the normal arachnoid cell itself rather than implying a different cytogenesis for each of the subtypes described. Previously complicated histologic classifications (Cushing and Eisenhart recognized 9 major types and 20 subtypes) can be reduced to two basic types and transitional forms between these two. No prognostic significance can be attached to any type, and mixture of two or more subtypes and all stages of transition can be seen. In the final analysis, a meningioma is a meningioma.

1. A meningothelial (meningotheliomatous, syncytial) type shows a uniform and moderately lobulated arrangement of compact masses of tumor cells with ill-defined cell membranes, the fibrous stroma being confined to trabeculae that separate them.

2. A fibroblastic (fibrous) type has elongated spindle cells that form closely interwoven bundles with numerous reticulin and collagen fibers separating the individual cells. This may occasionally result in dense areas of hyalinized connective tissue. Streaming cell patterns seen on routine H&E sections, however, are not necessarily accompanied by collagen or reticulin fibers.

3. A transitional (mixed) type constitutes an intermediate form between (1) and (2) with lobules composed centrally of syncytial cells and peripherally of elongated forms. There is often a conspicuous arrangement of cells to form concentric whorls.

The following secondary features are noted:

1. Psammoma bodies (from the Greek word psammos = sand) are concentric lamina of calcium salts, associated primarily with degeneration in the central portion of whorls but also arising from thickened and obliterated hyaline blood vessels or thickened fibrous connective tissue. When these bodies are found in profusion, the tumor may be termed "psammomatous meningioma." Occasional meningiomas, even though small, are composed largely of hyalinized whorls with heavy calcification.

2. Pseudopsammoma bodies are PAS-positive, small intracellular, and later large extracellular protein droplets thought to be secreted by meningothelial cells.

3. Karyomegaly and nuclear pleomorphism and giant cells are all considered degenerative processes rather than anaplastic ones.

4. Xanthomatous cells are foamy cells that are thought to represent a storage phenomenon rather than macrophages; they appear in degenerated areas in most instances. Grossly, they appear as yellow areas.

5. Areas of necrosis occasionally occur, usually in the central portion, and result in fibrosis. Rarely, they undergo cystic degeneration.

6. Spontaneous hemorrhages of significant size may rarely occur in large but clinically dormant meningiomas, suddenly unmasking their presence.

Special forms also occur:

1. Bone, fatty tissue, and cartilage can rarely be found in any of the above subtypes of meningiomas, and these forms are referred to as osteoblastic, lipoblastic, and chondroblastic meningiomas, respectively.

2. Rare variants with melanin pigment, "pigmented meningiomas," occur mostly in the posterior fossa and cervical regions, where the leptomeninges are normally rich in meningeal melanocytes. They may actually be melanotic neoplasms related to cutaneous nevocellular nevi.

3. The term "angioblastic meningioma" has, confusingly, been used to describe at least three different types of tumors as follows:

    a. Tumors with large numbers of nonneoplastic, thick, hyalinized blood vessels, but otherwise containing the usual meningioma cells, are at times erroneously labeled as angioblastic.

b. There is increasing evidence that some are, in fact, examples of hemangiopericytoma unrelated to meningeal cells (see below), although the tumors are often located in the meninges and behave very much like meningiomas.

c. Others are said to be very similar to, if not identical with, cerebellar hemangioblastomas.

4. Rare meningiomas containing areas of papillary arrangement are described which have a more aggressive behavior than the usual types.

5. Malignant meningiomas are a rare group of meningiomas (with usual gross and clinical features) showing varying degrees of anaplasia, including increased cellularity, nuclear atypism, mitoses, and local invasiveness. They tend to invade the brain parenchyma, which often shows conspicuous astrocytic proliferation. Some may give rise to extracranial metastases (see primary meningeal sarcoma). For other malignant meningeal tumors, see under "Sarcoma" (section 7.4, D).

When a meningioma-like tumor mass shows little or no histologic features of meningioma and instead clearly resembles a fibrosarcoma, it should properly be called such.

A diffusely infiltrating malignant neoplasm within the leptomeninges is usually referred to as "meningeal sarcoma" or "primary sarcoma" (−tosis) of the meninges. Component cells are undifferentiated in appearance, and their histogenesis has not been clearly established.

B. Xanthomatous tumors

These occur mainly as meningioma-like tumors attached to the dura in young persons.

1. Benign form: fibroxanthoma or fibrous histiocytoma

The tumor is identical to the tumor of the same name found elsewhere in the body and is composed of uni- or multinucleated cells with the morphologic features of histiocytes, Touton-type giant cells, and a storiform pattern in areas of spindle-shaped tumor cells, are characteristic.

2. Malignant form: xanthosarcoma, malignant fibroxanthoma, or malignant fibrous histiocytoma. The lesion is again identical to those found elsewhere in the body. Only a few cases have been reported.

C. (Capillary) hemangioblastoma (capillary hemangioendothelioma) (Fig. 7–38)

Young and middle-aged adults are primarily affected, most commonly in the fourth and sixth decades; 10 to 20% occur as part of von Hippel-Lindau disease (see below). The following sites are favored.

1. The cerebellum, especially in the paramedian hemispheric area. Tumors are almost always well-delineated reddish lesions appearing either solid (40%) or cystic with a mural tumor nodule (60% or more) and always in contact with the leptomeninges at some point. The cystic content is yellowish viscous fluid, which gels at room temperature.

2. The medulla. This is a rare but characteristic site, the solid tumor arising in the area postrema.

3. The spinal cord. The majority of these tumors occur in the cervical and thoracic regions of the cord. The tumors are usually single and solid. They are entirely intramedullary (60%) or extend into the pial surface, often (50%) accompanied by enlarged leptomeningeal vessels. A few (10%) are multiple. In more than two-thirds of intramedullary cases, a syrinx (see section 8.1, D) is associated with a tumor either at the same level or above or below. This may be regarded as the counterpart of a large cerebellar cyst.

4. Rare supratentorial lesions. As stated above (see meningioma), some "angioblastic" meningiomas are reported to be histologically similar, or identical, to the hemangioblastoma.

Histologically, these are benign tumors composed of thin-walled blood vessels enclosing islands of larger, pale cells, so-called stromal cells of mesenchymal and, presumably, of angiogenic ancestry; they contain varying numbers of sudanophilic lipid droplets ("xanthoma" or foam cells when loaded with lipid). Occasional hyperchromatic, multinucleated cells are seen among them, with no indication of malignancy.

D. Sarcomas (Fig. 7–39)

These are rare malignant neoplasms arising from connective tissue elements and their derivatives (dura and leptomeninges and their perivascular extension in the parenchyma, tela choroidea, and stroma of the choroid plexus). Considerable disagreement exists in their delineation and subclassification.

1. Fibrosarcoma

These tumors constitute the single largest group of sarcomas of the CNS. They are large, firm, homogeneous masses, well circumscribed but not encapsulated, mostly arising from and attached to the dura (i.e., a form of meningeal sarcoma); some arise within the brain substance without reaching the surface. Necrosis, hemorrhage, and cyst formation are common in more rapidly growing examples.

The most malignant and undifferentiated examples tend to occur at an early age, but otherwise no obvious correlation exists between age incidence and cellular differentiation. Some examples have developed 5 to 10 years after the course of radiation therapy to the head, especially for pituitary adenoma.

Histologically, the tumor resembles fibrosarcoma originating elsewhere in the body and is composed of long, parallel, intersecting bundles of elongated spindle cells with a rich network of intercellular connective tissue fibers (largely reticulin, some collagen) aligned along the long axes of the cells. Mitotic fibers are usually present. Variable grades of anaplasia and malignancy are present, with decreasing numbers of reticulin fibers. Higher grades of tumors in which the fibroblastic lineage cannot be demonstrated may be designated simply spindle cell sarcoma and polymorphic cell sarcoma (Rubinstein).

Rarely, fibrosarcoma arises from malignant degeneration of preexisting meningiomas.

A rare variant, which is seen predominantly in infants and children, infiltrates the leptomeninges diffusely in the absence of a definite mass. It is presumed to derive from the mesenchymal element in the meninges and is termed "meningeal sarcomatosis" or "primary diffuse sarcomatosis of the meninges." Histologically, the tumor resembles spindle cell sarcoma or polymorphic cell sarcoma. Medulloblas-

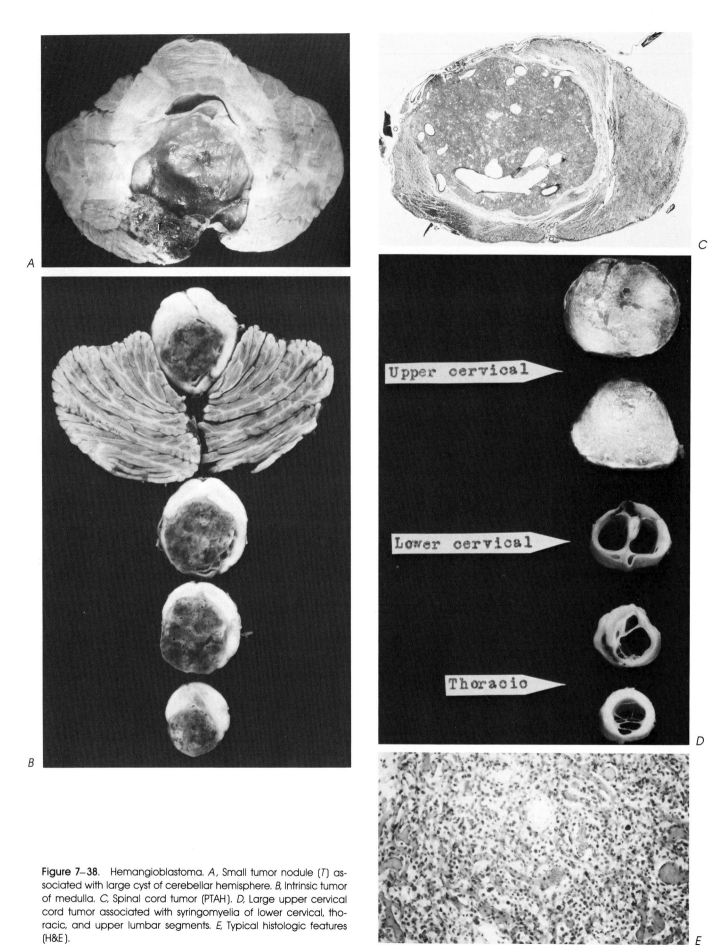

Figure 7–38. Hemangioblastoma. *A,* Small tumor nodule (*T*) associated with large cyst of cerebellar hemisphere. *B,* Intrinsic tumor of medulla. *C,* Spinal cord tumor (PTAH). *D,* Large upper cervical cord tumor associated with syringomyelia of lower cervical, thoracic, and upper lumbar segments. *E,* Typical histologic features (H&E).

222

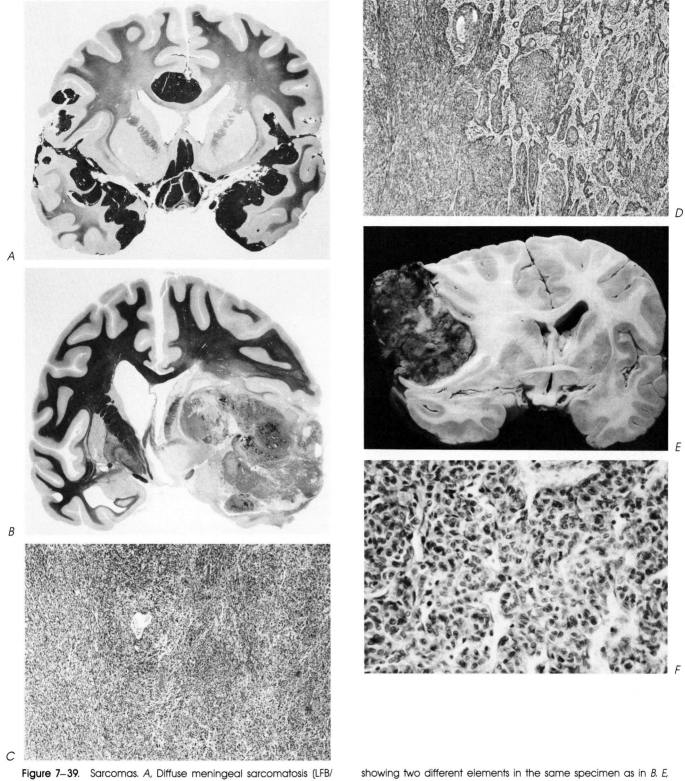

Figure 7–39. Sarcomas. *A,* Diffuse meningeal sarcomatosis (LFB/CV). *B,* Mixed malignant astrocytoma and fibrosarcoma (LFB/CV). *C* and *D,* Histologic features—H&E (*C*) and reticulin (*D*) stain—

showing two different elements in the same specimen as in *B. E,* Hemangiopericytoma of lateral convexity. *F* and *G,* Typical histo-

(Continued)

223

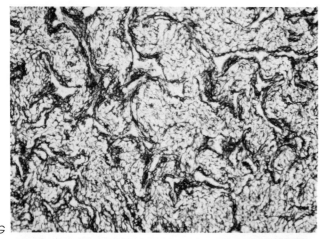

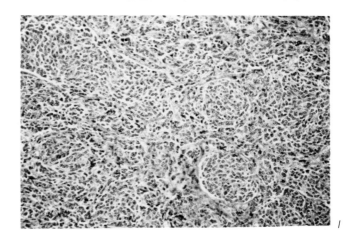

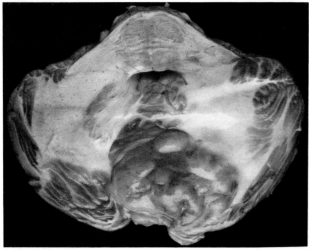

Figure 7–39. (Continued)
logic features with H&E (*F*) and reticulin (*G*) staining. *H* and *I*, "Circumscribed sarcoma of cerebellum" and its histologic features (H&E).

toma, leukemia, and lymphomas must be considered in the differential diagnosis.

2. Other rare sarcomas include myosarcoma, chondrosarcoma, and osteogenic sarcoma, which usually arise from and are attached to the meninges. Some are merely part of the more common fibrosarcomas. These and those designated as rhabdomyosarcoma may also represent embryonal tumors with chondroblastic or rhabdomyoblastic differentiation.

3. Mixed (or combined) sarcoma and glioma
Different modes of development are presented to explain the occurrence of these tumors.
   a. Sarcomas arising in a glioblastoma multiforme (malignant astrocytoma). This is a relatively common phenomenon and represents a logical extension of often extremely reactive vascular hyperplasia in the glioma into true neoplasia. The line of distinction is, in fact, difficult to draw. The resulting picture resembles that of a fibrosarcoma, and glial and mesenchymal elements often intermingle intimately and make identification of individual cells difficult or arbitrary. Reticulin stain often aids in differentiation. In other instances, the sarcomatous element may dominate the histologic picture.
   b. Malignant transformation of reactive astrocytes adjacent to a sarcoma. This form is considered to be extremely rare.
   c. The possibility must also be considered that a single carcinogenic agent is capable of transforming both glial and mesenchymal cells into neoplasia more or less simultaneously. This is suggested from evidence obtained in animal experiments with the use of chemical or viral agents. Furthermore, there exists a more remote or limited possibility of a glioma and a sarcoma arising independently and colliding within the cranial cavity.

4. Hemangiopericytoma
These tumors are in part identical to those described as angioblastic meningiomas (by Bailey, Cushing, and Eisenhardt, 1928) as previously stated (see section 7.4, A).
Histologically, the tumor consists of sheets of tightly aligned elongated cells with relatively sparse cytoplasm and large oval or polyhedral nuclei pointing in varying directions

and of numerous interposed endothelial-lined vascular channels and endothelial sprouts; an abundant network of reticulin is present throughout the tumor.

Increasing evidence indicates that pericytes (which are modified smooth muscle cells) and not meningothelial cells constitute the principal cell of origin for these tumors. They appear and behave very much like meningiomas except for their tendency to bleed profusely during surgery and, notably, a tendency toward recurrence and, in a few, definitely malignant behavior. Some are said to arise within the brain substance unattached to the dura.

5. Controversial entities

Controversy persists in the classification of a group of malignant tumors seen in young adults which are located in the lateral portion of the cerebellum. They are viewed (1) as an independent sarcomatous tumor designated as "circumscribed (or arachnoid) sarcoma of the cerebellum" (see medulloblastoma), which is rich in reticulin fibers and contains occasional islands of reticulin-free cell nests that the proponents of this entity consider to be mesenchymal in origin; or (2) as a desmoplastic, laterally placed variant of medulloblastoma with no clear distinction basically from the more typical (in younger patients) midline medulloblastomas. It appears at present more important simply to be aware of the special clinical behavior of this group of tumors until more definitive evidence of their distinct identity has been established.

Another, not so infrequent, type of tumor is known as "monstrocellular sarcoma" and "giant cell fibrosarcoma" or "giant cell glioblastoma." These are so distinctive histologically that they permit easy recognition. There are two different schools of thought regarding the cell of origin, as reflected in the terminology and classification. Each school claims the presence or coexistence of and transition to a mesenchymal sarcoma or a glioblastoma, respectively. These tumors behave like malignant astrocytomas (glioblastoma multiforme). In fact, more recent investigations appear to support the glial (astrocytic) origin of these tumors. It may be recalled that fibrosarcomas elsewhere in the body are not characterized by the presence of giant cells of this type. A conciliatory view that this group of tumors might represent a mixed mesenchymal and glial neoplasm is also offered. Recently, an immunohistochemical method for demonstrating glial fibrillary acidic protein (GFAP) of astrocytes in fixed paraffin sections by means of immunohistochemistry has become commercially available. This has facilitated the separation of many glial (astrocytic) tumors from the previously reported cases of giant cell fibrosarcoma in our own material.

7.5 TUMORS OF THE LYMPHORETICULAR SYSTEM AND LEUKEMIA (FIG. 7–40 TO 7–44)

Approximately 50% of the intracranial malignant lymphomas are primary neoplasms proved at autopsy to be confined to the brain or its coverings. In contrast, nearly all of the spinal cord or spinal root lesions occur as part of systemic disease.

Among numerous classifications of lymphomas, the one offered by Rappaport (1966) has gained wide usage. More recently, new cytochemical and immunologic techniques have made possible further categorization and identification of cells in the lymphoreticular system. Studies utilizing these techniques suggest that the currently recognized histopathologic entities of lymphoreticular malignancies are heterogeneous and that some of the histopathologic terminology of Rappaport requires modification. Until a more definitive universally accepted classification is arrived at, a more conventional terminology, as used in the neurologic literature, is retained here for various histopathologic entities. Histiocytosis X is included here because of its resemblance in some respect to lymphomas despite the uncertainty regarding its nosologic position and etiology.

It is convenient to discuss direct and indirect involvement of the nervous system by lymphoproliferative disorders in terms of the secondary and primary types.

Secondary Type	*Primary Type*
Lesions that are part of the generalized disease. The overall reported incidence of nervous system involvement is up to 25%. The spinal cord is the most commonly affected tissue. The peripheral nerves appear to be infrequently involved.	Lesions that are solely or largely limited to the CNS.
A. Hodgkin's disease The most frequent lesions are in the spinal epidural space, with extrinsic compression of the spinal cord itself. Occasionally, the disease process breaks through the dura and involves the	Independent cerebral parenchymal lesions are infrequent and may take the form of either a localized tumor mass or diffuse infiltrative lesions.

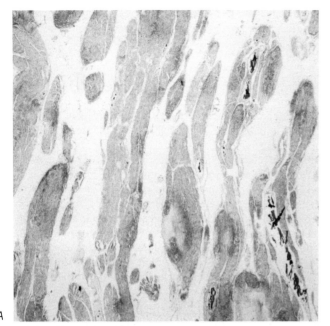

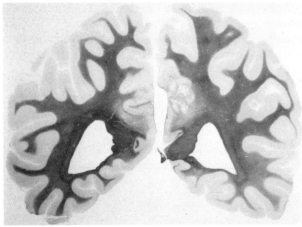

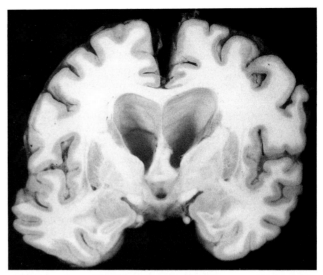

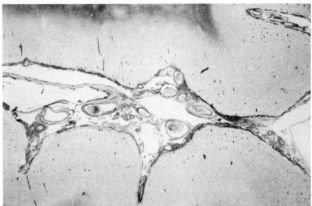

Figure 7–41. Systemic lymphosarcoma. A, Internal hydrocephalus secondary to diffuse leptomeningeal infiltration. B, Diffuse infiltration of leptomeninges at the level of the cerebral leptomeninges (LFB/CV).

Figure 7–40. Systemic Hodgkin's disease. A, Low-power histologic (LFB/CV) features of diffuse and nodular involvement of cauda equina roots. B, Focal infiltrative lesions in cunei (LFB).

leptomeninges and the spinal roots diffusely, but actual parenchymal invasion is uncommon. Infrequently, focal brain involvement may occur as an extension from lesions of the adjacent bone and meninges.

B. Lymphosarcoma (lymphocytic lymphoma)

The main type is spinal epidural involvement with cord compression.

Spinal and cranial nerve roots within the subarachnoid space may be diffusely infiltrated without significant epidural involvement.

Occasionally, intracranial dural lesions occur, with subsequent focal invasion of the underlying brain parenchyma, initially through extension along the perivascular spaces.

Focal cerebral lesions are infrequently observed.

Rare examples of primary diffuse leptomeningeal involvement have also been reported. These are difficult to separate from primary diffuse sarcoma of leptomeninges (see section 7.4, D).

C. Reticulum cell sarcoma (histiocytic lymphoma, immunoblastic sarcoma)

The patterns of CNS involvement are similar to those discussed above.

Simultaneous involvement of the CNS parenchyma and other organs is infrequent.

Primary lesions of the brain are relatively frequent, mainly in the cerebral hemispheres and rarely in the spinal cord. All ages are affected; the maximal incidence is in the fifth and sixth decades. A large separate group occurs in the first decade.

They occur in two main forms: (1) localized tumor masses and (2) diffusely infiltrative lesions without formation of a definite mass. In both types, the primarily perivascular origin of the tumor cells with subsequent invasion is apparent, particularly with the aid of a reticulin stain. Pronounced hypertrophic reaction of astrocytes in the intervening tissue is common at times, to the extent that it can cause confusion with malignant astrocytoma (this holds true to some extent in the other forms of cerebral lymphomas, primary or secondary). Lymphocytes may also be present in the lesion. Rod-shaped microglial cells are not infrequently found at the periphery, mainly in the gray matter, but rarely to an extent that warrants the term "microglioma" to describe the entire lesion, as had been popular in the past. Some authors consider these cells to be merely reactive.

Multiple lesions are relatively frequent.

An increased incidence of reticulum cell sarcoma is noted among patients receiving immunosuppressive treatment for renal transplantation.

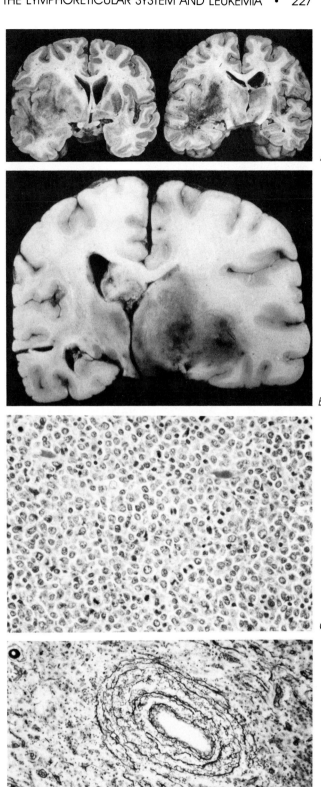

Figure 7–42. Primary cerebral reticulum cell sarcoma. A, Diffusely infiltrating form in left temporal lobe. B, Nodular lesion in fornices and diffuse lesion in right thalamus and hippocampus. C, Histologic features of compact cellular portion of tumor (H&E). D, Typical perivascular pattern of tumor cell infiltration associated with "reduplication" of reticulin fibers in diffuse type (reticulin stain). (B courtesy of Dr. Bruno Volk.)

D. Multiple myeloma

Vertebral and epidural involvement with cord compression is the most common mode (6% of cases).

Secondary intracranial dural involvement occasionally occurs, but actual brain invasion is rarely seen, although the skull is involved rather frequently (up to 70%).

Parenchymal cerebral or spinal lesions are rarely observed.

E. Histiocytosis X

Secondary invasion of the pituitary-hypothalamic region from bony lesions at the base of the skull is well recognized.

Localized masses occur which are not associated with basal skull involvement in the hypothalamic-infundibular region (Ayala's disease or Gagel's granuloma).

Separation of this form from a slowly evolving neoplastic proliferation of the reticuloendothelial system (malignant lymphomas) is not easy, and intermediate forms that appear to bridge these two conditions have been reported.

The nosologic placement of this enigmatic entity, like that of histiocytosis X in general, remains to be determined.

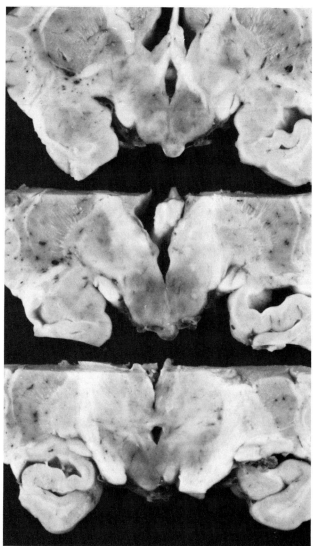

A

F. Leukemia

Hemorrhagic lesions associated with leukemic disorders have been discussed in section 1.6. In this segment, infiltration of the nervous parenchyma and its coverings will be dealt with. In general, hemorrhagic phenomena are more commonly observed among adults, whereas significant infiltrative lesions are more common among children.

More commonly, CNS infiltrative lesions take the form of diffuse infiltration of the spinal and cranial leptomeningeal spaces, with concomitant involvement of spinal and cranial nerve roots in a manner similar to that of malignant lymphoma. The CNS parenchyma is, as a rule, secondarily involved by perivascular extension of cellular infiltration from the leptomeninges and ventricles. In recent years, the frequency of leukemic infiltration of this type has increased, as many more remissions and longer survival have become possible with more aggressive chemotherapy. The cerebrospinal fluid space appears to give sanctuary to leukemic cells from the effect of systemic therapy and allows them to proliferate while the neoplastic cells elsewhere are succumbing to it.

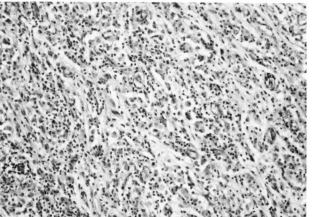

B

Figure 7–43. Histiocytosis X confirmed in hypothalamic region. *A,* Gross appearance. *B,* Typical histologic (H&E) appearance.

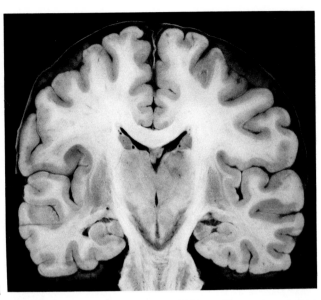

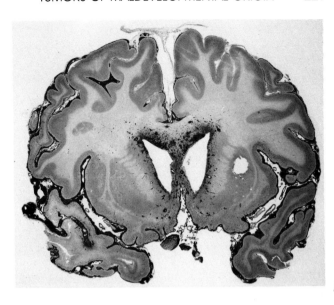

Figure 7–44. Leukemic infiltration of CNS and its coverings. *A*, Thick pancake-like subdural infiltration (chloroma). *B*, Brain of a child who finally succumbed to diffuse spinal, leptomeningeal, and periven- tricular infiltration after more than 10 years of survival with acute lymphocytic leukemia (remission in bone marrow and viscera) (CV).

This phenomenon is sometimes referred to as colonization. Thus a pronounced infiltration of the leptomeningeal space may be seen in the face of marrow and systemic remission, particularly among young patients with acute lymphocytic leukemia, who now enjoy long remissions in a high percentage of cases.

Isolated focal, primarily intraparenchymal infiltrative lesions are rarely encountered.

Clinically significant infiltration of the peripheral nervous system is relatively infrequent; the precise incidence is difficult to establish.

Spinal epidural and intracranial subdural infiltrations may be clinically significant.

7.6 TUMORS OF MALDEVELOPMENTAL ORIGIN

Included here are the following:

A. Primary germ cell tumors
1. Germinoma
2. Teratomatous group
   a. Embryonal carcinoma
   b. Teratoma
   c. Choriocarcinoma

B. Dermoid and epidermoid

C. Lipoma

D. Neuroepithelial ectopic tumors and hamartoma
1. Ectopic glioma
2. Hypothalamic ganglionic hamartoma
3. Granular cell tumors of the neurohypophysis
4. Craniopharyngioma
5. Intrasellar Rathke's pouch cleft cyst
6. Leptomeningal (or arachnoid) cyst
7. Enterogenic cyst

A. Primary intracranial (and spinal) germ cell neoplasms and tumors (Fig. 7–45 to 7–47)

The modern classification of germ cell neoplasms and tumors first adopted for testicular tumors by Dixon and Moore (1952) has now been applied to the CNS as well. A modified flow sheet is presented in Figure 7–45 to illustrate the interrelationship of the various subtypes.

Any mixture of the component types can be seen. Roughly grouped, reported incidences are germinomatous, 60%; teratomatous, 20% (all nongerminomatous forms included); and mixed, 20%. There is no intermediate form between the germinomatous and teratomatous forms; apparently both are formed by two distinct populations of cells. It must, however, be remembered that the transitions are fluid for the teratomatous tumors.

Grossly, they form large masses, the benign varieties being well circumscribed and firm, whereas the more malignant ones are infiltrative at the border and soft, hemorrhagic, and necrotic. The latter have a tendency to disseminate throughout the cerebrospinal fluid space.

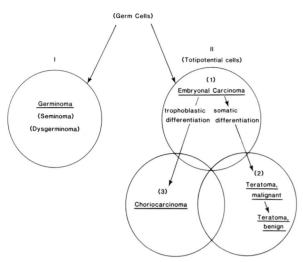

Figure 7–45. Schematic representation of the interrelationships among various types of "germ cell tumors."

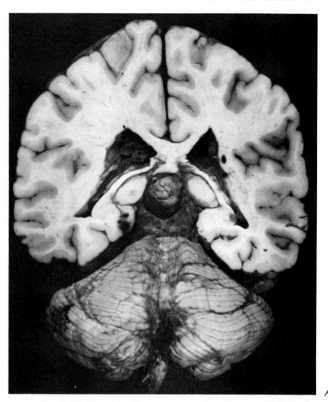

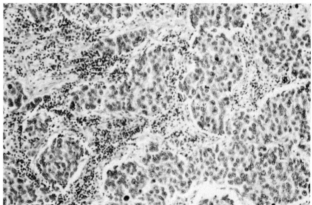

Figure 7–46. Germinoma. *A,* Pineal tumor. *B,* Typical histologic (H&E) features.

1. Germinoma

These tumors are histologically identical to seminomas of the testis and dysgerminomas of the ovary and are composed of characteristic large, uniform cells with clear cytoplasm that resembles primordial germ cells, supported by varying amounts of lymphoid or granulomatous stroma. They are of a relatively low grade of malignancy and are highly radiosensitive.

The pineal region is most often involved (60 to 80%), and the suprasellar region is second in frequency.

Their sites of predilection are as follows:

a. The pineal gland

This is the most frequent site of involvement by intracranial germinomas, which account for more than 50% of all tumors in this region. As such, pineal germinomas were previously known simply as "pinealoma" (see section 7.2, D). Occasionally, they arise not in the pineal gland but in the adjacent tissue.

b. The midline hypothalamic (or suprasellar) region

Germinomas in this region were previously called "ectopic pinealomas."

Initially, germinomas appear as well-defined, soft, friable, granular, and grayish red tumors, but they soon begin to disseminate through the cerebrospinal fluid pathway and infiltrate the adjacent tissue.

The neoplasms and tumors discussed here are relatively rare, constituting only 1 to 2% of intracranial tumors of all ages. In childhood, their frequency is roughly 2 to 4%.

A pronounced male preponderance is well known. The peak incidence is in the latter half of the second decade.

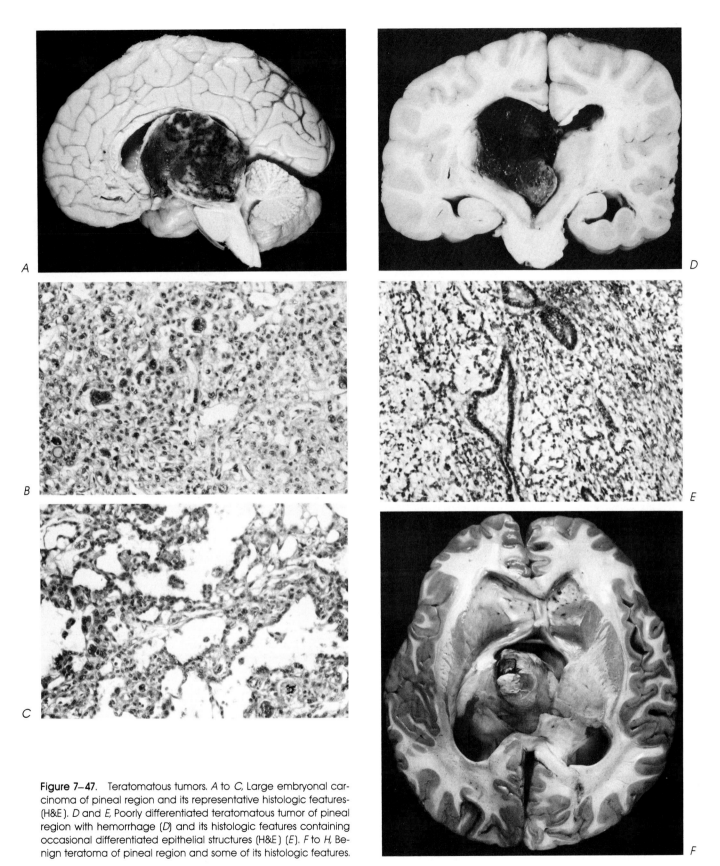

Figure 7–47. Teratomatous tumors. *A* to *C,* Large embryonal carcinoma of pineal region and its representative histologic features (H&E). *D* and *E,* Poorly differentiated teratomatous tumor of pineal region with hemorrhage (*D*) and its histologic features containing occasional differentiated epithelial structures (H&E) (*E*). *F* to *H,* Benign teratoma of pineal region and some of its histologic features.

(Continued)

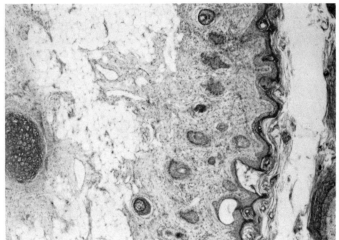

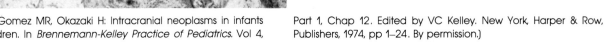

G

H

(A From Gomez MR, Okazaki H: Intracranial neoplasms in infants and children. In *Brennemann-Kelley Practice of Pediatrics*. Vol 4, Part 1, Chap 12. Edited by VC Kelley. New York, Harper & Row, Publishers, 1974, pp 1–24. By permission.)

2. "Teratomatous" group

These encompass three subgroups, all being derived from totipotential cells. Mixtures are not uncommon, and the entire group should be considered as the expression of a continuum of differentiation.

a. Embryonal carcinomas are undifferentiated tumors composed of cells that have an embryonic and anaplastic epithelial appearance and show a variable pattern of acinar, tubular, papillary, or solid and reticular structures. The tumors mimic different stages of embryonal development—being completely undifferentiated, having early somatic differentiation, having early trophoblastic differentiation, or being mixed.

b. Teratomas represent lesions that have differentiated along embryonic lines. They are complex tumors with recognizable elements of more than one germ layer in various stages of maturation: (1) immature—composed of primitive neuroectoderm, entoderm, or mesoderm tissues; (2) intermediate—with maturation to the tissue level (cartilage, bone, etc.); (3) differentiated (organoid)—tumors with areas that show abortive organ formation (e.g., neural, gastrointestinal, respiratory); and (4) mixed (more frequent).

Note: Commonly and for the sake of simplicity, teratomas are considered in terms of the malignant-benign continuums, since the more immature the components of a tumor are, the more likely it is to behave like a malignant one. However, considerable confusion exists in the teratoma terminology, particularly in the usage of the following terms, which have been used to mean different conditions by different authors.

• "Malignant teratomas" may mean embryonal carcinoma, which in turn is synonymous with teratocarcinoma (see below) to some authors; teratoma, with more primitive tissue (= "teratoid," see below); or malignancy in teratoma (as used here), which may be total or nearly total malignancy, but sometimes with one or two differentiated elements (e.g., so-called rhabdomyo-

sarcoma, in which differentiation toward striated muscle occurs among otherwise undifferentiated cells), or malignancy of one component only—for example, overgrowth of the epithelial component—which results in a teratocarcinoma.

• Many authors advocate abandonment of the term "teratoid" because of the vagueness of its definition. The term has been used to designate mixed tumor containing elements of one or two embryonic layers, in contrast to all three layers required for the old definition of a teratoma; teratomas with more primitive elements, which confer malignant features (including germinomas); or the entire group of germ cell tumors listed above, except for those composed of mature elements (that is, mature or benign teratomas).

c. Choriocarcinomas are examples of differentiation along the extraembryonic pathways and are composed solely of cytotrophoblastic and syncytiotrophoblastic cells without true villous formation. Yolk sac carcinoma is a recently recognized (though still controversial) entity and also belongs to this subgroup. It is histologically characterized by the presence of "endodermal sinuses," perivascular endodermal cells, and many thin-walled cystic spaces (synonym: endodermal sinus tumor).

B. Dermoid and epidermoid (or dermoid cyst and epidermoid cyst) (Fig. 7–48)

Some authors include these lesions in the group of teratomatous tumors discussed above as being examples of one-sided development within originally more complex (multiple germ layers) tumors. In fact, on occasion, as in the ovaries, more careful search will reveal other tissue elements in small amounts elsewhere in what are thought to be dermoids and epidermoids. Other authors consider them to be unrelated to teratomas and prefer to classify them separately, as resulting from inclusion of the epithelial elements at the time of closure of the neural groove (between the third and fifth weeks of gestation).

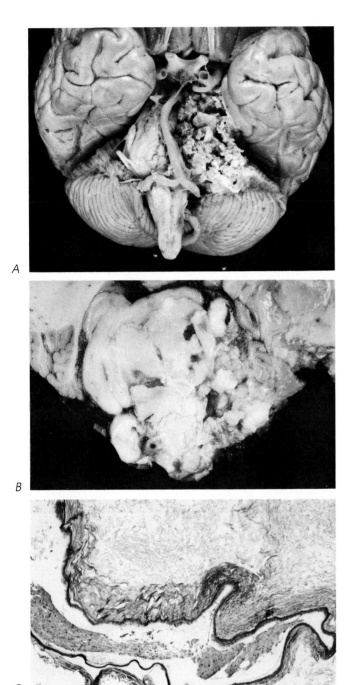

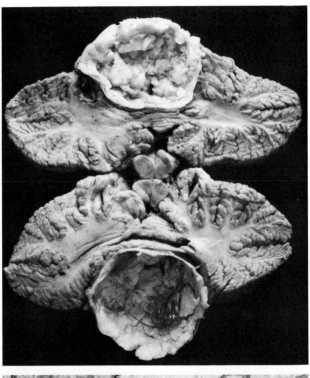

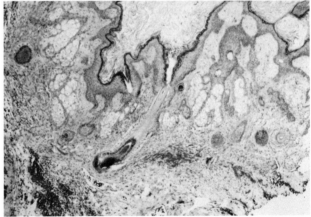

Figure 7–48. Epidermoid and dermoid. *A*, Epidermoid of left cerebellopontine angle with upward extension. *B*, Cross section of medulla with multiple indentations by an epidermoid of the cerebellopontine angle. *C*, Close-up of histologic appearance. *D*, Dermoid of midline posterior cerebellum (note hair inside cyst). *E*, Histologic (H&E) features of dermoid (with skin adnexae).

Although these two lesions are often grouped together under the name of "pearly tumors" because of desquamated keratin, which gives a "sheen" to the gross appearance of these tumors, there are enough differences in the clinical and anatomic patterns between the two types to warrant separate but contrasting descriptions.

Dermoid

These are well-defined lobulated masses containing thick, butter-yellow mate-rial. A dermal sinus may be present in the spinal and occipital regions.

The lining of the cysts is a stratified squamous epithelium with dermal appendages (hair follicles and sebaceous and sweat glands). The content is secretions of sebaceous glands and desquamated epithelium.

Epidermoid

These are well-defined masses (mainly extra-axial) with an irregular outer surface and a shiny "mother-of-pearl" appearance. Inside, they are filled with soft, flaky material that is rich in cholesterol crystals.

The lining is a simple, stratified squamous epithelium with a variable degree of keratinization (which fills the cyst) on a thin connective tissue layer. Desqua-

It occurs principally in the third decade in its intraspinal form. The sites of involvement are as follows:

(1) The spinal canal, mainly lumbosacral (intra- or extramedullary). Spina bifida may coexist. Some of the lesions may be produced by repeated lumbar puncture, which carries elements of skin intrathecally, as in the case of tuberculous meningitis in children.

(2) The posterior fossa, in the midline vermis or in the fourth ventricle

(3) Infrequently in other intracranial locations, mainly at the base of the brain

mated epithelium fills the cyst.

The portion adjacent to the brain tissue often shows an extensive and complicated pattern of invagination into the parenchyma.

It occurs in highest incidence in the fourth, fifth, and sixth decades. Sites of involvement (in order of frequency) show a large variation of locations and deviation from the midline:

(1) cerebellopontine angle
(2) parapituitary region (middle fossa, embedded in the temporal lobe)
(3) cranial diploes (mainly frontal and parietal)
(4) spinal (at all levels with or without a defect in the spine and a dermal sinus)

The spilling of the contents of the cyst (such as during surgery) in both lesions will elicit "chemical" meningitis, sometimes with fatal outcome.

C. Lipoma (Fig. 7–49)

These are rare and often clinically silent tumors, except in the spinal canal; they have been found in all age ranges. They are composed of adipose tissue and a variable amount

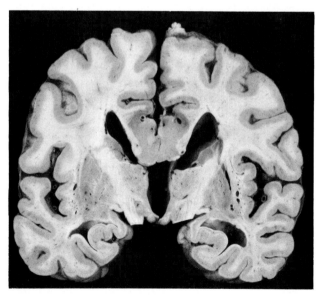

Figure 7–49. Lipoma. Large tumor is associated with partial (posterior) absence of corpus callosum.

of vascular elements, collagen and muscle fibers, glial cells, and ganglion cells, which are indicative of their malformative nature. Calcification and ossification are not infrequent.

Sites of involvement are as follows:
1. Intracranial

They occur most commonly in the midline, especially over the corpus callosum (which often shows partial or complete agenesis), the tuber cinereum, and the midbrain tectum (quadrigeminal plate).

2. Spinal (representing about 1% of all spinal tumors)

The majority occur in the thoracic region (intradural and extramedullary, occasionally intramedullary), commonly in the second and third decades. In one-third of cases these tumors are associated with other congenital abnormalities, for example spina bifida, bifid spinal cord, and meningomyelocele.

D. Neuroepithelial ectopic tumors and hamartomas

Note: Hamartomas are essentially nonneoplastic malformations that are characterized by an abnormal mixture of tissue indigenous to the site, grow much slower than true neoplasms, and generally do not display a potential for malignancy. The separation from true neoplasm is often difficult, as in neurofibromatosis (see section 7.7), and the classification may be considered as flexible and arbitrary at present.

1. Ectopic gliomas
   a. Cranial examples

   These are tumors occurring at the bridge of the nose ("nasal glioma") or, more rarely, in the soft palate and associated with an underlying bony defect in the cribriform plate, through which the tumors are attached to the interior of the cranium. These lesions are regarded by most authors as essentially hamartomatous and are composed of a mixture of fibrillary glial tissue and vascular connective tissue.

   b. Spinal examples
   • Intradural-extramedullary

   They are, histologically, astrocytomas or ependymomas, usually in the lumbosacral region, and they are often associated with spina bifida occulta.
   • Extraspinal

   They are usually ependymomas capable of producing considerable erosion of the sacral bone and further anterior extension (presacral ependymoma). They are symptomatic in adult life.

2. Hypothalamic ganglionic hamartoma

This is redundant gray matter usually (but not always) attached to the tuber or the mamillary bodies. It shows male preponderance with precocious puberty (probably by mechanical effects on the hypothalamus).

3. Granular cell tumor of the neurohypophysis (choristoma)

This is usually a microscopic tumor found incidentally in the pituitary stalk and the pars nervosa, especially in the older age group. The tumor is composed of large cells with finely granular cytoplasm, whose nature and origin are uncertain. Identical tumors are well known in the soft tissue elsewhere in the body.

Occasionally, larger tumors, which may compress the optic chiasm or invade the floor of the third ventricle, are reported.

4. Craniopharyngioma (Fig. 7–50)

This is one of the most common supratentorial neoplasms in childhood; 50% of cases occur in the first and second decades, and there is a second peak in the fifth decade.

They are well-defined tumors of varying size in the suprasellar region, being either largely cystic (containing straw-colored, motor-oil-like fluid rich in cholesterol) or partially solid and cystic. Gritty foci of calcification are frequent. They may elevate and infiltrate the chiasmatic and hypothalamic regions or grow primarily inside the third ventricle. Less often, they extend into the pituitary fossa or project posteriorly along the ventral aspect of the pons. Exceptionally, they directly invade the basal ganglia, the frontal or temporal lobes, or the brainstem parenchyma.

The tumor is basically composed of epithelial cells, the outside layer being formed by uniform columnar cells resting on a collagen basement membrane and the internal portions being either squamous with pearly keratin formations (with subsequent calcification) or composed of loosely arranged stellate cells. Between the cords is loose stromal tissue, which often degenerates and becomes hemorrhagic; microcysts and, later, large, confluent cysts result. Some examples appear simply to consist of a large cyst lined by stratified squamous keratinizing epithelium, indistinguishable from the epidermoid cysts discussed previously. The term "suprasellar cysts" is often applied to these lesions. At the margins of the tumor, there is a pronounced tendency for the epithelial fronds to penetrate deep into the brain tissue; this makes complete tumor resection difficult. An intense reactive gliosis rich in Rosenthal fibers is seen in the invaded brain tissue.

The origin of the tumor cells is undetermined. Proposed cell origins include (1) ? simply another form of midline congenital tumor not fundamentally different from epidermoid cysts; (2) ? inclusion of the dental anlage tissue (identical to "adamantinoma" or ameloblastoma of the jaw); and (3) ? squamous cell nests normally found at the junction of the pituitary stalk and the pars distalis, considered to be remnants of Rathke's pouch (Erdheim's rests). Many authors now regard these as metaplastic in nature.

5. Intrasellar Rathke pouch cleft cysts (intrasellar cysts of Rathke pouch origin)

These represent an enlarged version of the cleft often normally found between the pars distalis and the pars intermedialis, lined by cuboidal and occasionally ciliated epithelium and considered to be the genuine remnants of the original Rathke pouch. The term has been erroneously applied by some authors to craniopharyngiomas. Occasional examples extend beyond the diaphragma sellae and compress the rest of the pituitary gland. Spontaneous hemorrhage may

occur into the cystic space. They are, however, rarely symptomatic.

6. Leptomeningeal (or arachnoid) cyst (Fig. 7–51)

These are considered by most as being developmental in origin—that is, a malformation, not a neoplasm—but are discussed here with tumors for convenience. They often present as space-occupying lesions.

The lesions consist of a sac filled with cerebrospinal fluid-like fluid. The sac is produced by splitting of the arachnoid membrane, and it causes varying degrees of compression of the brain tissue underneath.

Characteristic locations are (1) the anterior portion of the sylvian tissue, commonly associated with a malformed or poorly developed temporal lobe, with few clinical signs; (2) the paracollicular region or cisterna ambiens, commonly associated with compression of the aqueduct and resulting in hydrocephalus; (3) the cerebellopontine angle; (4) the region of the cisterna magna; and (5) the cerebellar hemisphere.

7. Enterogenic cyst

This lesion is usually intraspinal in location and is composed of a cyst lined by mucin-secreting epithelium resembling that of the gastrointestinal tract.

7.7 PHAKOMATOSES

This is a group of diseases that are genetically determined and familial and that have in common an association of distinctive malformations of the neuraxis with small tumors (phakomas = lentil-like neoplasias). These involve the skin, the nervous system, and the eye. They are also collectively referred to as "neurocutaneous syndrome," a term that is too restrictive because dysplastic processes are more widespread in most instances than the term indicates. The following relatively common conditions are considered here:

A. Tuberous sclerosis
B. Multiple neurofibromatosis (Recklinghausen's disease)
C. Sturge-Weber disease
D. Von Hippel-Lindau disease
E. Neurocutaneous melanoma and primary meningeal melanoma

A. Tuberous sclerosis (tuberous sclerosis complex; Bourneville's disease) (Fig. 7–52)

The disease is transmitted as a mendelian dominant trait with clinical manifestations appearing in childhood or adolescence. Occasionally, mental retardation and epilepsy begin early in life.

Pathologic lesions include the following:

1. Cortical nodules (tubera or tubers)

These are superficial foci of cortical gliosis containing abnormal (large, bizarre) neuronal and glial cells with abnormal cyto-architecture. They occur mostly in the cerebral, infrequently in the cerebellar, cortices.

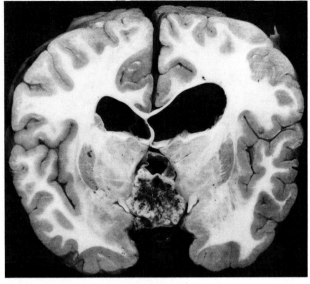

A

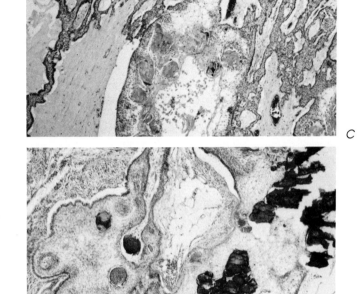

C

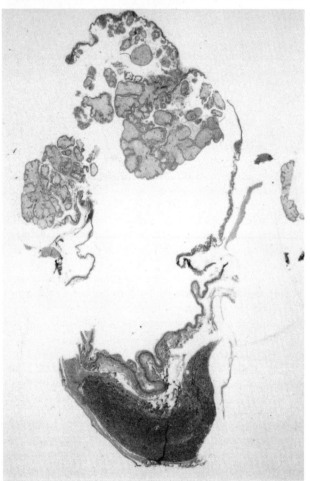

B

D

Figure 7–50. Craniopharyngioma. *A,* Partially (dorsal portion) cystic tumor projecting into third ventricle. *B,* Photomacrograph of cystic tumor in midsagittal section, compressing pituitary gland. *C* and *D,* Two views of histologic features of tumor with degenerative changes and foci of calcification within epithelial cords (H&E).

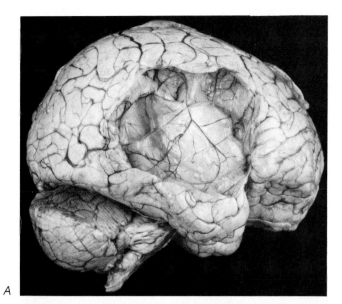

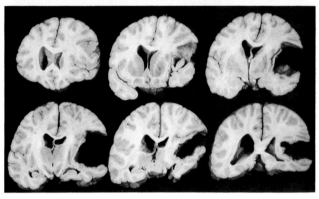

A

B

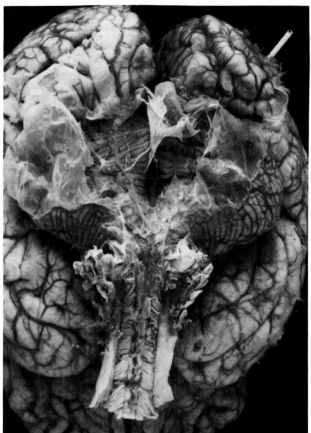

C

Figure 7–51. Leptomeningeal cyst. *A* and *B,* External (*A*) and cross-sectional (*B*) views of large cyst in right temporal lobe; outer membrane has been torn away. *C.* Posterior fossa cyst (underwater photograph) with outer membrane partially torn.

2. Glial nodules in the white matter
These are nests of atypical gemistocytic astrocytes.

3. Subependymal nodules
These are small, hard nodules that project into the lateral ventricles along the sulcus terminalis; they are partially embedded in the thalamus or caudate nucleus, and they have the characteristic gross appearance of "candle gutterings." Histologically, they consist of elongated, fibrillated, and gemistocytic astrocytes and are often calcified.

4. True neoplasms (relatively rare in the syndrome as a whole)
Giant cell astrocytomas arise from the above-mentioned subependymal lesions and are therefore mostly subependymal and intraventricular in location. Other tumors include malignant giant cell astrocytomas (glioblastomas), ependymomas, and diffuse gliomatosis of the cerebral hemispheres and brainstem.

5. A large gangliogliomatous tumor (essentially malformative in nature) replacing a cerebral hemisphere (rare).
Somatic lesions include (1) cutaneous lesions—peau de chagrin, subungual fibromas, adenoma sebaceum, and molluscum fibrosum pendulum; (2) visceral hamartomas—angiofibromas (kidney) and rhabdomyomas (myocardium); and (3) small retinal tumors, usually astrocytic.

B. Multiple neurofibromatosis (Recklinghausen's disease) (Fig. 7–53) (also see Fig. 7–30)

This is the commonest and the most varied of the phakomatoses. It is an autosomal dominant condition with highly variable phenotypic expression; it is relatively rare in the fully developed form, whereas abortive forms are most common.

The basic pathologic lesions are foci of hyperplasia and neoplasia of the supportive derivatives of the primitive ectoderm. Commonly added to this basic pathologic process are hyperplasia of nutritive elements (blood vessels) and, in rare instances, hyperplasia of parenchymatous elements.

Clinicopathologic varieties include:

1. Peripheral forms—peripheral and subcutaneous nerve sheath tumors and café-au-lait spots (multiple cutaneous tumors and large plexiform neurofibromas dominate)

2. Central forms—intracranial and spinal tumors (CNS

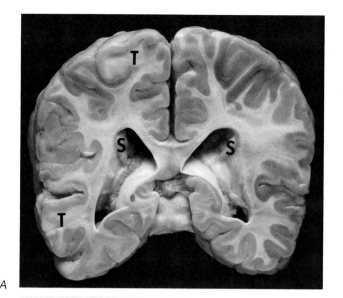

A

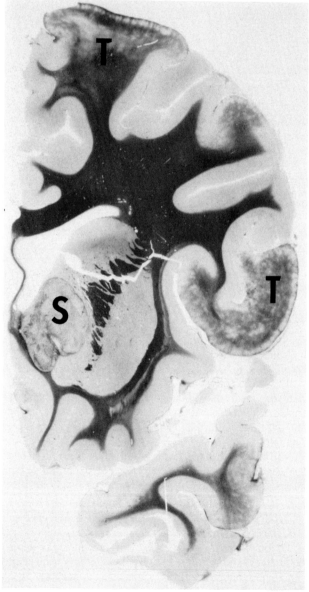

B

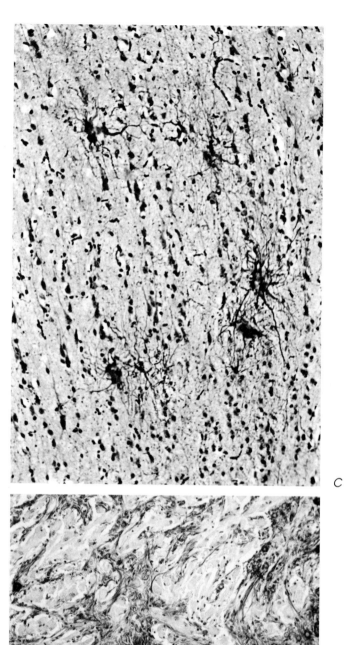

C

D

Figure 7–52. Tuberous sclerosis. *A*, Gross appearance of cortical tubera (*T*) and candle gutterings (i.e., subependymal nodules, *S*). *B*, Cortical (*T*) and subcortical (*S*) nodules, rich in glial fibers, of right frontal lobe are demonstrated by PTAH. *C*, Giant neurons in cortical nodule (Bodian). *D*, Clusters of gemistocytic astrocytes and their fibrous processes, constituting subependymal nodule (PTAH).

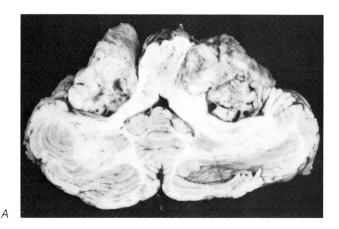

A

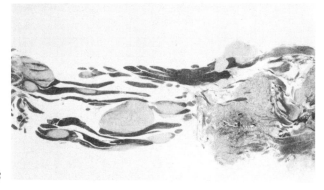

B

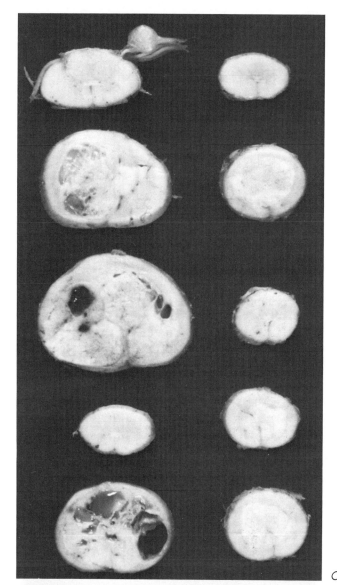

C

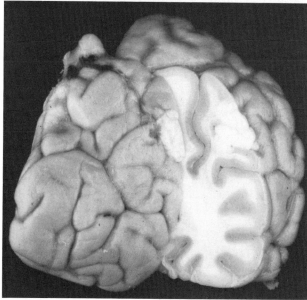

D

Figure 7–53. Multiple neurofibromatosis. *A*, Bilateral acoustic schwannomas. *B*, Multiple schwannomas (pale areas) along trigeminal nerve and gasserian ganglion (LFB/CV). *C*, Multiple (four) ependymomas of spinal cord. Note a small schwannoma in posterior root of an upper cervical segment. *D* and *E*, Meningioangiomatosis in right parietal lobe in gross (*D*) and histologic (H&E)

(Continued)

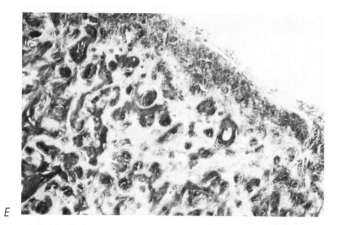

E

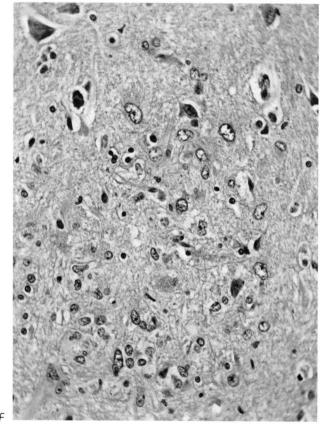

F

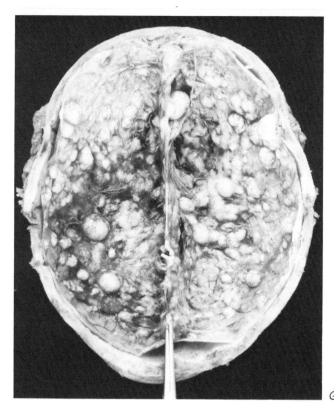

G

Figure 7–53. (Continued)

(*E*) appearance. *F,* Cortical nest of abnormal astrocytes (H&E). Meningiomatosis: inside view of convexity dura (*G*). (*F,* from Harlan WL, Okazaki H: Neurocutaneous diseases. In *Skin, Hereditary, and Malignant Neoplasms.* Edited by HT Lynch. Garden City, New York, Medical Examination Publishing Company, 1972, pp 104–148. By permission; *G,* previously published in Kepes JJ: *Meningiomas: Biology, Pathology, and Differential Diagnosis.* New York, Masson Publishing USA, 1982.)

parenchyma, coverings, and nerve roots) with few cutaneous manifestations

3. Visceral forms—neurofibromas and ganglioneuromas of the visceral or autonomic nervous system, especially in the mediastinum, mesentery, and retroperitoneal region; schwannomas occur as single or multiple tumors in the intestinal tract

4. Forme fruste—lesions limited in number
Pathologic features are as follows.

Peripheral lesions
a. Plexiform neurofibromas (characteristic of the disease)

These are circumscribed or poorly defined tumors occurring in any location (of the skin and deep tissue), often attaining a massive size, which feel like a "bag of worms" on palpation and tend to involve progressively the nerve of origin and grow toward the spinal cord and brain. These are associated with diffuse proliferation of compactly arranged spindle cells, apparently of perineurial or epineurial origin, into the surrounding tissue. Diffuse fibroblastic infiltration of the dermis and subcutis may also occur (neurofibrolipomatosis). The cutaneous hyperplasia has received the names "dermatolysis," "pachydermatocele," and "elephantiasis neuromatosa." The commonest sites are the temple, upper lid, and back of the neck.

b. Nonplexiform cutaneous neurofibromas (or molluscum fibrosum, fibroma molluscum)

These are sessile or pedunculated skin nodules; histologically, they are identical to solitary tumors. The presence of a few of these nodules does not necessarily constitute the syndrome.

c. Single or multiple schwannomas of the intestinal tract

d. Skin lesions—café-au-lait hyperpigmentation

e. Bone lesions, in the absence of any tumor in the region

They cause pressure, erosion, or destruction of the bone, including scoliosis and radiolucent lesions (fibrosis), pseudoarthrosis, and irregular cortical thickening.

f. Visceral lesions

There is local overgrowth of the soft tissue, causing hemihypertrophy, for example of the tongue, face, extremities, or viscera.

g. Glaucoma, buphthalmos, and involvement of the uveal coat are occasionally seen.

h. Pheochromocytoma

Central lesions

a. Schwannoma

These may be bilateral acoustic schwannomas (characteristic) or multiple other cranial and spinal nerve root schwannomas of varying sizes. Microscopic lesions may be considered as a form of schwannosis (see below).

b. Meningioma

These are characteristically multiple (and often diffuse); there is an unusually high frequency of choroid plexus meningiomas.

c. Glioma

• Pilocytic astrocytoma of the third ventricle and optic nerve glioma (astrocytoma)

Ten percent of all cases of these lesions occur in association with Recklinghausen's disease. Retinal astrocytomas also occur.

• Ependymoma

These are often multiple tumors and they usually occur in the spinal cord with or without syringomyelia; occasionally, they occur in the brainstem.

d. Malformations (hamartomas), which are often microscopic and diffuse

• Marginal gliosis and glial nests composed of pleomorphic, atypical glial cells, seen mainly in the cerebral cortex

• Subependymal nodules (such as those found in tuberous sclerosis)

• Ectopic ependymal cell nests mainly in the spinal cord

• Meningiomatosis or meningioangiomatosis

This is an indurated plaque in the cortex (and occasionally elsewhere), consisting of compact arrays of psammomatous meningeal elements, which appear to grow along, or are even incorporated among, the intersecting stroma of greatly thickened blood vessels

• Cortical angiomatosis

This is a simple vascular lesion without meningeal involvement in the cortex or the leptomeninges.

• Schwannosis

In this disorder, irregular extensions of Schwann cells occur within the spinal cord (and occasionally medulla), usually at dorsal nerve root entry sites (adjacent to schwannomatous nodules of the corresponding dorsal roots). Multiple, small, microscopic proliferations of this type are common in the cranial and spinal roots.

• Syringomyelia

• Disturbed cortical architecture and neuronal heterotopia

C. Sturge-Weber disease (Sturge-Weber-Dimitri disease, encephalo-trigeminal or meningofacial angiomatosis) (Fig. 7–54)

This sporadic disease is regarded as a malformation of the embryo's primitive vascular plexus, which precedes the formation of separate vessels for the supply of the integumentum, skull, and meninges. The basic pathology is as follows:

1. Leptomeningeal vascular malformation

This is composed of capillary and venous channels ("sinusoidal," "embryonal") with or without secondary degenerative fibrotic changes in their walls. Although the cortex is free of gross vascular malformation, occasional large blood vessels enter it and run toward the ventricular wall. Angiographically, these are functional, whereas the flow to the superior sagittal sinus over the surface is minimal.

2. Cortical calcification

It occurs first in and around capillaries and apparently is not preceded by other degenerative changes in the blood vessels or parenchyma. Its pathogenesis is uncertain.

3. Ipsilateral facial angiomatosis

Associated changes include (1) angiomatosis of choroid plexuses, pituitary stalk, and choroid of the eye, (2) neuronal heterotopia in the brain, (3) capsular cell proliferation and ectopic ganglion cells in the gasserian and spinal ganglia, and (4) angiomas of the lungs, intestine, and ovary.

D. Von Hippel-Lindau disease (Fig. 7–55)

This is a dominant or irregularly dominant disease, usually manifest in adulthood. It consists of the following triad:

1. Hemangioblastoma (hemangioendothelioma), at times multiple in the cerebellum, medulla (dorsal), and spinal cord (with or without syringomyelia)

2. Hemangioblastoma of the retina

3. Renal tumors, consisting of (a) simple cysts or polycystic kidneys or (b) adenoma or hypernephroma.

Associated lesions are pancreatic cyst, cysts or hemangioma of the liver, simple cyst and cystadenoma of the epididymis, and pheochromocytoma.

E. Neurocutaneous melanoma and primary meningeal melanoma (Fig. 7–56)

The following variants are recognized:

1. Neurocutaneous pigmentation

This is a rare, familial, nonneoplastic diffuse hyperpigmentation of the leptomeninges associated with cutaneous pigmented nevi.

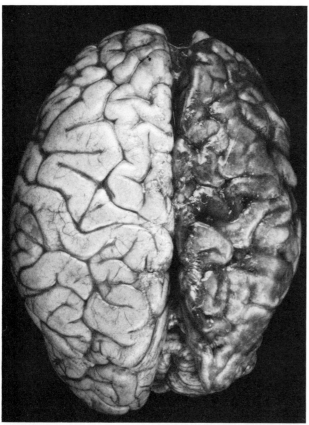

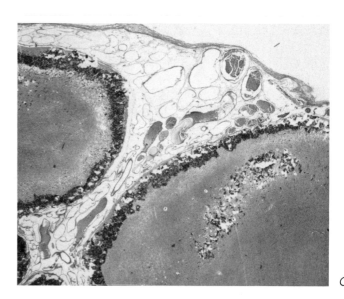

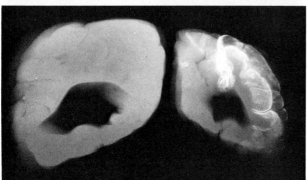

Figure 7–54. Sturge-Weber disease. *A*, Dorsal view of cerebral hemispheres. The right side is smaller and is covered with numerous small blood vessels, which give rise to a darker appearance. *B*, Roentgenograms of parietal brain slices with calcification of right side. *C*, Low-power view of leptomeninges filled with thin-walled vessels and layers of cortical calcification. (*A* from and *B* modified from Harlan WL, Okazaki H: Neurocutaneous diseases. In *Skin, Hereditary, and Malignant Neoplasms.* Edited by HT Lynch. Garden City, New York, Medical Examination Publishing Company, 1972, pp 104–148. By permission.)

2. Neurocutaneous melanosis

This form consists of a nonfamilial diffuse and often frankly invasive proliferation of melanin-containing cells throughout the leptomeninges, associated with giant cutaneous nevi. Most cases occur in infants under 2 years of age.

3. Primary meningeal melanoma

These tumors may or may not be associated with cutaneous nevi, and they occur either as circumscribed tumors or as a diffuse neoplastic process involving wide areas of the leptomeninges and often spreading through the cerebrospinal fluid space. At times, they show the appearance of primary tumors of intracerebral or spinal parenchyma.

Note: Tumors in the skin are often extensive, tending to localize over the posterior surface of the trunk. Two types are recognized: (1) benign lesions, which show features of ordinary cellular nevus, blue nevus, neurofibroma, and melanotic neurofibroma, and (2) malignant tumors, such as malignant melanomas.

7.8 SECONDARY NEOPLASMS OF THE CNS—DIRECT EXTENSION OF LOCAL TUMORS AFFECTING THE CRANIUM AND SPINE

A. Pituitary adenoma (Fig. 7–57)

When pituitary adenomas were originally classified by histologic features on the basis of relatively simple staining methods, three tumor cell types were recognized: eosino-

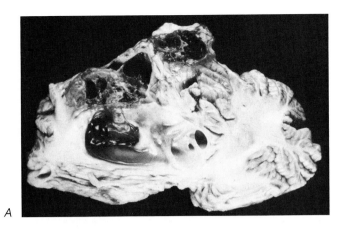

A

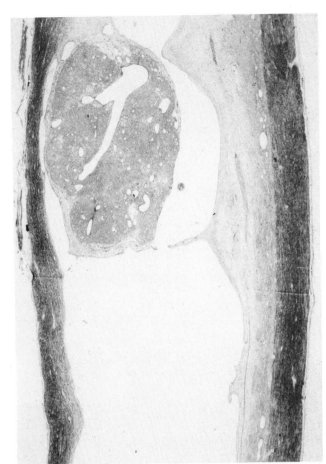

B

Figure 7–55. Von Hippel-Lindau disease. *A,* Multiple (three) hemangioblastomas of cerebellum, *B,* Longitudinal section (LFB/PAS/H) of spinal hemangioblastoma associated with syrinx.

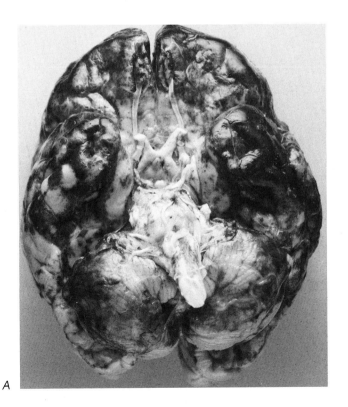

A

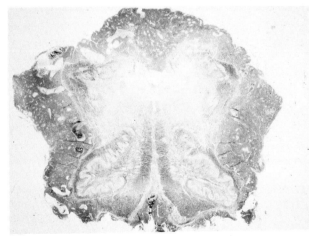

B

Figure 7–56. Diffuse meningeal melanomas. *A,* Basal view of brain. *B,* Diffuse infiltration of leptomeninges at level of medulla (LFB/CV).

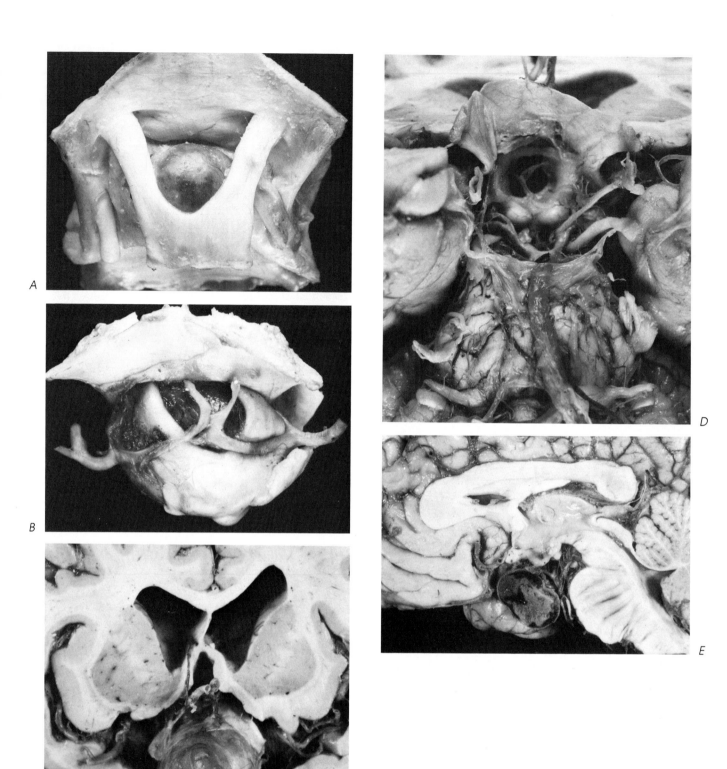

Figure 7–57. "Chromophobe" pituitary adenoma. *A*, Small tumor with prechiasmatic presentation. *B*, Medium-size tumor with asymmetric elevation and stretching of optic chiasm and A₁ segment of each anterior cerebral artery cutting into proximal optic nerves. *C* and *D*, Pronounced membranous stretching of optic chiasm as viewed (*C*) from front (with tumor) and (*D*) from below (without

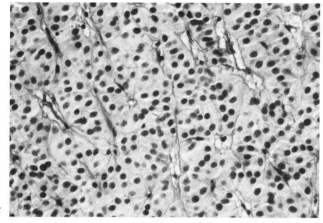

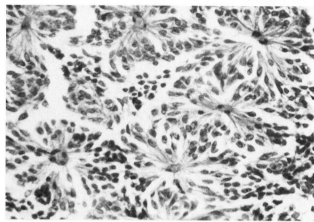

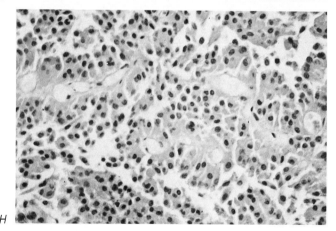

tumor). *E,* Small tumor with "pituitary apoplexy." *F* to *H,* Some of the histologic patterns of tumor cells (H&E). (*C, D,* and *E* courtesy of Kings County Hospital, Brooklyn, New York.)

philic, basophilic, and chromophobe cells. These were correlated with acromegaly and pituitary gigantism, Cushing's disease, and hypopituitary manifestations, respectively. It later became evident that the range of hormonal and clinical manifestations was much more complex, particularly as many so-called chromophobe adenomas were found to be associated with endocrine function.

More recently, the parallel development of radioimmunoassay for the detection of serum hormone levels and of safe and practical transsphenoidal hypophysectomy has made it possible to uncover and surgically treat many instances of functioning microadenomas of the anterior pituitary while these lesions are still intrasellar and lack clear radiologic findings. Recent advances in immunocytochemistry, particularly the immunoperoxidase technique, have given the pathologist methods for identifying hormones within cells. Electron microscopy has disclosed certain unusual ultrastructural features of pituitary tumor cells, but the functional importance of these structures is unclear.

On the basis of these new discoveries, more refined functional-morphologic classifications have been offered, such as that of Kovacs et al. (1980), which recognizes five main types: (1) prolactin (PRL) cell, (2) growth hormone (GH) cell, (3) mixed GH-PRL cell, (4) ACTH cell, and (5) undifferentiated cell adenomas (and their subtypes). In some cases, however, certain discrepancies may be found between hormonal levels and morphologic findings, because of biologic complexity and technical problems at surgery and in the laboratory.

Functionally active tumors manifest themselves by their hormonal activities before their size is significantly large, whereas tumors with little or no functional activity become clinically manifest only after their large size causes significant compression of the functioning pituitary cells and the surrounding nervous structures. The latter group of tumors has traditionally been called "chromophobe" because the tumor cells contain few if any granules stainable by conventional staining methods.

1. Pituitary adenomas with little or no recognizable functional activities ("chromophobe" adenomas)

These tumors are most commonly symptomatic in middle age and are very uncommon in children before adolescence. They are composed of cells without definite tinctorial affinity, arranged in a diffuse, sinusoidal, trabecular, or papillary pattern. They are not encapsulated within the anterior lobe but compress the normal cells toward the periphery. Hypopituitarism, however, develops rarely, and only after rather extensive compression and loss of the normal pituitary cells. Sparse secretory granules are present in many "chromophobe" adenomas under the electron microscope.

These tumors have a notorious tendency to expand beyond the confines of the sella after enlarging it. They may expand primarily in the cranial portion but eventually grow beyond the diaphragma sellae as a thinly encapsulated lobular mass. This may cause a number of changes, as follows:

a. Elevation and stretching of the optic chiasm, whose central crossed fibers suffer most (resulting in bitemporal hemianopsia). Occasionally, the A_1 segments of the anterior cerebral arteries cut into the optic nerves on their dorsal aspect. Approximately 85% of cases show some visual impairment at the time of diagnosis.

b. Compression of the hypothalamus and adjacent tissue (e.g., the basal ganglia), causing sympathetic disturbances or interruption of the hypothalamo-hypophyseal axis

c. Invasion into the third ventricle, causing obstructive hydrocephalus

With respect to malignancy, carcinomas are rarely reported. Since benign tumors often exhibit cellular atypism (probably "degenerative" in nature), the histologic diagnosis of carcinoma is sometimes uncertain. Some authors insist on evidence of extracranial metastasis before making the diagnosis of malignancy.

2. Functional (hormone-secreting) adenomas

Some of these tumors are "chromophobe" by conventional staining techniques. They are rarely large enough to cause compressive effects on the nervous tissues, although the sella may be enlarged roentgenographically. Many are "microadenomas." These tumors are notorious for their tendency to show cellular pleomorphism, nuclear hyperchromatism, and local venous permeation.

Depending on the hormones secreted, the following signs and symptoms are commonly encountered:

a. Gigantism and acromegaly (somatotropic [growth] hormone)

Most (some 90%) acromegalic patients have enlarged sellae. Histologically, "eosinophilic adenomas" are the tissue substrate.

b. Amenorrhea and galactorrhea complex or Forbes-Albright syndrome (prolactin)

Usually, microadenomas of the "chromophobe" type are found.

c. Cushing's syndrome (ACTH)

"Basophilic" microadenomas may be found.

Note: Questions have long been raised concerning the relationship between Cushing's syndrome (due to hypercortisolism) and pituitary dysfunction since Harvey Cushing (1932) concluded, in a review of 12 patients, that basophilic pituitary adenomas were responsible in well over half the clinical cases. Recent reports appear to vindicate his conclusion. Nearly 70% of patients were found to have pituitary dysfunction or "pituitary-dependent" Cushing's syndrome (i.e., Cushing's disease), and 40 to 50% of these cases involved microadenomas of the basophilic type. The remainder of the cases were due equally to primary adrenal hyperplasia or tumor and to ectopic production of ACTH by nonpituitary tumors (the most frequent cause being carcinoma of the lung). A 90 to 95% remission rate is reported after transsphenoidal microadenomectomy.

It must be remembered that many basophilic microadenomas are seen at autopsy as an incidental finding, and it remains possible that the primary error lies in the hypothalamus, where an excess of corticotropin-releasing factor is secreted. It has also been suggested that when "chromophobe" adenomas display an increasing degree of aggressiveness, the association with Cushing's syndrome becomes progressively more common. Such association was noted in almost half of the reported cases of pituitary adenomas with extracranial dissemination.

Even in patients having predominantly neurologic symptoms, some degree of endocrine dysfunction can be demonstrated by appropriate testing. Clinical syndromes resulting from pituitary hormone hypersecretion are not in-variably accompanied by the presence of an adenoma, roentgenographically or histologically. In general, children and young adults more readily demonstrate endocrine abnormalities, whereas older patients more often present with symptoms due to pressure from the expanding mass.

B. Paraganglioma (chemodectoma) of the glomus jugulare (Fig. 7–58)

These tumors originate in the middle ear from the glomus jugulare and are capable of invading the posterior fossa. Up to 40% of patients with this tumor present with neuro-

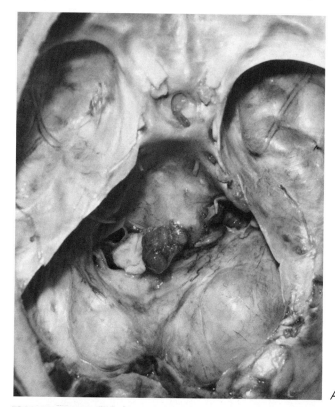

A

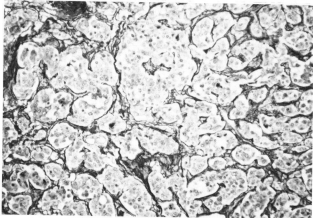

B

Figure 7–58. Chemodectoma of glomus jugulare. *A,* Right-sided tumor projecting into foramen magnum and causing compression of lower medulla. *B,* Typical histologic appearance with "Zellballen" (reticulin).

logic symptoms referrable to a posterior fossa or cerebellopontine angle mass.

The architecture of the tumor resembles that of the normal organ but in a state of glandular hyperplasia or "proliferative caricature." Ovoid to polygonal cells with a more than usual degree of pleomorphism are partitioned into cell clusters ("Zellballen") by vascular connective tissue stroma.

C. Chordoma (Fig. 7–59)

These tumors originate from intraosseous vestigial remnants of the notochord and are composed of compact masses or cords of cells containing PAS- and mucicarmine-positive material surrounded by a basophilic matrix separated into lobules by fibrous connective tissue septa. They appear as a soft or firm, lobulated, partially hemorrhagic mass, which is locally invasive and capable of extensive bone destruction. Sites of predilection are the following:

1. Sacrococcygeal

This is the most common site (roughly 50%). The tumors may extend into the epidural space, invade the dura, and surround the cauda equina roots.

2. Clivus (spheno-occipital region)

Tumors in this location often project intracranially, causing compression of the pons and medulla. Otherwise, they grow into the nasopharynx or paranasal sinuses.

3. Spinal column (15%)

A histopathologically separate group (approximately one-third) of spheno-occipital chordomas has been recognized which have a surprisingly better prognosis. These tumors show combinations of chordoid and chondroid elements, which may bear a striking histologic resemblance to chondromas or chondrosarcoma and are designated "chondroid" chordoma.

D. Carcinoma arising in the ear, mastoid cavity, and nasopharynx

Carcinomas may become neurologically manifest by (1) affecting multiple cranial nerves as they traverse the affected areas of the bone, (2) penetrating the base of the skull and infiltrating the leptomeninges and cranial nerve roots, or (3) disseminating throughout the cerebrospinal fluid spaces (less frequently).

7.9 METASTATIC NEOPLASMS (FIG. 7–60 TO 7–62)

Involvement of the nervous system by metastasizing neoplasms arising elsewhere in the body may, for convenience, be divided into two categories.

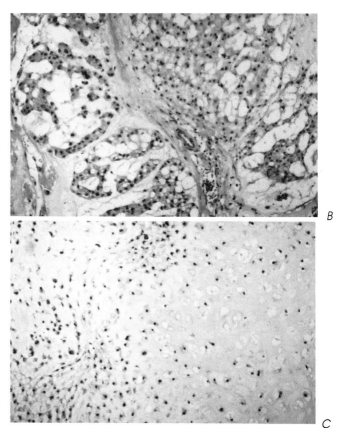

Figure 7–59. Chordoma of base of brain. *A,* Dorsal view of larger tumor of clivus. *B,* Histologic features of tumor (H&E). *C,* Chondroid chordoma variety of tumor (H&E).

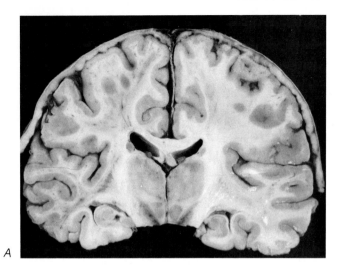

A

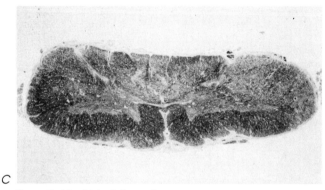

C

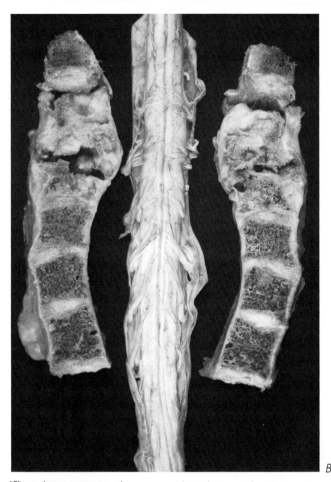

B

Figure 7–60. Metastatic malignancies to bone and dura. A, Diffuse subdural deposits of carcinoma of lung. B and C, Focal metastatic encroachment on cervical cord by adenocarcinoma of lung (B), and appearance of compressed cord segment on cross section (LFB/CV) (C).

Indirect involvement by metastatic foci outside the nervous tissue, which act as compressing masses. Lesions in the cranial and vertebral bones and the dura are considered to be in this category.

Direct hematogenous involvement of the nervous system (mainly the central nervous system) parenchyma and its leptomeningeal covering. Direct parenchymal involvement of the peripheral nervous system is rarely seen and will not be considered further.

Malignant lymphomas have already been considered in both of the above categories (see section 7.5), in part because of the possibility that multiple lesions are multicentric in origin rather than metastatic from one focus to others.

A. Metastatic neoplasms in the skull, spine, and dura mater

These may be neuropathologically significant in the following manners.

1. Spinal

Compression of the spinal cord or nerve roots by growth of tumors into the epidural space or by collapse of the vertebral column is frequent. Carcinomas of the breast, lung, and prostate are common primary lesions. Transgression of the dura is very unusual, and direct involvement of the spinal cord rarely occurs. Pathologic changes seen in the cord parenchyma are discussed in section 2.7.

2. Cranial

Involvement of the dura and formation of subdural deposits can cause varying degrees of brain compression. Here too, the leptomeninges tend to act as a barrier against contiguous involvement of the brain substance.

a. Nodular forms, often multiple, cause usually mild cerebral compression. Carcinomas of the breast and, to a lesser extent, of the lung are frequent primary lesions. Obliteration of venous sinuses, either by direct tumor invasion alone or by a complication of thrombosis, may occur.

b. Diffuse forms, which are often hemorrhagic, occasionally lead to the formation of a subdural hematoma (particularly with carcinomas of the breast or stomach with extensive bony metastasis and myelophthisic anemia), which in turn causes cerebral compression.

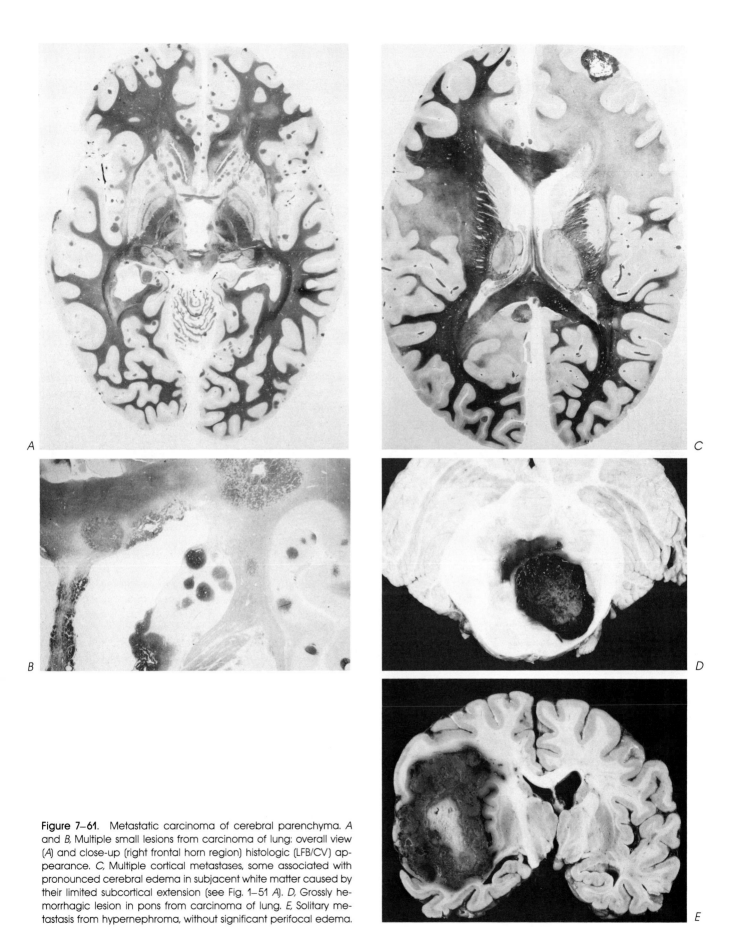

Figure 7–61. Metastatic carcinoma of cerebral parenchyma. *A* and *B,* Multiple small lesions from carcinoma of lung: overall view (*A*) and close-up (right frontal horn region) histologic (LFB/CV) appearance. *C,* Multiple cortical metastases, some associated with pronounced cerebral edema in subjacent white matter caused by their limited subcortical extension (see Fig. 1–51 *A*). *D,* Grossly hemorrhagic lesion in pons from carcinoma of lung. *E,* Solitary metastasis from hypernephroma, without significant perifocal edema.

(Continued)

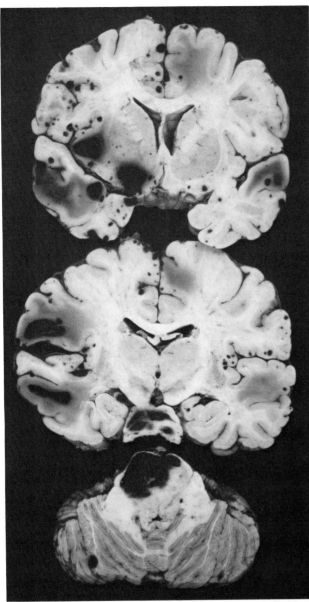

F

Figure 7–61. *F,* Multiple metastatic melanomas, most of them with gross hemorrhage.

B. Direct hematogenous metastases to the CNS and its coverings

The incidence of metastatic malignancies (mostly carcinomas, rarely sarcomas) among brain tumors (they are rare in the spinal cord) varies according to the sources (autopsy versus surgical material; general versus specialty institutions; symptomatic versus incidental cases, and so on), ranging from 4.0 to 37%. A rough estimate is that 20% of clinically significant brain tumors are metastatic in origin. It is also estimated that roughly 10 to 15% of all fatal malignancies have cerebral metastases.

1. The following are the most important sources in neurologic practice:
   a. Lung
   Tumors of the lung are particularly important because of the frequency (up to 30%) with which the primary carcinomas are silent when CNS signs and symptoms first emerge. Roughly 40% of lung cancers will metastasize to the brain.
   b. Breast
   Roughly 25% of breast tumors will metastasize to the brain. Together with lung cancers, they constitute roughly 60% of the metastatic primaries.
   c. Kidney (renal cell carcinoma)
   d. Gastrointestinal tract (mainly the colon)
   e. Melanoma (up to 15% of all metastatic carcinomas in the CNS in some series)

Note: 1. Primary sites stressed in the literature but rarely encountered in our practice are the stomach, prostate, and thyroid gland.
   2. It is not always possible to determine the site of primary tumor from the microscopic appearance of metastasis.

2. Several patterns, not mutually exclusive, are recognized as follows:
   a. Parenchymal nodular implantation
   Well-defined, circumscribed nodules of varying size, either solid or partially cystic (filled with mucinous material, necrotic debris, or hemorrhagic fluid). Most of these are multiple (80%), but in some series, a third to a half of symptomatic metastatic tumors are said to be single. Tumors with a high predilection for CNS spread tend to be multiple and others, such as renal and gastrointestinal malignancies, are more often solitary. The embolic origin of these nodules is rarely demonstrable even in small lesions, which are assumed to begin with small numbers of cells being arrested in the capillaries. It is believed that many of these tumor cells die or fail to establish a nidus; some cause infarction of the surrounding brain tissue (see d below).

   All the areas of the brain may be affected; the corticomedullary junction appears to be the favored starting point. The spinal parenchyma is rarely involved. The relative incidence in the various regions of the brain appears to be proportionate to their volumes. When the white matter is involved, perifocal edema is often present and is sometimes quite extensive, disproportionate to the size of the metastatic nodule.

   Extensive hemorrhage into metastatic nodules may occur, most characteristically with metastatic melanomas (frequent) and choriocarcinomas (with a low overall incidence). Lung carcinomas are also often hemorrhagic.
   b. Leptomeningeal carcinomatosis (''carcinomatous meningitis'')
   The pure form of this disorder is relatively infrequent; nodular parenchymal lesions are often found elsewhere to account for focal clinical symptoms.
   Diffuse infiltration of the subarachnoid space is

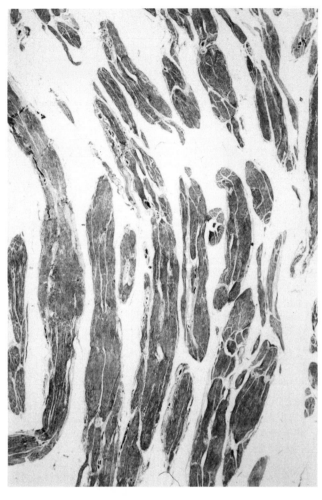

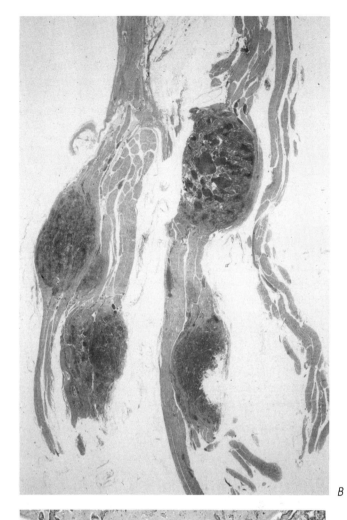

A

B

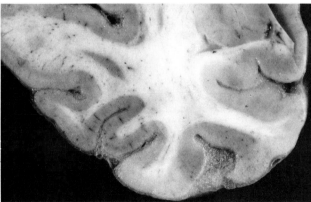

C

D

Figure 7–62. Diffuse metastatic carcinomatosis. *A*, Histologic (H&E) features of diffuse involvement of cauda equina roots. *B*, Histologic (H&E) features of more nodular involvement of cauda equina roots. *C* and *D*, Meningeal carcinomatosis to temporal lobe from adenocarcinoma of lung: close-up gross view (*C*) and histologic (H&E) appearance (*D*).

maximal over the base of the brain and in the posterior aspect of the spinal cord, with concomitant involvement of cranial and spinal nerve roots in it. The involvement may be quite subtle macroscopically, and its presence may be signalled by internal hydrocephalus, which it

produces. More apparent infiltration is usually found in the lumbosacral-cauda equina region.

The walls of the ventricular system may become involved, presumably as an extension of the meningeal spread. Commonly, further invasion into the CNS substance takes place via the perivascular spaces for a varying distance.

Adenocarcinomas, particularly from the lungs, gastrointestinal tract, breast, and ovaries, are most commonly responsible. Melanomas may be involved.

c. Parenchymal "encephalitic" type

This lesion consists of a diffuse perivascular pattern of infiltration, usually within relatively circumscribed areas of the parenchyma but also over a wide area and often in association with leptomeningeal carcinomatosis. It is sometimes referred to as "metastatic meningoencephalitic carcinomas without tumefaction."

d. Tumor embolism

This process was discussed with the vascular diseases. The parenchymal lesions, which are often multiple, consist almost exclusively of infarcts of various sizes distal to the occluded arteries. Intravascular and eventually extravascular proliferation of embolized tumor cells may occur secondarily to form metastatic nodules. Primary tumors tend to be those that retain cohesiveness of neoplastic cells, such as better-differentiated squamous cell carcinomas or adenocarcinomas. In contrast, the usual metastatic nodules are not preceded by histologically recognizable embolic vascular occlusion; this indicates that they are probably a result of small groups of isolated malignant cells, or even isolated ones, caught in capillary-size vessels.

Note: The pituitary gland is often shown to be involved when routine histologic examination of this tissue is performed. However, this is usually in the form of incidental microscopic lesions, which rarely produce clinical hypopituitary symptoms. Clinically more significant is involvement of the pituitary stalk, alone or in combination with that of the hypothalamus, which results in signs and symptoms of diabetes insipidus.

REFERENCES

Bailey P, Cushing H, Eisenhardt L: Angioblastic meningiomas. *Arch Pathol* 6:953–990, 1928.

Cushing H: The basophil adenomas of the pituitary body and their clinical manifestations (pituitary basophilism). *Bull Johns Hopkins Hosp* 50:137–195, 1932.

Dixon FJ, Moore RA: Tumors of the male sex organs. *In* Atlas of Tumor Pathology, Fascicles 31b and 32. Washington DC, Armed Forces Institute of Pathology, 1952.

Kovacs K, Ezrin C, Weiss MH, et al: *Pituitary Diseases.* Boca Raton, Florida, CRC Press, 1980.

Rappaport H: Tumors of the hematopoietic system. *In* Atlas of Tumor Pathology, Fascicle 8. Washington DC, Armed Forces Institute of Pathology, 1966.

8. *Perinatal Nervous System Damage and Malformations*

The lesions to be discussed in this chapter may be divided for convenience into two broad categories:

I. Congenital malformations
II. Perinatal encephaloclastic lesions

For the perinatal encephaloclastic lesions, the exogenous factor(s) responsible for the destruction of normally matured brain up to that point is more readily recognized or inferred. The majority of these lesions were previously lumped together under the term "birth injuries" and emphasis was placed on mechanical obstetric difficulties as the cause. In recent years, the greater importance of cerebral anoxia and ischemia has been recognized. "Cerebral palsies" is another term that is commonly used to cover the conditions under discussion, because it is the cerebral damage and its clinical manifestations that are most frequent and most prominent. The precise timing of the causative pathologic process is often difficult to determine, and the term "perinatal" conveniently encompasses the general time frame. The cause(s) of the malformation is often obscure. Some appear to be due to disturbances of genes and others are probably a result of exogenous factors (e.g., maternal measles infection) that affect the fetus in its early embryonic stage. When external abnormalities in the head or spine are absent, basically malformative lesions are likely to be lumped together with the "birth injury group." "Cerebral palsies" as a clinical term thus encompasses both malformations and encephaloclastic lesions. Table 8–1 summarizes the clinical and pathologic spectrum of the conditions under discussion.

I. Congenital malformation (8.1–8.6)

An etiologic classification of CNS malformations is not possible at present because in only a few instances are specific etiologic factors known. Therefore, one has to be content with a purely morphologic classification aided by the available information regarding normal fetal development, which might help us reconstruct the "when" and "how" of various malformative end results. Although this too is possible only on a limited scale, the following tentative scheme is employed in order to gain some insight into the morphogenesis (or formal pathogenesis) of these disorders (Table 8–2).

8.1 DISORDERS OF CLOSURE: DYSRAPHIC STATES

A spectrum exists between the two forms described below, and individual lesions are seen in all degrees of severity.

A. The major forms of dysraphism (Fig. 8–1)

1. Craniorachischisis totalis (cranio + rachis [= spine] + schisis [= fissure or cleft]), or total failure of closure of the neural tube

2. Anencephaly (exencephalia acrania)

Defective closure of the anterior end of the neural tube—a partial (cerebral) form of craniorachischisis totalis. Many of the anencephalic fetuses are spontaneously aborted in prematurity. There are associated defects of the cranial vault and scalp. The brain is absent or rudimentary and is represented by fibroglial tissue containing islands of neural elements and networks of thin-walled, small and large vascular channels (the area cerebrovasculosa) resting on the base of the skull. Cystic spaces lined by ependymal cells or containing the choroidal tissue are not uncommon. At times, the brainstem and cerebellum may be spared or less severely involved. The eyes are, as a rule, well formed, although the optic nerves are rudimentary or cannot be traced. This indicates that part of this malformation is secondary to destruction of the previously formed portions of the brain, rather than being purely dysplastic. Fifty percent of the cases show absence and hypoplasia of the pituitary gland associated with hypoplasia of the adrenal glands.

3. Amyelia

Total absence of the spinal cord, found only in association with anencephaly.

B. More limited forms of dysraphism

1. Cranium bifidum with (meningo-) encephalocele (= exencephalus) (Fig. 8–2)

Protrusion of brain substance or portion of brain and meninges through a congenital opening of the skull. This disorder is really due to failure of development of the overlying mesenchymal tissue, with a local cerebral "blow out"; the brain itself is not truly dysraphic. The posterior (midoc-

TABLE 8–1. Clinical and Pathologic Spectrum of Cerebral Palsies

I. Clinical	Time of inception of disease	Prenatal (50–70%)	"Perinatal"
		Natal (30%)	
		Postnatal (the rest)	
	Basic symptoms	Spastic paresis	approx 50%
		Dyskinesias	approx 40%
		Chorea	
		Athetosis	
		Dystonia	
		Tremor	
		Rigidity	
		Ataxia	approx 10%
		Combinations	common
	Commonly associated symptoms	Mental deficiency	
		Severe	30%
		Significant	>50%
		Convulsive disorders	about 35%
	Course	Essentially nonprogressive	
II. Neuroanatomic	Localization of lesions	Pyramidal system	
		Extrapyramidal system	
		Cerebellum (infrequent)	
		(Spinal and peripheral)	
III. Pathologic			
Type and origin	Pathologic processes	Morphologic conditions	
Systemic disorders producing brain lesions	Anoxia neonatorum	Elective parenchymal necrosis	
		Lobar sclerosis	
		Ulegyria	
		Leukomalacia	
		Status marmoratus	
		Hemorrhage (matrix and ventricular)	
	Erythroblastosis	Kernicterus	
	Toxic (carbon monoxide, alcoholism)		
Local intracranial pathogenetic processes	Mechanical injuries	Meningeal hemorrhage; contusion and laceration of brain	
	Circulatory disorders	Hemorrhages	
		Ischemia/infarct	
	Infections	Herpes simplex virus, cytomegalovirus, and *Toxoplasma* encephalitides	
	Hydrocephalus	Compressive parenchymal damage	
Developmental defects of brain	Arrest of growth and differentiation	Cerebral hypogenesis and dysgenesis (rarely hypergenesis)	

cipital and occipitocervical) type is by far the commonest in fatal cases. The herniated portions may include not only the posterior cerebral hemispheres (with or without the ventricular cavities and often dysplastic) but also the brainstem (with the aqueduct) and cerebellum.

2. Spina bifida (Fig. 8–3) with:
  a. Meningocele
    Subcutaneous herniation of the meninges through a defective closure of the vertebral arch
  b. Meningomyelocele
    Herniation of both the leptomeninges and the spinal cord
  c. Myelocystocele
    Myelomeningocele with dilatation of the central canal and thinning of the posterior portion of the cord

  d. Myeloschisis (with rachischis)
    The spinal cord forms a flat disk of vascular tissue that contains remnants of the neural tissue (the area medullovasculosa, equivalent of the pseudoencephalic mass or area cerebrovasculosa). This represents a spinally localized component of craniorachischisis totalis described above. It may involve the entire length of spinal cord or only a part of it.
  e. Diastematomyelia
    Two cord segments are separated by a spur of fibrous collagenous or bony tissue. Fifty percent of cases are associated with myelocystocele and myeloschisis (cleft spinal cord).

Also probably belonging to the category of dysraphic states are the following disorders.

TABLE 8-2. Morphogenesis of Congenital Malformations

Major Events*	Types of Malformation
1. Closure of the neural tube (during the fourth week)	Disorders of closure
2. Enlargement of the prosencephalon to form the telencephalic vesicles, which will later expand dramatically. The right and left ridges each grow forward and backward above and lateral to the upper brainstem as the enormously enlarged cerebral hemispheres.	Disorders of diverticulation
3. Proliferation of the undifferentiated cells destined to give rise to neurons at all levels of the neuraxis (the germinal matrix in the cerebrum) as the neural plate is rounding up to form a tube and for several weeks thereafter	Disorders of proliferation
4. Migration of neuroblasts in the germinal matrix laterally to form the mantle zone, which is the anlage of the gray matter (the earliest arriving in the seventh week but the last of them not reaching their destination until after birth)	Disorders of migration
5. Thickening of the cortical plate. The first fissures now demarcate the previously smooth outer surface by the fifth month; the secondary sulci develop during the final trimester; the tertiary ones begin to appear before birth and are completed by the sixth postnatal month.	Disorders of sulcation
6. The corpus callosum develops between the 12th and 22nd weeks.	Disorders of commissuration

*These events occur in normal fetal development during which the pathologic process is presumed to take effect.

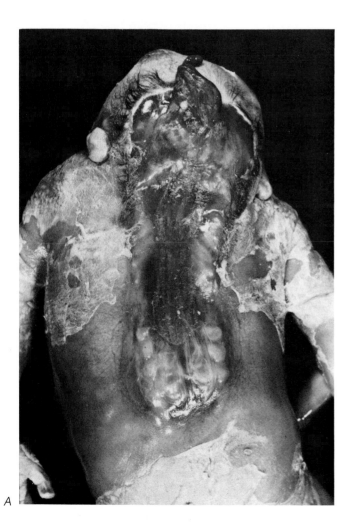

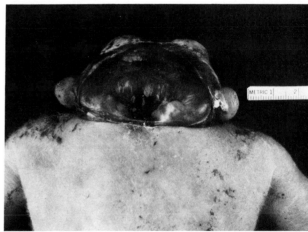

Figure 8-1. Major forms of dysraphism. *A,* Craniorachischisis totalis, dorsal view. *B,* Anencephaly, posterior (occipital) view.

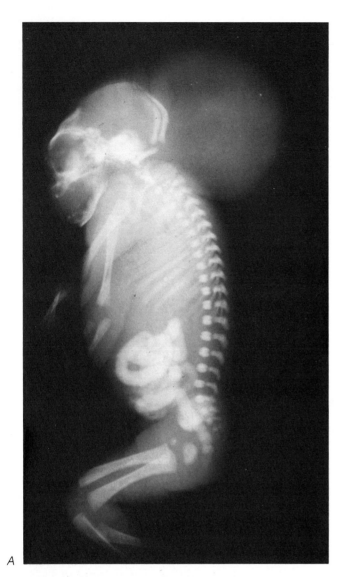

A

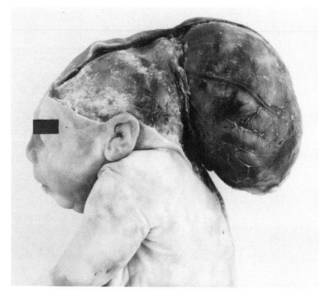

C

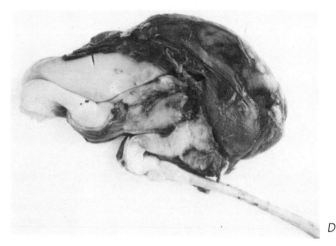

D

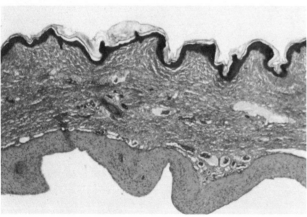

B

Figure 8–2. Meningoencephalocele. *A*, Largely cystic occipital lesion is seen on a lateral roentgenogram of the head (bony defect is not demonstrated because of overlap of bones). *B*, Histologic section of "sac" shows (from top to bottom) skin and subcutaneous tissue of the scalp and a thin layer of gliotic tissue. *C* and *D*, Left lateral view (*C*) and midsagittal view of right side of brain (*D*), showing a large "solid" lesion through a large occipital cranial defect, containing much of the cerebrum, upper brainstem, and cerebellum.

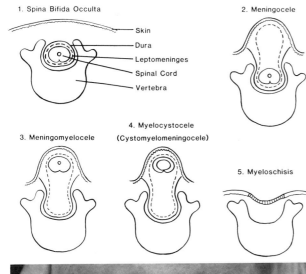

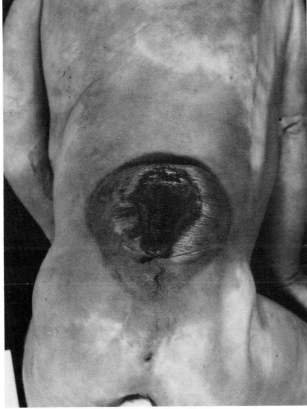

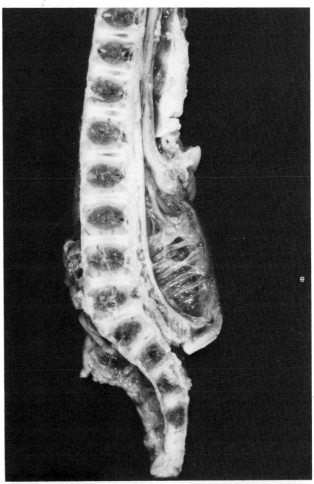

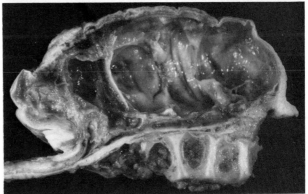

Figure 8–3. Spinal dysraphism. *A*, Diagrammatic presentation of various forms of spinal dysraphism. *B* and *C*, Lumbar myeloschisis on dorsal (*B*) and lateral midsagittal (*C*) views of dissected spec-

imen. *D*, Meningomyelocele in midsagittal plane of dissected specimen, with spinal cord entering in sac (left side of photo).

C. Aqueductal malformations (four main types) (Fig. 8–4)

1. Stenosis

Narrowing without abnormal gliosis in the surrounding tissue (a rare hereditary variant is known)

2. Forking

Two main, reduced channels, the dorsal one showing considerable branching and the ventral one being represented by a narrow slit. These two channels may communicate with each other and with the ventricle or may end

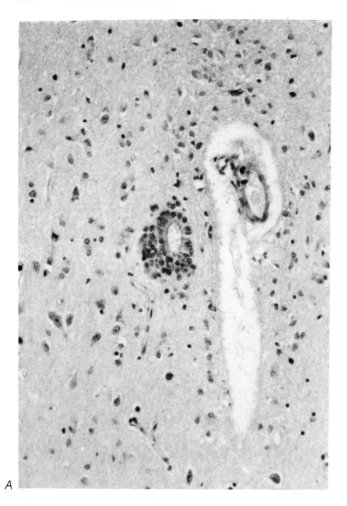

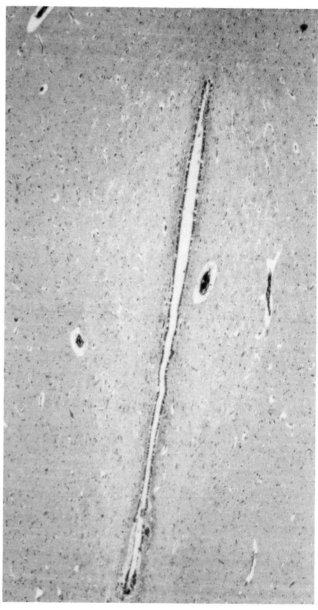

Figure 8-4. Aqueductal malformations (all in cross section of midbrain). *A,* Single, minute channel without gliosis (H&E). *B,* Long vertical slit without gliosis (H&E). *C and D,* Two different levels of cases with forking. One level shows multiple small channels only, and the other level has a ventral long channel. No gliosis is seen at either level (H&E).

B

(Continued)

blindly (atresia). Associated malformations include fusion of the quadrigeminal plate or of the oculomotor nuclei, and spina bifida.

3. Septum formation

A thin neuroglial membrane occluding or partially obstructing the caudal end of the aqueduct (rare). Some are associated with granular ependymitis (as a result of an infection during fetal life ?).

4. Gliosis

A narrowing of the aqueduct or its subdivision into two or more smaller channels in conjunction with well-marked gliosis, the margin of which evidently marks out the previous outline of the aqueduct and contains disorderly groups of

ependymal cells. Gliosis may involve only one part of the aqueduct; the other (usually anterior) portion shows dilatation. This form is not associated with other malformations.

Although stenosis and forking are considered to be due to dysplasia, septum formation and gliosis are thought to result from acquired conditions. There are, however, cases with mixed features which cast doubt about the validity of the above simple, clear-cut classification. Whether one could confidently distinguish between congenital and acquired forms is questioned by these observations. Recently, a view was even expressed that in some cases aqueductal stenosis could be a result of, rather than the cause of, hydrocephalus. The term "atresia" (nonpassage at birth), used in the sense of aplasia (nonformation), is inappropriate here, because the

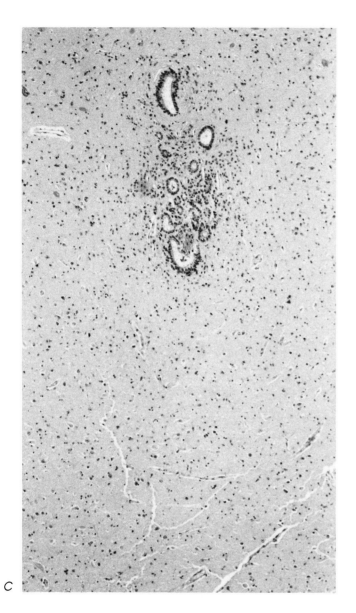

C

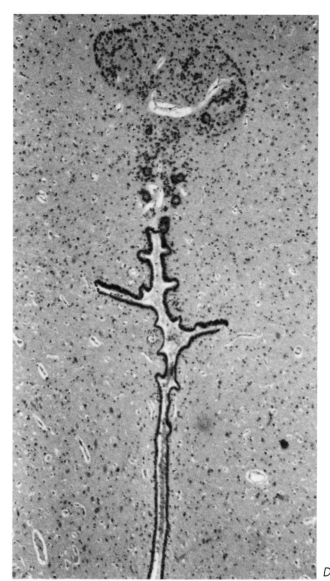

D

(Continued)

neural tube has a lumen from its very origin, and therefore all strictures of this lumen must be secondary and acquired. The difference between "congenital" and "acquired" obstructions has probably more to do with the timing of the disease process than with any basic difference of pathogenesis. As stated earlier, this principle probably applies to many conditions under discussion in this chapter.

D. Hydromyelia (Fig. 8–5)

This disorder represents congenital dilatation of the central canal, which normally becomes obliterated postnatally. Most often it is associated with meningomyelocele and Chiari malformation. Otherwise, it occurs only as an incidental finding, often over a relatively few segments at autopsy; it rarely causes symptoms.

E. Syringomyelia (Fig. 8–6)

The lesion consists of a slit or tubular cavitation of the spinal cord (syrinx = tube), presumably representing a dysraphic process related to fusion of the alar and basal wings of the spinal cord anlage. As such, this is fundamentally different from hydromyelia as described above. It occurs mainly in the cervical and thoracic regions of the cord, and the lumbar and sacral portions are rarely affected.

The cavities may be multiple or irregular in their course. In the cervical cord, the lesion closely resembles the cruciform shape of the fetal central canal before the fusion of the alar and basal laminae and is situated in the dorsal horns and behind the central canal, where a midline ventral extension of the cavity often destroys the anterior commissure. The central canal may become incorporated into the syrinx.

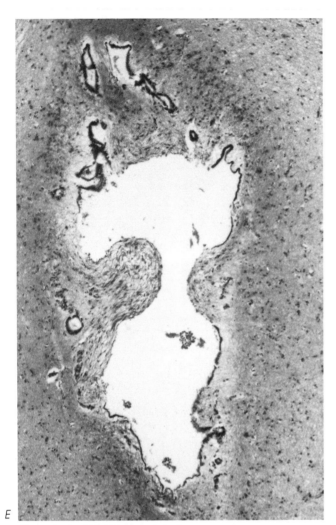

E

Figure 8–4. *E,* Subependymal gliosis partially destroying lumen (H&E).

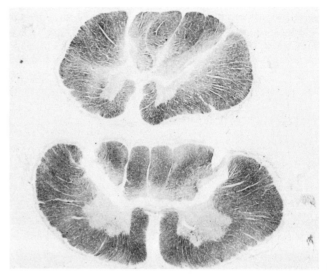

A

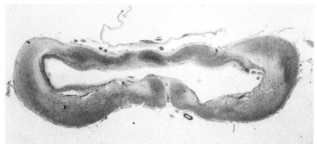

B

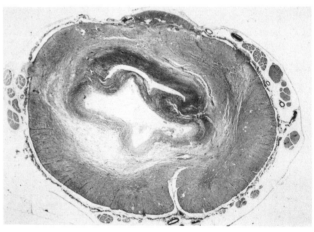

C

Figure 8–6. Syringomyelia. *A,* Narrow slit from one posterior root entry zone to another without gliosis in cervical cord (LFB/CV). *B,* Large cervical cavity with considerable parenchymal damage (LFB/PAS/H). *C,* Unilateral double cavities with considerable gliosis and (mainly ventral) parenchymal rarefaction in low-thoracic cord, associated with hemangioblastoma at higher level (PTAH).

The syrinx may be filled with clear, slightly yellow fluid, which gives the affected cord segment a swollen appearance. Compressive damage to the surrounding tissues, including the anterior horns, may result. The cavity usually extends up to the level of C-2 without communicating with the fourth ventricle.

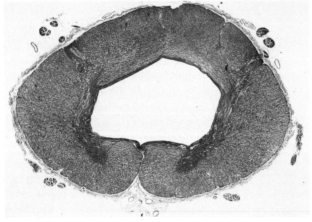

Figure 8–5. Hydromyelia. Larger yet asymptomatic cavity is shown (H&E).

In the thoracic cord, the cavities may be present unilaterally in one dorsal horn or occur bilaterally but at different levels. Usually these fuse into a single cavity at a higher level.

The histologic appearance of the cavities varies from one resembling a simple tear of the tissue to one with walls of fibrous astrocytosis of varying width. A thin layer of collagen fibers may be seen.

An association of syringomyelia with intramedullary spinal cord tumors is well known, particularly with astrocytomas, ependymomas, and hemangioblastomas.

The relative relationships of syrinx and tumors are variable, as demonstrated below.

Similar cavities in the medulla, often in association with cervical syringomyelia, are known as "syringobulbia" and may be seen in three different forms (Fig. 8–7), as follows.

1. A slit running out in a ventrolateral direction from the floor of the fourth ventricle external to the nucleus of the 12th nerve (with or without connection with the ventricle). It is located mainly in the lower half or two-thirds of the medulla and is more often bilateral than unilateral. The nucleus gracilis and nucleus cuneatus and the medial lemniscus are often interrupted.

2. Extension of the fourth ventricle along the median raphe, lined by ependyma and occasionally showing neuroglial scar. It interrupts the connection between the descending vestibular tract and the medial longitudinal fasciculus.

3. A slit between the pyramid and the inferior olive. It interrupts the nucleus of the 12th nerve (unilateral).

8.2 DISORDERS OF DIVERTICULATION: FAILURE OF CLEAVAGE

A. Holoprosencephaly (= holotelencephaly) (Fig. 8–8)

This disorder represents a tendency for the prosencephalon to remain whole as a single, simple, more or less undifferentiated bulb. It may be divided into three subtypes, as follows.

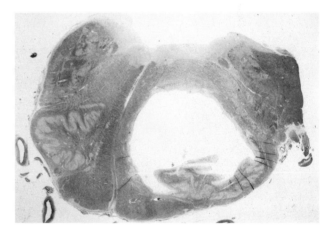

B

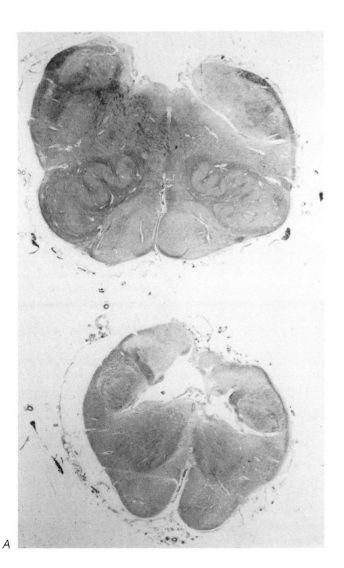

A

Figure 8–7. Syringobulbia. *A,* Type 1 lesions, unilateral at upper and bilateral at lower level (LFB/PAS/H). *B,* Markedly dilated type 1 unilateral lesion (LFB/PAS/H).

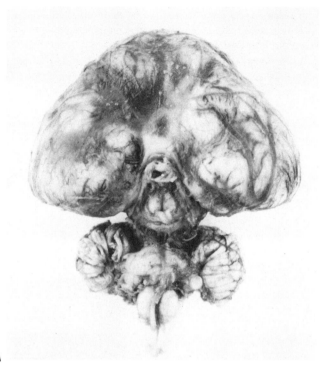

A

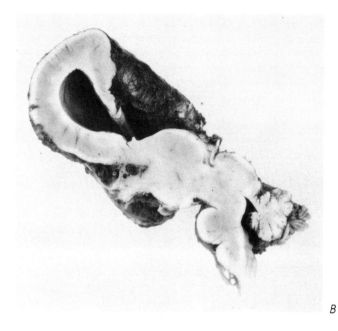

B

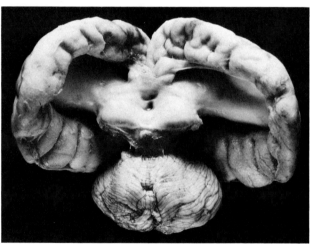

C

Figure 8–8. Holoprosencephaly. *A* and *B,* Anterior (*A*) and mid-sagittal (*B*) views of the brain of a cyclops. Thin (and easily torn at removal) dysplastic membrane covering posterior portion of cerebral mantle is not shown. *C,* Posteroanterior view of somewhat better developed brain, again with thin membrane missing from specimen.

1. Alobar holoprosencephaly

A small monoventricular cerebrum remains undivided into lobes or hemispheres. A thin membrane forms a portion (usually posterior) of the roof of the cerebral ventricles, which may balloon out dorsally to form a cyst. Olfactory bulbs and tracts are always absent. Facionasal malformations are invariably present.

2. Semilobar holoprosencephaly

Lobe formation and an interhemispheric fissure are indicated but are incomplete. Olfactory bulbs and tracts are usually absent. Corpora striata are continuous across the midline. Facionasal malformations are often present.

3. Lobar holoprosencephaly

The lobes and interhemispheric fissure are well formed.

Note: 1. Ocular abnormalities arise early and may range in severity from a single median eye (cyclopia) to a relatively mild bilateral coloboma.

2. A normal karyotype is the rule but 13–15 trisomy has been reported in some instances of holoprosencephaly.

B. Chiari (Arnold-Chiari) malformations (Fig. 8–9)

Originally, four types of malformations were described by Chiari, but the following two types are of importance.

1. Type I (adult type)

This type consists of variable downward herniation of cerebellar tonsils (the vermis is normally shaped) without elongation of the medulla and fourth ventricle; it is compatible with survival into adult life. Usually no associated spina

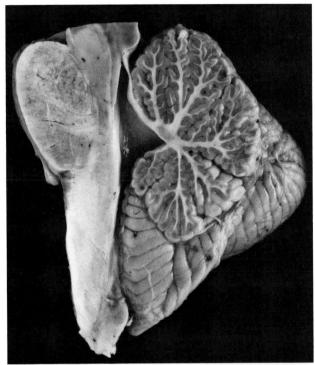

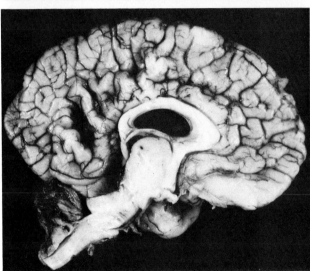

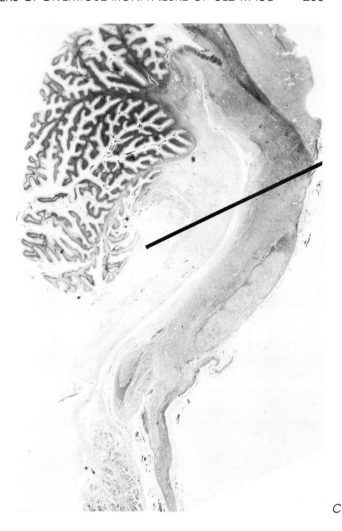

Figure 8–9. Chiari malformation. *A,* Incidental type I (adult) with tonsillar herniation without abnormality of vermis. *B,* Type II (infantile), midsagittal view. *C,* Type II (infantile) with pronounced elongation of medulla accompanied by herniating, sclerotic caudal midline cerebellar structure (vermis) and prolapsed choroid plexus of caudal fourth ventricle. *Line* indicates level of foramen magnum (Weil).

bifida is present. However, arachnoidal adhesions may develop around the tonsils, and they may cause symptoms.

Syringomyelia frequently (nearly 50%) coexists and this rather than the herniated tonsils is often responsible for the clinical symptoms.

2. Type II (infantile type)

This complex malformation probably arises during the early inductive period but has additional features, which imply a more prolonged causation. It consists of the following components, which are usually conjoined.

   a. Malformation of the basocranial bones
     • Platybasia (flattening at the base)
     • Occipito-atlantal assimilation (fusion of the occipital bone with the atlas)

     • Shallow posterior fossa and small foramen magnum
     • Defects in the occipital squama or cervical spina bifida
     • Klippel-Feil abnormality (fusion of several vertebrae)
   b. Malformations of the cerebellum

     Hypoplasia and vertical elongation ("peg shaped" or "fingerlike") of the inferior vermis into the cervical canal (as low as the level of C-3 vertebra) posterior to the spinal cord.

   c. Persistence of embryonic cervical flexure
     • Foreshortening of the hindbrain and ventral juxtaposition of the pons and inferior olives
     • Elongation and downward displacement of the

medulla (elongated fourth ventricle) and cervical cord with cervical nerve roots running upward to their foramina of exit

d. Other frequently associated features (Peach, 1965)
• Lumbar meningocele or meningomyelocele (95%)
• Hydrocephalus (95%, many with ventricular neuronal heterotopia), fused thalamus (90%), and absent septum (40%)
• Microgyria (55%)
• Tectal malformation (75%)
• Aqueductal atresia (>35%)

Note: Certain features of this malformation must be induced in the earliest stages of embryonal development (first several weeks), long before the purely mechanical factors, such as fixation of roots (by meningomyelocele) and downward pull on the cord by the growing spine.

C. Dandy-Walker syndrome (Fig. 8–10)
This is a complex malformation of the rostral part of the roof of the fourth ventricle comprising the following features.

1. Hypoplasia and aplasia of the cerebellar vermis (chiefly the inferior portion)

2. A cyst of the fourth ventricle formed above the median aperture and involving the inferior medullary velum. The wall of the cyst is composed of a layer of pia-arachnoid and an attenuated glial-ependymal membrane. The latter may contain recognizable cerebellar cortical tissue for a variable length, usually at the beginning of the cystic wall. The cyst is accommodated by a large posterior fossa with a high tentorium and associated sinuses.

3. Hydrocephalus, which is not dependent on atresia of the outlets of the fourth ventricle. This atresia is absent in some examples.

4. Other, less frequent, anomalies, including agenesis of the corpus callosum, neuronal heterotopia, spinal dysplasia, renal defects, and polydactylism.

It appears that components (1) and (2) appearing alone may allow a patient to lead a normal life, whereas the additional defects, especially (3), usually account for the prominent clinical and pathologic features of this syndrome. This syndrome probably begins later in the embryonic period than does the Chiari malformation but before the seventh week. It seems to begin in the rostral membrane area where the cerebellar plates meet.

8.3 DISORDERS OF MIGRATION AND SULCATION

This category encompasses disorders ranging from complete failure of migrating neurons to reach the cerebral cortex to

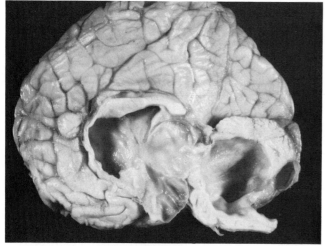

A

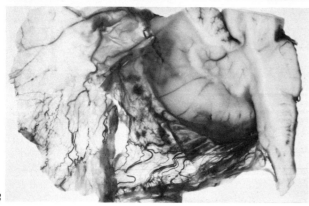

B

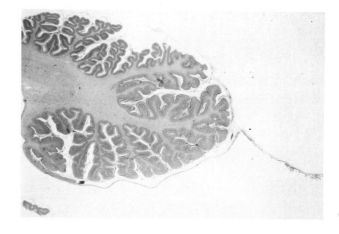

C

Figure 8–10. Dandy-Walker syndrome. *A,* Midsagittal view of entire right side of brain with large fourth, third, and lateral ventricles. *B,* Isolated posterior fossa structure photographed under water with dysplastic membrane indirectly transluminated. *C,* Histologic section of paramedian plane through cerebellar hemisphere and dysplastic membrane (H&E). (*A* courtesy of Kings County Hospital, Brooklyn, New York.)

localized failures of cortical formation and quantitative abnormalities of the cortical structure (cortical dysgenesis). Similar disturbances of migration may be expected in any part of the nervous system. Some of the more frequent examples (occurring in various combinations) follow.

A. Neuronal heterotopia (Fig. 8–11)

This disorder is characterized by abnormal accumulation of nerve cells in abnormal positions, due to impaired (arrested) migration of neuroblasts. These accumulations may take the form of nodular masses of varying size about the ventricular walls or a more diffuse form involving the centrum semiovale and composed of small columnar masses of neurons separated by bundles of myelinated fibers.

B. Lissencephaly (agyria) and pachygyria (Fig. 8–12)

These two terms are often used synonymously, but by traditional definition, pachygyria shows relatively few broad gyri (a reduction in the number of secondary gyri), whereas lissencephaly ("smooth brain" or agyria) is characterized by an absence of cerebral convolution. However, even in lissencephaly a short sylvian fissure is often recognizable, and the presence of primary fissures and a few sulci is not unusual. Therefore, these conditions may conveniently be regarded as differing only in degree.

The abnormality may be bilateral, but it is not uncommonly confined to one hemisphere. The hemispheric walls beneath the smooth surface have a molecular layer of normal proportions, a neuronal layer representing the true cortex (often shallower and more densely packed than normal), and a deep layer of neurons often arranged in broad columns (representing neurons arrested in migration, see above) separated by bundles of myelinated fibers radiating from the fourth, thin periventricular layer of white matter. The lesion is thought to represent retardation of the normal development to the level of a 12-week-old embryo brain.

The brain as a whole is usually small and underweight ("microcephalia vera"), but the lateral ventricles are relatively larger. When only a small area is involved (one or two broad gyri = macrogyria), the change superficially resembles tuberous sclerosis.

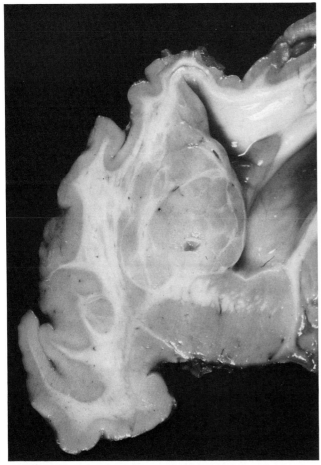

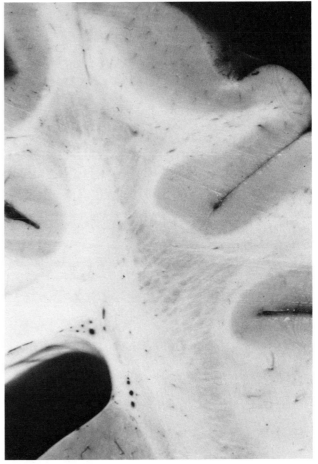

A

B

Figure 8–11. Neuronal heterotopia. *A,* Multiple large, complex (over caudate nucleus) gray matter heterotopia in neonatal hydrocephalic brain. *B,* Right frontal white matter with clusters of gray matter separated by bundles of white matter. (*A* courtesy of Dr. Bruno Volk; *B* courtesy of Kings County Hospital, Brooklyn, New York.)

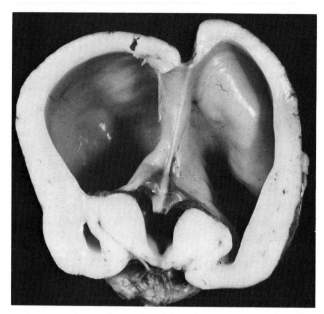

Figure 8–12. Lissencephaly (agyria) and pachygyria. Neonate brain has little evidence of sulcal development and shows large lateral (and to a lesser extent, third) ventricles. (Courtesy of Dr. Abner Wolf.)

C. Micropolygyria (synonym, polymicrogyria) (Fig. 8–13)

This disorder consists of a collection of miniature convolutions without sulci but with a characteristic bossed external appearance.

The extent of the abnormality varies from brain to brain. Histologic features are also variable. Usually there are no indications of differentiated lamination or formation of radial bundles; abnormal tangles of myelinated fibers are seen in molecular layers or elsewhere. Several subtypes are recognized: (1) a wavy, festoon-like arrangement of the nerve cell ribbon, with no separation of the molecular layer (the commonest form); (2) a more complex "glandular" formation with tubular columns of cells ramifying in tortuous plications; (3) a multifoliate structure; and (4) a four-layered type composed of (a) a molecular layer, (b) a nerve cell layer, (c) an acellular layer with myelinated fibers, and (d) a nerve cell layer.

Micropolygyria is often associated with "cerebellar microgyria" (see D below). Some examples are associated with fetal anoxia and fetal infections, as in maternal carbon monoxide poisoning and cytomegalovirus and rubella infections. Minor vascular malformations in the micropolygyric cortex have been reported. "Brain warts" (or nodular dysgenesis) are minor malformations consisting of elevated nodular collections of fusiform and stellar neurons, usually in the crown of the frontal gyri. These occur in isolation or in conjunction with deeper cortical architectural abnormalities.

Note: The term "microgyria" is loosely applied to any type of abnormally small convolution irrespective of cause, including ulegyria. "Polygyria" signifies excessive formation of secondary sulci in the otherwise normal convolutional pattern of the brain, without necessarily involving gliosis or

shrinkage. Chiari type II malformation is characteristically associated with hydrocephalic cerebral hemispheres with polygyria.

D. "**Cerebellar microgyria**" is a complex and anarchic arrangement of neurons between patches of smooth cerebellar cortex; the disordered ("scrambled") architecture has no relation to any normal stage of development.

8.4 DISORDERS OF PROLIFERATION (DISORDERS OF SIZE)

A. Megalencephaly (Fig. 8–14)

This term is used to signify brains with simple excessive weights (1,600 to 2,850 g) recorded in persons of normal or exceptional intelligence and in epileptics and mentally defective persons. It is also used in restricted and preferred connotations, such as for heavy brains with additional structural anomalies, including the following three (really two) main varieties.

1. Brains with diffuse blastomatous glial (astrocytic) overgrowth, which may undergo a malignant transformation. Associated nerve cell malformations include irregularities of stratification, cells of abnormally large size—isolated or in groups (as in pachygyria)—and heterotopia in the white matter.

2. Generalized increase in size without glial proliferation (with or without minor neuronal abnormalities)

3. Increased size occurring as an incidental feature of some other malformations or "degenerative" conditions, such as tuberous sclerosis, Tay-Sachs disease, metachromatic leukodystrophy, and spongy degeneration. This last category does not properly belong here except as a purely descriptive term.

Note: The term "megalocephaly" refers to the enlargement of the head irrespective of the types of lesions in the underlying brain, including hydrocephalus, neoplasms, and so on, and should not be confused with megalencephaly, with small brain substance, discussed above.

B. Micrencephaly (= small brain) (Fig. 8–14)

This term may be defined arbitrarily as signifying a small brain—less than 900 g in adulthood. In association with the small brain, the cranium is usually small—microcephaly = small head. This term is sometimes used synonymously with "micrencephaly."

In most cases the condition is a result of various perinatal destructive processes (e.g., anoxia, infection) rather than a true malformation.

A substantial portion of severe cases of microcephaly (and micrencephaly), estimated to be about 50%, belong in the category of familial micrencephaly (brain weight usually 500 to 600 g), a distinctive clinical entity with a mendelian recessive mode of inheritance. The cerebral convolutional pattern is greatly simplified, as in higher apes, with relatively broad gyri showing numerous minor anomalies of architectronics—for example, irregularly oriented and abnormally

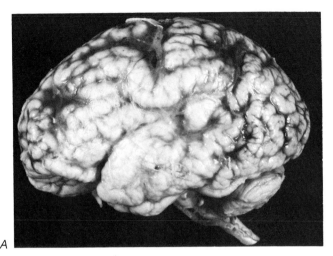

A

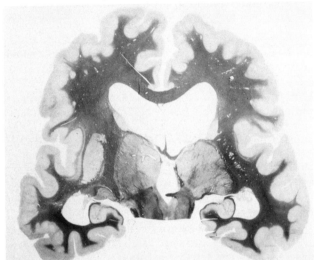

B

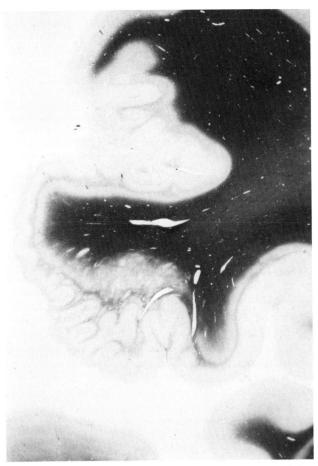

C

Figure 8–13. Micropolygyria. *A* and *B,* External (*A*) and histologic section (LFB/CV) (*B*) views of diffuse micropolygyria. *C,* Closer-up view of focal micropolygyria (Weil) (same case as in Figure 8–15 *A*).

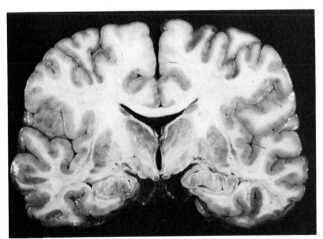

A

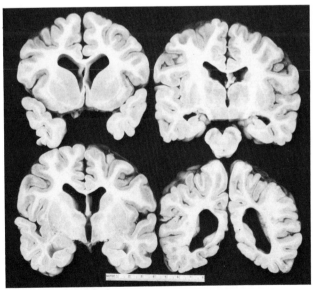

B

Figure 8–14. Megalencephaly and micrencephaly. *A,* Brain of 49-year-old man with mental retardation (IQ 27); weight of brain is 1,770 g. Except for absence of fornices and septum and small mammillary bodies, no gross or histologic changes are present. *B,* Brain of 13-year-old mentally retarded boy—brain weight, 965 g—with no histologic evidence of encephaloclastic or overt dysplastic process despite moderate ventricular dilatation.

large neurons or vertical columnar (instead of laminar) arrangement of neurons. Heterotopic nests of nerve cells are often noted in the white matter or along the ventricular wall.

C. Restricted forms of abnormal proliferation

These changes are discussed under phakomatosis (see section 7.7).

D. Schizencephaly (Fig. 8–15)

This is a special type of maldevelopment characterized by symmetrically placed clefts. These clefts are in the line of primary fissures and they involve the whole depth of the cerebral wall. The following two types are recognized, depending largely on whether hydrocephalus is present or absent.

1. Those in which the clefts are in contact with each other along a seam and directed toward the ventricles

2. Those in which the marginal layers of the malformed cortex covering the lips of the clefts are fused into a solid seam known as the "pia-ependymal ridge." This represents a stretched and outpouched pia-ependymal seam as a result of pressure from within the ventricle when hydrocephalus is severe and occurs early. The pia-ependymal seam (or ridge) may be absent in some severe examples and the result is a ventricular system that communicates with the outside. The leptomeninges are usually missing over this defect. The term "basket brain" is applied when the parasagittal tissues are present and the gaps in the central portion of each hemisphere communicate with one another and with the subdural space.

The morphogenesis (formal origin) of the clefts is fairly evident. However, the causal origin of these clefts is obscure.

The clefts are believed to arise at points of localized failure of growth and differentiation in the cerebral wall before the end of the second month, before closure of the roof of the prosencephalon. In support of this view is (1) the vesicular character of the ventricular cavities with a thick cortical plate and thin white matter, (2) the presence of cortical dysgenesis (micropolygyria) at the lips or elsewhere and subarachnoid heterotopia of the cerebral substance, and (3) the presence of hyperplasia of the rhinencephalon and striatum, premature myelination of some fiber systems, and complete agenesis of other systems of the telencephalon.

Characteristically, there is no evidence of previous necrosis, inflammation, or glial or connective tissue scar formation. However, circulatory disturbances may occur later and result in superimposed encephaloclastic changes.

Note: These and similar congenital cerebral defects are usually referred to as "porencephalies," the term that was first proposed in the mid-19th century. Yet it is an ill-defined term (a "brain with holes"), and it later acquired a latitude of meaning which defeats its usefulness by referring to most heterogeneous and dissimilar circumscribed defects in the cerebral wall. The vagueness in the original text (based only on gross specimens) and the insecurity of evidence for the alleged complete communication between the subarachnoid space and the ventricular cavity led gradually to an even broader interpretation of the term. The qualifications of

"complete" or "true," "incomplete," "partial," or "non-communicating" and "pseudo-porencephaly" came into use without contributing much to the clarity of the subject. The term "porencephaly" should therefore either be abandoned or be qualified in terms of the origin of the defects to which it is applied—for example, dysgenetic or encephaloclastic (due to infarct, hemorrhage, trauma, etc., including hydranencephaly). Dysplastic porencephaly may be equated with schizencephaly.

8.5 DISORDERS OF COMMISSURATION

A. Agenesis of the corpus callosum (Fig. 8–16)

The absence of the corpus callosum (which normally develops between 12 and 22 weeks) may be complete or it may be partial ("hypogenesis"), with the presence of a thin anterior portion.

The "stump" of the corpus callosum on each side is formed by fibers projecting in a fronto-occipital direction (the longitudinal callosal bundle of Probst). These apparently consist mainly of fibers intended to form at least part of the corpus callosum. The gyri on the medial surface above the Probst bundles have a radial arrangement, and the cingulate gyrus is buried beneath the surface.

The space between the hemispheres is usually occupied by the large third ventricle, but occasionally a lipoma, cyst, or meningioma takes its place.

The lesion may be part of more serious malformations, such as holoprosencephaly, pachygyria, and schizencephaly.

It may occur independently or in association with other anomalies, including webbed toes, funnel chest, spina bifida-meningomyelocele, persistent fontanelles, facial asymmetry, high arched palate, agenesis of the cerebellar vermis, and ventricular septal defect.

Clinically, it may be totally asymptomatic or associated with mental retardation, seizures, speech disturbance, and the like.

B. Agenesis or hypoplasia of the septum pellucidum (Fig. 8–17)

This change is regularly associated with agenesis of the corpus callosum, holoprosencephaly, and so on. It can occur independently as an isolated incidental finding or in conjunction with other minor developmental defects, primarily involving the lateral ventricles and the optic nerves and tracts ("septo-optic dysplasia").

C. Cavum septi pellucidi ("fifth ventricle") (Fig. 8–18)

In the newborn brain, this is a normal constant feature. Its persistence into childhood and adulthood constitutes, for the most part, a totally asymptomatic anomaly. Small cystic spaces are quite frequent in routine autopsies.

The cavity is typically located between the descending crura of the fornices, but it usually extends for variable distances posteriorly, even encompassing the entire length of the corpus callosum. When the posterior extremity is sep-

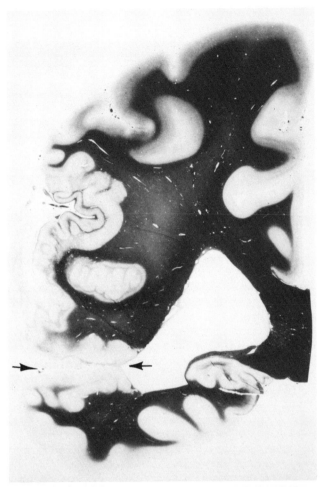

A

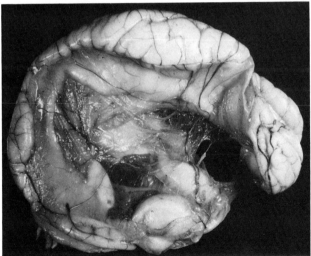

B

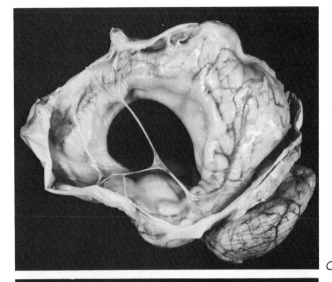

C

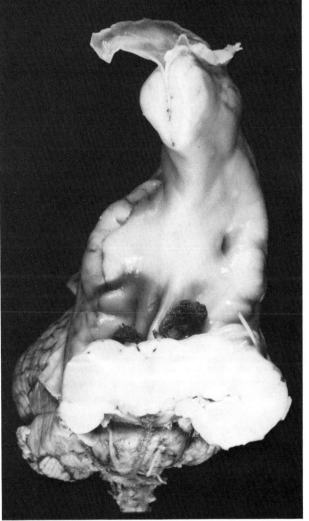

D

Figure 8–15. Schizencephaly. *A,* Closed form of schizencephaly in temporal lobe (*arrows*) with micropolygyria along defect and beyond (Weil). *B,* Right lateral view of infant brain, showing extensive but thin pia-ependymal membrane, through which enlarged ventricles and basal gray nuclei can be seen. *C* and *D,* Left lateral (*C*) and anteroposterior coronal section (*D*) views of "basket brain." Thin strands are only remnants of (meningeal)-pia-ependymal membrane. (*B* courtesy of Kings County Hospital, Brooklyn, New York; *C* and *D* courtesy of Dr. Emmanuel Stadlan.)

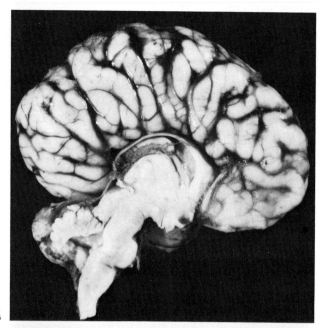

A

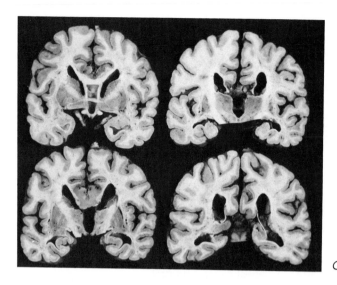

C

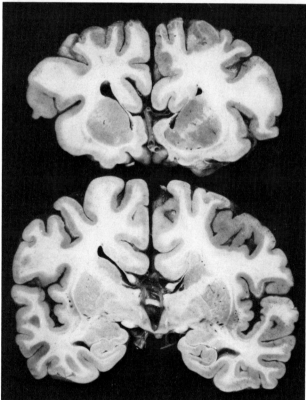

B

Figure 8–16. Agenesis of corpus callosum. *A*, Midsagittal view of neonate brain. *B*, Cross section of frontal lobes. *C*, Partial (posterior) agenesis associated with lipoma (in lower left slice).

arated from the anterior and more common cavity, it is referred to as cavum Vergae (''sixth ventricle''). The cavity is filled with cerebrospinal fluid-like fluid, and the septa are often fenestrated in late adulthood, particularly in association with dilatation of the lateral ventricles.

8.6 OTHER MALFORMATIONS: DOWN'S SYNDROME (TRISOMY 21) (FIG. 8–19)

This syndrome is responsible for nearly 20% of the severely retarded population. The neuropathologic alterations are

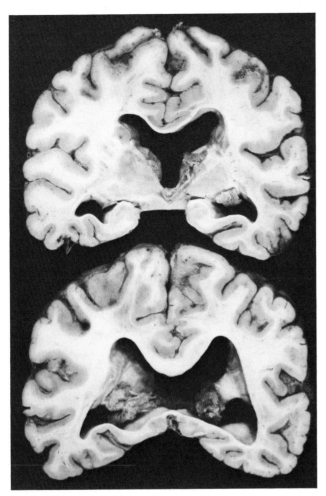

Figure 8–17. Agenesis of septum pellucidum. Mentally retarded 62-year-old man has absent fornices and septum, hypoplastic corpus callosum, conjoint cingulate gyrus across midline, and moderate ventricular dilatation.

usually diffuse and rather indefinite. Many subjective, unconfirmed, and contradictory statements are seen in the published descriptions.

The external features of the affected brain are more characteristic when present. The brain appears more rounded as viewed laterally and dorsally, mostly because the frontal lobes are reduced in all dimensions. The narrowing of the superior temporal convolution is another relatively constant feature. The brainstem and cerebellum are small in comparison with the cerebrum.

Histologic changes are indefinite. Minor microscopic anomalies that have been described are shared by other forms of severe oligophrenia. Some of these may be related to abnormal constitutional factors, such as congenital heart disease or general circulatory asthenia.

Middle-aged patients often show Alzheimer's tangles and senile plaques prematurely, identical to those found in Alzheimer's disease.

II. Perinatal lesions (8.7 and 8.8)

These lesions, as mentioned, correspond to conditions that have been known as "birth injuries." In recent years, the emphasis in the consideration of their cause has shifted from purely mechanical obstetric factors to anoxic-ischemic factors. The designation "perinatal" signifies the uncertainty that often exists in determining the precise time (or period) in which the damage is sustained. Therefore, the term covers the prenatal (or intrauterine), delivery and also postnatal periods.

8.7 ANOXIC-ISCHEMIC LESIONS

Abnormal conditions that are important with respect to the development of the CNS lesions to be described here include (1) during the prenatal period: maternal anemia, heart disease, pneumonia, shock of various causes, placental infarcts and infections and premature detachment, knots and compression of the umbilical cord, and oversedation and improper anesthesia during delivery (which can lead to primary apnea and difficulty in resuscitation of the neonate); and (2) during the postnatal period: aspiration, unrelieved airway obstruction, respiratory distress syndrome, and pneumonia.

A. Infarct-like lesions (Figs. 8–20 and 8–21)

These conditions are characterized by tissue necrosis with subsequent reactive glial scar formation (astrocytosis), in which circumstantial (or, rarely, concrete) evidence incriminates anoxia or ischemia (or both) as the causative factor.

Many of these lesions are found in the brains of older children and adults dying after a lifetime of mental deficiency or motor dysfunction of varying degrees. They are sometimes found in infants who died within the first few weeks of life but are rarely seen in those who died in the first few days. Therefore, the acute stage of these lesions is rarely

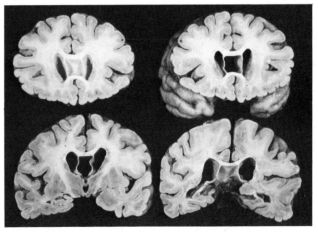

Figure 8–18. Cavum septi pellucidi. Large but asymptomatic cavum extends the entire length of the corpus callosum (left row in posteroanterior view; right row in anteroposterior view).

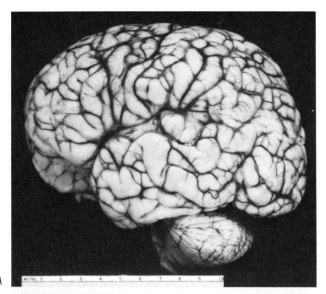

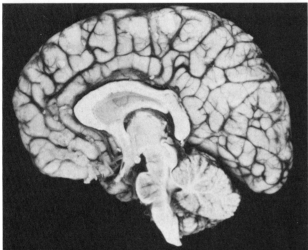

Figure 8–19. Down's syndrome. A and B, Left lateral (A) and midsagittal (B) views of brain.

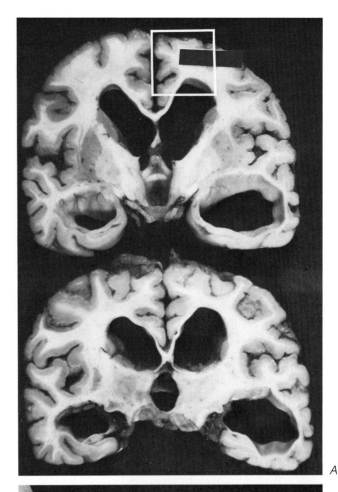

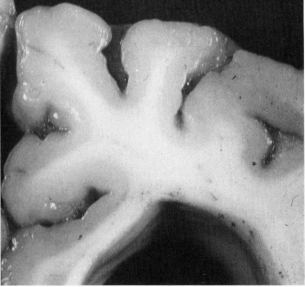

encountered. Even in severely affected brains, the brainstem is usually spared, or less severely involved, so that these conditions are not immediately life-threatening.

It is generally agreed that, in premature infants, the cerebral white matter tends to be more severely affected, whereas in full-term infants the cerebral cortical damage predominates.

Note: The immature brain reacts to tissue necrosis such as that brought about by hypoxia and ischemia differently from the mature brain. In the immature brain, the resolution of the necrotic tissue is more complete and reactive astrocytic scar formation is very subdued and results in a smooth-walled defect. Lesions occurring near the end of gestation, such as those of multilocular cystic encephalomalacia, result in regular, shaggy defects with gliotic intervening tissue, similar to the cystic stage of infarcts in adulthood.

Component lesions that make up individual examples in various combinations are as follows.

Figure 8–20. Predominantly gray matter lesions of perinatal hypoxia. A and B, Diffuse lobar sclerosis with relatively uniform involvement of cerebral cortex, although depths of sulci are more severely affected (thinner and paler in appearance). B is area marked by box in A.

(Continued)

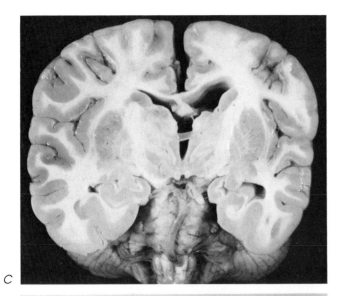

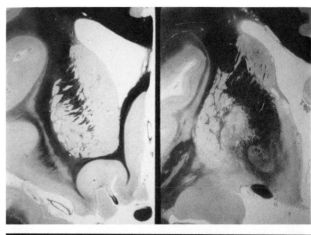

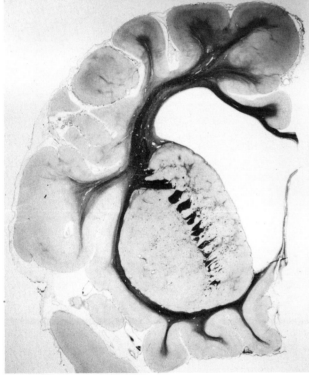

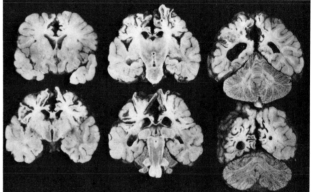

C and D, Cortical sclerosis more localized to arterial border zones bilaterally. Periphery of lesions shows "plaques fibromyeliques" on gross (C) and LFB/CV-stained (D) preparations. E, Status marmoratus of lateral portion of caudate and putamen (LFB/CV).

F, More extensive multifocal sclerosis with cortical and subcortical involvement. (A, B, and E courtesy of Kings County Hospital, Brooklyn, New York.)

1. Cortical changes (mostly cerebral but occasionally cerebellar)

   a. Ulegyria

     Individual or, more commonly, a group of shrunken sclerotic gyri are seen in which loss of tissue is maximal at the depth of the sulci. Extreme examples are known as "mushroom gyri." These changes tend to be more pronounced in the arterial border zones but may also be confined to an arterial territory. They are often flanked by gyri with lesser degrees of neuronal loss and irregular patches of myelinated axons; these are known as "plaques fibromyéliques," a change considered equivalent to status marmoratus (see below). There is corresponding atrophy of the subcortical white matter. The changes are often bilateral and symmetric but can be focal and unilateral.

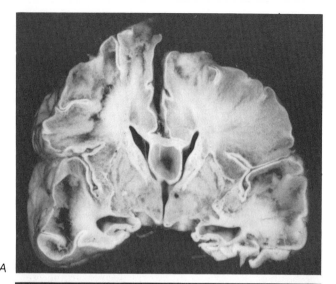

A

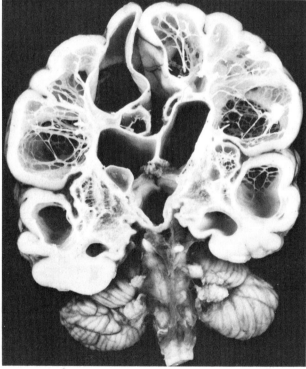

B

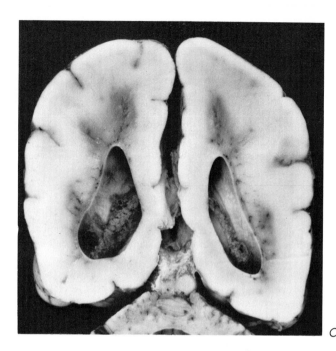

C

Figure 8–21. Predominantly white matter lesions of perinatal hypoxia. *A,* Diffuse white matter necrosis (also with thin, scarred cortex) due to abruptio placentae. *B,* Multilocular cystic encephalomalacia. *C,* Periventricular leukomalacia in parietotemporal regions.

b. Diffuse lobar sclerosis

Cortical atrophic change is evenly distributed over a wide area, usually bilaterally and symmetrically, resembling the pattern of pseudolaminar necrosis. When the change is diffuse throughout the hemispheres, the term "walnut kernel brain" is applicable.

2. Basal gray matter changes

a. Cystic necrosis

This change is usually seen in association with more extensive lesions elsewhere.

b. Partial necrosis

This disorder is characterized by more irregular and incomplete neuronal loss and astrocytosis, often but not always accompanied by irregular bundles of myelinated nerve fibers, particularly around small blood vessels. This gives rise to a mottled or marbled appearance of status marmoratus or état marbré.

3. White matter lesions

a. Multilocular cystic encephalomalacia

This lesion consists of multiple cystic cavities and intervening gliotic remnants of white matter similar to the appearance in old infarcts in adulthood. There is always some destruction of deeper gray matter. This change is more likely to be seen in infancy because this degree of tissue destruction is incompatible with long survival.

b. Periventricular leukomalacia

In this more restricted pattern of tissue damage, multiple, small foci of tissue necrosis within the periventricular white matter are seen either in the acute stage or in a subsequent scarred stage. Prematurity, respiratory distress syndrome, episodes of apnea, and cardiac arrest are the most frequent clinical correlates. Petechiae and at times confluent hemorrhage may complicate these ischemic lesions.

Note: Perinatal telencephalic leukoencephalopathy is a morphologic entity consisting of hypertrophic astrocytes and perivascular amphophilic globules in the cerebral white matter. It is postulated to represent the adverse effects of gram-negative endotoxin incident to bacteremia on myelogenesis in progress or some other maturational process unique to infant white matter. Its boundary with the white matter lesion described above is not always clear-cut, and coexistence of both may be suspected in a given case.

c. Centrilobular sclerosis

This extensive bilateral retractile glial scar was in the past confused with some of the demyelinating conditions of childhood.

4. Hydranencephaly (Fig. 8–22)

This condition is regarded as an extreme variety of the perinatal encephaloclastic process. The cerebral hemispheres, largely corresponding to the carotid artery territory, are reduced to membranous sacs, composed of leptomeninges and a thin gliotic remnant of the cerebral mantle. This encephaloclastic lesion should be separated from schizencephaly (see section 8.4, D) described above.

B. Hemorrhagic lesions (Fig. 8–23)

1. Germinal matrix hemorrhage

This is the major source of "intraventricular" hemorrhage, and it is now believed to be precipitated by perinatal anoxia (as in respiratory distress syndrome) in premature neonates (in whom there is persistence of the germinal matrix) rather than to be due to mechanical birth injury as was previously believed. Although the precise mechanism of the bleeding is unknown, rupture of thin-walled veins in this region incident to pronounced venous congestion appears to be the final step. There is little evidence to support the hypothesis that infarction of the matrix is the prerequisite. When the hemorrhage is extensive, the entire ventricular system distends with blood, which enters the subarachnoid space through the openings in the fourth ventricle. The hemorrhage may also dissect into the centrum semiovale. Occasionally, intraventricular hemorrhage appears to originate from the choroid plexus, particularly in full-term infants. Organization of the subarachnoid hemorrhage may result in progressive hydrocephalus among survivors.

2. Subarachnoid hemorrhage

Extensive subarachnoid hemorrhage may be the consequence of infarct-like lesions described above. Multiple patches of subarachnoid hemorrhage can occur as a result of perinatal anoxia; traumatic venous tear is thought to be responsible for a single large subarachnoid hemorrhage.

8.8 OTHER FORMS OF CNS DAMAGE DURING THE PERINATAL PERIOD

A. Focal circulatory disorders of the brain

1. Arterial lesions

Thrombotic occlusion of a major (mainly middle cerebral) artery in neonates and infants is rare. Occasional embolic occlusion may be seen in association with congenital heart disease. Focal arterial lesions are implicated in the production of localized (lobar or hemispheric) atrophy or hypoplasia, often with unconvincing evidence.

2. Venous lesions

Hypoxic systemic circulatory failure may lead to stasis-thrombosis of the intracranial venous system. In the premature fetus and neonate the deep internal venous system, and in the term infant the superficial cerebral veins and sinuses, are mainly affected, and hemorrhagic infarction of the corresponding drainage regions may result. Purulent leptomeningitis is another factor predisposing to venous thrombosis.

3. Congenital arteriovenous malformation, particularly involving the vein of Galen system, may be symptomatic in the early postnatal period (see section 1.4).

B. Traumatic lesions due to molding and other forceful cranial distortion during delivery: subdural hemorrhage

This is usually a complication of laceration of the falx or tentorium, with damage to bridging veins, the straight sinus, or the vein of Galen; it is classically seen in full-term infants with prolonged labor. Posterior fossa subdural hemorrhages are rare, but when they occur they are often fatal unless evacuated. Convexity lesions are less likely to be fatal. They may be bilateral and lead to enlargement of the head. Eventually, they become encased by neomembrane formation (subdural hygroma), as in adult subdural hemorrhage (see Chapter 2). The sac may increase in size as a result of fresh bleeding into it.

C. Perinatal infections

1. Premature infants are significantly more susceptible than full-term babies to neonatal leptomeningitis. Other predisposing factors are maternal infection and complications during labor or delivery. Gram-negative bacteria, particularly *Escherichia coli,* are the commonest offenders, and purulent meningitis is often part of a generalized septicemic process with a very high (to more than 80%) mortality. Endarteritis and widespread necrotizing vasculitis in the meninges and in the parenchyma lead to multiple infarcts with resultant serious neurologic complications among survivors. Obstructive hydrocephalus is also a well-recognized late complication.

2. Particularly devastating tissue damage often results from perinatal infections by herpes simplex virus (mainly type II) and cytomegalovirus (see section 3.5). Maternal rubella in

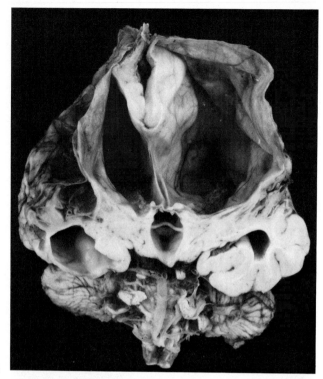

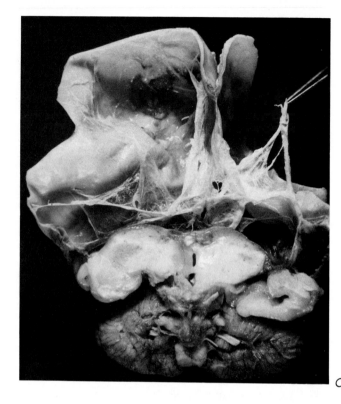

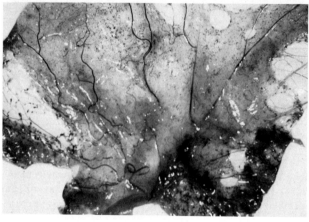

Figure 8–22. Hydranencephaly. *A,* Anteroposterior view of brain, showing cortical territory of middle cerebral artery reduced to thin semitranslucent gliotic membrane and ulegyria in adjacent areas. *B,* Transluminated gliotic membrane. *C,* Involvement of territories of middle cerebral artery and anterior cerebral artery bilaterally with gliotic membrane adherent to dura. (*B* and *C* courtesy of Kings County Hospital, Brooklyn, New York.)

the first trimester is known to result (in 10 to 12% of cases) in congenital heart disease, cataracts, deafness, and mental retardation. The frequent neuropathologic substrate is microcephaly with micropolygyria.

3. Congenital toxoplasmosis also results in granulomatous meningoencephalitis with severe parenchymal damage leading to late calcification in the cortex and periventricular tissue, similar to that seen in the residual lesions of congenital cytomegalovirus infection.

D. Toxic metabolic conditions

1. Bilirubin encephalopathy (kernicterus, literally nuclear jaundice)

The major etiologic factor in neonatal hyperbilirubinemia is recognized to be a lack of or deficiency in bilirubin conjugation in the liver, seen in erythroblastosis fetalis or hemolytic anemias due to isoimmunization—80% by Rh incompatibility and 20% by ABO system incompatibility. The frequency of blood group incompatibility as a cause diminished drastically after the advent of exchange transfusion in 1950. Currently, kernicterus is more commonly seen in infants with relatively low bilirubin levels (<20 mg/dl) but with one or more predisposing factors, including prematurity, low birth weight, hypoxia, acidosis, or septicemia. Under these conditions, damage to the normal blood-brain barrier is considered to be of primary importance.

Already as early as 1903, two types of brain tissue staining by bilirubin were recognized. The first occurs symmetrically in certain selected nuclear groups, most often including the pallidum, substantia nigra, Ammon's horn, certain cranial nerve nuclei (particularly the III, VIII, and XII), inferior olive, and dentate nucleus (kernicterus).

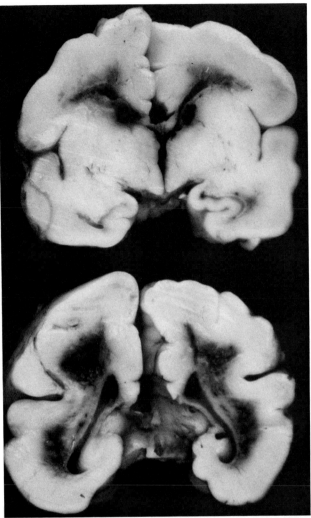

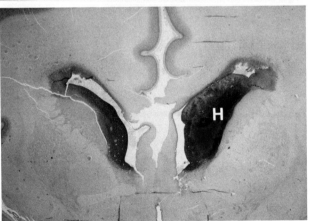

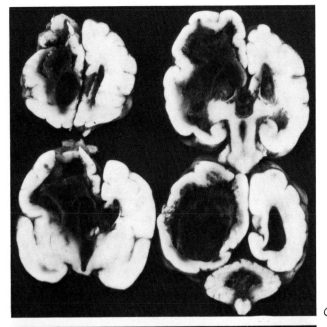

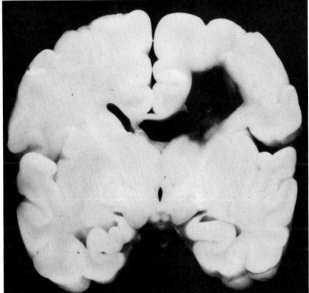

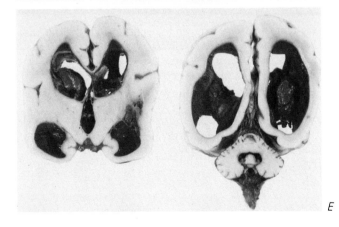

Figure 8–23. Germinal matrix hemorrhage. *A*, Bilateral, small matrix hemorrhages associated with leukomalacia complicated by hemorrhages. *B*, Small hemorrhage with rupture into lateral ventricle (*H*). *C*, Massive hemorrhage with ventricular and white matter extension. *D*, Cavitary remnant of previous matrix hemorrhage extending into frontal white matter. *E*, Hydrocephalus secondary to organization of ventricular and subarachnoid hemorrhage.

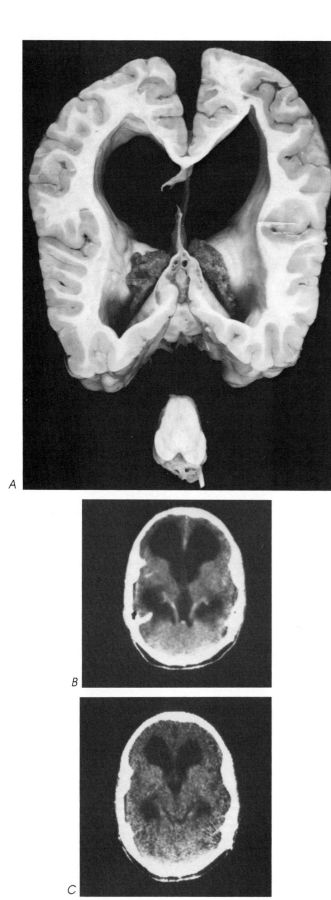

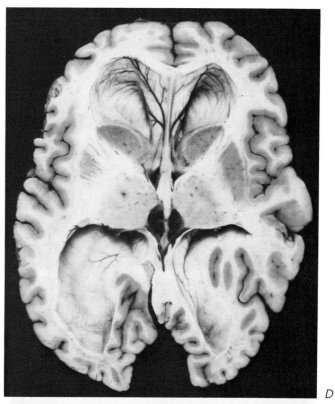

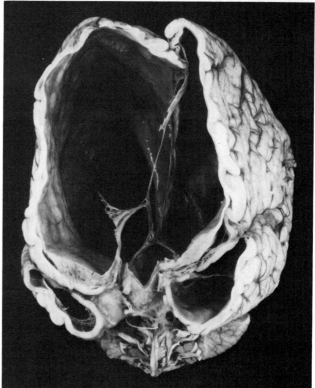

Figure 8–24. Hydrocephalus. *A*, A 4-year-old boy with "obstructive" hydrocephalus due to aqueductal stenosis and lumbar meningo-cele (not shown) was treated with many shunting procedures. Death was due to purulent meningitis. *B*, A 17-year-old girl with hydro-cephalus secondary to aqueductal stenosis was diagnosed and

The second type is more diffuse and is seen in association with such destructive lesions as periventricular leukomalacia. This type has rarely been reported in the subsequent literature, and the term "kernicterus" is now generally used to designate the pathologic lesions as well as the clinical features of the disease. Microscopically, yellow discoloration of neurons and their processes by unconjugated bilirubin is seen best when viewed on frozen section. Many of these neurons show signs of necrobiosis, such as pyknosis and eosinophilic degeneration.

Among those who survive, atrophy (neuronal loss and glial scarring) of the pallidum, subthalamic nucleus, and Ammon's horn is fairly consistently seen (posticteric encephalopathy), although other areas may show milder changes. No residual pigmentation is evident.

2. More recently, deleterious effects of maternal alcohol abuse during pregnancy have been recognized. Excessive numbers of stillbirths, shorter gestation, and decreased birth weight have been reported. Maternal alcoholism may have teratogenic effects and produce the so-called fetal alcohol syndrome. The reported spectrum of neuropathologic changes ranges from severe dysraphic state, holoprosencephaly, "porencephaly," agenesis of corpus callosum, and hydranencephaly to only biochemical (subanatomic) abnormalities.

E. Special note on hydrocephalus (Fig. 8–24)

Hydrocephalus in modern usage refers to a condition in which there is an excess quantity of cerebrospinal fluid (CSF) under pressure, either intermittently or persistently and currently or in the past. In the vast majority of cases it is due to relative or absolute obstruction of the normal flow of CSF somewhere between the sites of formation and the sites of absorption. The only recognized nonobstructive cause of hydrocephalus is excess formation of CSF by papilloma of the choroid plexus.

Note: 1. Ventricular dilatation due to primary atrophy or congenital hypoplasia of the cerebral parenchyma has traditionally been called "hydrocephalus ex vacuo" and as such is not related to pressure factors in the vast majority of cases. Commonly, there is also enlargement of the CSF-filled subarachnoid space. Therefore, hydrocephalus ex vacuo generally shows features of both "internal" and "external" hydrocephalus, in terms of the previously common terminology. This form is not considered further here.

2. Traditionally, hydrocephalus was classified either as communicating or as noncommunicating. This distinction is not synonymous with the obstructive-nonobstructive classification of the modern writers.

The following is a tabular presentation of types of hydrocephalus and some of the common causes.

Noncommunicating		Communicating	
Obstructive (relative or absolute)			Nonobstructive
Intraventricular	Extraventricular		
Congenital or acquired obstruction usually occurs at sites where the caliber of the CSF pathways is naturally narrow, particularly at the aqueduct of Sylvius, the fourth ventricle, and the foramen of Monro.	Obstruction occurs distal to the outlet foramina of the fourth ventricle, usually at the level of the basal cistern, within the subarachnoid space over the lateral surface of the brain, or at the absorption sites (the arachnoid villi).		There is excess formation of CSF.
Common causes include malformations (aqueductal atresia or stenosis, Arnold-Chiari and Dandy-Walker malformations), mass lesions (neoplasms, cysts, aneurysms), and ependymal changes secondary to inflammation (infectious or otherwise) or hemorrhage.	Postinfectious or hemorrhagic fibrosis of the subarachnoid CSF pathway is the common cause. Dysplasia such as Arnold-Chiari malformation can be considered to have mechanical features of extraventricular CSF pathway obstruction.		Some papillomas of the choroid plexus are responsible for this type of hydrocephalus.

treated with shunts at age 5 months. The computed tomography image shows pronounced ventricular dilatation at the time of clinical deterioration 9 months before death. Clinical improvement followed revision of the shunt. C, This computed tomography image in the same case as B was made at the time of a recent episode of rapid clinical deterioration associated with markedly rising ventricular pressure (more than 400 mm Hg). Note the less pronounced ventricular dilatation as compared with B. Death occurred within 2 days. D, Gross appearance of fixed brain specimen in same case as B and C. Medullary infarction secondary to tonsillar herniation (not shown) was the immediate cause of death. E, A 25-year-old institutionalized man had extreme hydrocephalus associated with lumbar meningomyelocele (repaired in infancy). Profound mental retardation, seizure disorders, blindness, deafness, and contracture in flexion of the extremities characterized his clinical course. Death was due to aspiration pneumonia.

The compressive effects of hydrocephalus on the brain parenchyma affect largely the white matter, and the cerebral cortex is quite resistant. Progressive thinning of the white matter is accompanied by progressive chronic edema due to seepage of CSF into the periventricular white matter. This seepage is a result of stretching of and eventual damage to the ependymal lining. Chronically compressed and edematous white matter shows reduction in oligodendroglial cells and fibrous gliosis. Occasional macrophages may be seen. Smooth-walled cystic cavities may be formed within the white matter after focal rupture of the ventricular wall. It goes without saying that infant skulls with unclosed sutures will allow enlargement of the vault of the cranium and extreme dilatation of the ventricular system.

REFERENCE

Peach B: Arnold-Chiari malformation: anatomic features of 20 cases. *Arch Neurol* 12:613–621, 1965.

General Reading References

Asbury AK, Johnson PC: Pathology of peripheral nerve. *Major Probl Pathol* 9:1–301, 1978.

Blackwood W, Corsellis JAN (eds): *Greenfield's Neuropathology*. Third edition. London, Edward Arnold (Publishers), 1976.

Burger PC, Vogel FS: *Surgical Pathology of the Nervous System and Its Coverings*. Second edition. New York, John Wiley & Sons, 1982.

Dyck PJ, Thomas PK, Lambert EH (eds): *Peripheral Neuropathy*. Vols 1 and 2. Philadelphia, WB Saunders Company, 1975.

Friede RL: *Developmental Neuropathology*. New York, Springer-Verlag, 1975.

Harkin JC, Reed RJ: *Tumors of the peripheral nervous system. In* Atlas of Tumor Pathology, Second Series, Fascicle 3. Washington DC, Armed Forces Institute of Pathology, 1969.

Haymaker W, Adams RD (eds): *Histology and Histopathology of the Nervous System*. Vols 1 and 2. Springfield, Illinois, Charles C Thomas, Publisher, 1982.

Hirano A: *A Guide to Neuropathology*. Tokyo, Igaku-Shoin, 1981.

Johannessen JV (ed): *Electron Microscopy in Human Medicine*. Vol 6: Nervous System, Sensory Organs, and Respiratory Tract. New York, McGraw-Hill International Book Company, 1979.

Kernohan JW: Primary tumors of the spinal cord and intradural filum terminale. In *Cytology & Cellular Pathology of the Nervous System*. Vol 3. Edited by W Penfield. New York, Paul B Hoeber, 1932, pp 993–1025. Cited by Rubinstein LJ.

Kernohan JW, Sayre GP: *Tumors of the central nervous system. In* Atlas of Tumor Pathology, Fascicle 35. Washington DC, Armed Forces Institute of Pathology, 1952. Cited by Rubinstein LJ.

Lemire RJ, Loeser JD, Leech RW, et al: *Normal and Abnormal Development of the Human Nervous System*. Hagerstown, Maryland, Harper & Row, Publishers, 1975.

Rubinstein LJ: *Tumors of the central nervous system. In* Atlas of Tumor Pathology, Second Series, Fascicle 6. Washington DC, Armed Forces Institute of Pathology, 1972.

Russell DS, Rubinstein LJ: *Pathology of Tumours of the Nervous System*. Fourth edition. Baltimore, Williams & Wilkins Company, 1977.

Vinken PJ, Bruyn GW (eds): *Handbook of Clinical Neurology*. Vols 1–36. Amsterdam, North-Holland Publishing Company, 1969–1979.

Walton JN (ed): *Disorders of Voluntary Muscle*. Fourth edition. Edinburgh, Churchill Livingstone, 1981.

Zülch KJ: *Brain Tumors: Their Biology and Pathology*. Second edition. (Translated by AB Rothballer, J Olszewski.) New York, Springer Publishing Company, 1965.

Index

Abscess
  brain, 109
  epidural, 107
  subdural, 107
Acromegaly, 246
Actinomycosis, 125
Acute cell disease of neuron, 12
Acute swelling of neuron, 12
Adenoma, pituitary, 242–246
Adrenoleukodystrophy, 150
Agenesis
  corpus callosum, 258
  septum pellucidum, 268
Agyria, 265
Alcoholism, chronic, 174
Alexander's disease, 150–151
Alzheimer
  astrocytes, types I and II, 18, 172
  disease, 153
  neurofibrillary degeneration, 12–13, 153
  tangles, 12–13, 153
Amebiasis, 140
Amenorrhea-galactorrhea complex, 246
Amino acid metabolism disorders, 172
Amputation neuroma, 105
Amyelia, 253
Amyloid angiopathy, primary cerebral, 157
Amyloidosis, 179
Amyotrophic lateral sclerosis, 163–164
Anastomosis, 36
Anencephaly, 253
Aneurysms
  atherosclerotic, 70–71
  carotid-cavernous sinus, 72
  congenital, 62–63
  dissecting, 71
  fusiform, 70
  giant, 65
  saccular, 62–63
  septic, 111
Angiitis, granulomatous, 75–76
Angiomatosis
  cortical, 241
  encephalo-trigeminal, 241
  meningofacial, 241
  meningioangiomatosis, 241

Angiospasm, 49
Anoxia
  ischemic, 25
  stagnation, 25
Anoxic-ischemic lesions, perinatal, 271–275
Aqueductal malformations, 257–259
Arachnoid cyst, 235
Arterial infarction, 25
  boundary, 38–39
  border zone, 38–39
  partial, 38
  total, 38
Arteriosclerosis, 29, 55–56
Arteriovenous vascular malformations, 67–70
  of spinal cord, 70
Arteritis
  giant cell, 75
  panarteritis, 72–74
  periarteritis nodosa, 72–74
  temporal, 75
Artery
  anterior cerebral, 41
  anterior choroid, 41
  basilar, 43–46
  internal carotid, 39–41
  middle cerebral, 41
  posterior cerebral, 46
  posterior inferior cerebellar, 43–44
  superior cerebellar, 44
  vertebral, 41–43
Arthritis, rheumatoid, 75
Aseptic meningitis, 131
Aspergillosis, 124
Astroblastoma, 187
Astrocytes
  acute necrosis of, 16
  alterations of, 16–18
  Alzheimer types I and II, 18, 172
Astrocytoma, 185–196
  pilocytic, 187
  piloid, 187
Astrocytosis, 18
Astroglyosis, 18
Ataxia-telangiectasia, 162

Atherosclerosis, 27–29, 55
Atrophy
  cerebellar, alcoholic, 174
  cerebral, alcoholic, 174
  cribriform, 57
  granular, 32
  infantile spinal muscular, 164–165
  lobar, 155
  multiple system, 162
  olivopontocerebellar, 162
  optic, 163
  peroneal muscular, 164–165
  simple cerebral, 153
  simple neuronal, 12, 14
  syphilitic optic, 123
Austin's disease, 170
Axonal reaction, 9
Axons, alteration of, 13–14

Ballooned cell, 13, 155
Binswanger's disease, 57
Bleeding globes, 59
Blood vessel-connective tissue, alterations of, 20
Bourneville's disease, 235–237
Brain abscess, 109
Bunina body, 13

Calcification
  cerebral idiopathic nonarteriosclerotic, 173
  pineal gland, 23
Canavan's spongy sclerosis, 151
Candidiasis, 124
Capillary hemangioblastoma, 22█
Capillary telangiectasia, 65–█
Carcinomatosis, leptomen█
Carcinomatous menin█
Cavum septi pellu█
Cell sclerosis, █
Central ner█
  dama█
  ne█
C█

Cerebral atrophy, 174
  presenile, 153
  senile, 153
  simple, 153
Cerebral edema, 79–81
Cerebral herniations, 81
Cerebral infarction, 30–32
  anemic, 30
  arterial, 25
  arterial border zone, 38–39
  boundary zone, 38–39
  encephalomalacia, 30
  granular atrophy, 32
  hemorrhagic, 30
  ischemic, 30
  laminar necrosis, 32
  partial, 38
  red, 30
  softening, 30
  total, 38
  white, 30
Cerebral infarcts, morphology
  absorption, 34
  cavitation, 34–36
  coagulation necrosis, 32–34
  liquefaction, 34
Cerebral neuroblastoma, 206
Cerebral-parenchymal damage, focal,
    93–98
Cerebral vascular disease, 46–51
Cerebrosidoses, 167–169
Ceramide trihexosidosis, 170
Ceroid-lipofuscinoses, neuronal, 167
Charcot-Marie-Tooth disease, 165
Chemodectoma, 246–247
Chiari malformation, 262–264
Chordoma, 247
Choriocarcinomas, 282
Choroid plexus, 18–19
Chromatolysis
  central, 9
  peripheral, 9–12
Chronic cell dise~
Circ~

Cyst formation, 23
Cysticercosis, 140
Cytomegalovirus, 135–136, 275–276
Cytoplasmic bodies, membranous, 167

Dandy-Walker syndrome, 264
Degeneration
  Alzheimer's neurofibrillary, 12–13, 153
  cerebellar cortical, 178
  cerebello-olivary, 162
  eosinophilic, 12
  hepatolenticular, 172–173
  heterogeneous system, 159
  retrograde, 12
  Simchowicz's granular vacuolar, 13
  spinocerebellar, 160–163
  spongy, of nervous system, 151
  transsynaptic, 12
  Wallerian, 13–14
Dejerine-Sottas disease, 165
Dementia, multi-infarct, 156–158
Demyelinating disease, 141–151
Dermoid tumors, 235
Derry's disease, 168
Devic's disease, 145–146
Diabetes mellitus, 177
Diastematomyelia, 254
Down's syndrome, 270
Dura, alterations of, 23
Duret hemorrhages, 82
Dysraphic states, 253–261
Dystonia musculorum deformans, 158
Dystrophy, neuroaxonal, 14

Ectasia, 29
Ectopic gliomas, 234
Edema
  cerebral, 79–81
  traumatic, 99–100
Embolism, 29–30, 49
  fat, 30
  septic, 111
~bryonal carcinoma, 232
  ~halitis
    ~rnia virus, 132
    ~quine, 131–132
    ~'s lethargica, 137
    ~elitis, 130–131

Encephalopathy
  anoxic, 51
  bilirubin, 276
  dialysis, 176–177
  hepatic, 175–176
  hypertensive, 62
  hypoglycemic, 51, 54–55, 177–178
  hypoxic, 51
  progressive multifocal
    leukoencephalopathy, 136
  subacute necrotizing, 171
  subcortical arteriosclerotic, 57
  uremic, 176–177
  Wernicke's, 174
Encephalo-trigeminal angiomatosis, 241
Enterogenic cyst, 235
Eosinophilic degeneration, 12
Eosinophilic intracytoplasmic inclusion, 13
Ependymal cells, alteration of, 18
Ependymoblastoma, 197, 207
Ependymoma, 196–197
Epidemic typhus, 138
Epidermoid tumor, 233–234
Epidural abscess, 107
Epidural hemorrhage, 89
Epilepsy, myoclonus, 162–163
État criblé, 57
État lacunaire, 57
Exencephalus, 253–254

Fabry's disease, 170
Fahr's disease, 173
Fat embolism, 100
Ferrugination, 13
Fifth ventricle, 268–270
Fibrosarcoma, 221–224
Fibrosarcoma of the nerve, 214
Fibrosis, 20–21
Fibrous histiocytoma, 221
  malignant, 221
Fibroxanthoma, 221
  malignant, 221
Foix-Alajouanine, subacute necrotic
    myelitis, 70
Forbes-Albright syndrome, 246
Friedreich's ataxia, 162
Fungal infections, 124–125
Fungus cerebri, 84
Fusiform aneurysm, 70

Galactocerebrosidosis, 169
Galactosemia, 171
Gangliocytoma, 206
Ganglioglioma, 206
Gangliosidoses, 167
  infantile G_{M2} gangliosidosis, 167
Gaucher's disease, 167–169
Germinal matrix hemorrhage, 275
Germinoma, 230
Giant cell arteritis, 75
Giant cell fibrosarcoma, 225
Giant cell glioblastoma, 225
Gigantism, 246
Gitter cells, 20

Glial shrub, 20
Glioblastoma multiforme, 186
Gliomas, 183–202
    ectopic, 234
    ganglioglioma, 206
    mixed, 185
    nasal, 234
Gliomatosis cerebri, 191
Gliosis
    anisomorphic, 18
    astrogliosis, 18
    isomorphic, 18
Globes, bleeding, 59
Globoid cell leukodystrophy, 148
Glucocerebroside lipidosis, 167–169
Glycogen storage disease, 171
Glycogenoses, 171
Granular cell tumor of the
    neurohypophysis, 234
Granulomatous angiitis, 75–76
Grinker, leukoencephalopathy of, 180
Guillaine-Barré syndrome, 142
Gunshot wounds, 98–99, 102

Hallervorden-Spatz disease, 159–160
Hamartoma, hypothalamic ganglionic, 234
Hartnup's disease, 172
Hemangioblastoma, capillary, 221
Hemangioendothelioma, 221
Hemangiopericytoma, 224–225
Hematin pigment, 13, 154
Hematomyelia, traumatic, 102–103
Hemorrhage
    Duret, 82
    epidural, 89
    germinal matrix, 275
    hypertensive, 58–62
    subarachnoid, 64, 89–92, 275
    subdural, 89, 275
    subdural perinatal, 275
    traumatic, 96
Hepatolenticular degeneration, 172–173
Heredopathia atactica polyneuritiformis,
    170
Herniations, cerebral, 81
Herpes simplex encephalitis,134
Herpes simplex virus, 134, 275–276
Herpes zoster, 135
Heterogeneous system degeneration, 159
Heterotopia, neuronal, 265
Hippocampal sclerosis, 53
Hirano body, 13
Histiocytoma
    fibrous, 221
    malignant, 221
Histiocytosis X, 228
Holoprosencephaly, 261–262
Holotelencephaly, 261–262
Homocystinuria, 172
Hunter's disease, 170
Huntington's chorea, 158
Hurler's disease, 170
Hyalin body, intracytoplasmic, 13
Hydranencephaly, 275

Hydrocephalus, 81, 279–280
    normal-pressure, 156
Hydromyelia, 259
Hypertrophic interstitial neuritis, 165
Hypertrophic interstitial neuropathy, 165
Hypertrophy, onion-bulb of Schwann
    cells, 15
Hypoglycemic encephalopathy, 51, 54–
    55, 177–178
Hypoparathyroidism, 172
Hypoplasia of septum pellucidum, 268
Hypothalamic ganglionic hamartoma, 234

Idiopathic nonarteriosclerotic cerebral
    calcification, 173
Infantile G$_{M2}$ gangliosidosis, 167
Infantile spinal muscular atrophy, 164–165
Infarct, 25 (see also Cerebral and Arterial
    Infarctions)
    septic, 111
Influenza encephalitis, 132
Internal carotid system, 39–41
Intracytoplasmic hyalin body, 13
Intracytoplasmic inclusion, eosinophilic, 13
Iron incrustation, 13
Ischemic attacks, prolonged, 49
Ischemic cerebral vascular disease, natural
    history, 46–51
Ischemic nerve cell change, 12
Ischemic neurologic deficits, reversible, 49
Isomorphic gliosis, 18

Japanese B encephalitis, 132

Kayser-Fleischer ring, 172
Kernicterus, 276
Kernohan's notch, 82
Korsakoff's disease, 174
Krabbe's disease, 148, 169
Kuru, 138

Lacerations, 96
Lacunar state, 57
Lacunes, 57
Lafora's amyloid inclusion, 13
Laminar necrosis, 53
Leigh's disease, 171
Leptomeningeal carcinomatosis, 252
Leptomeningeal cyst, 235
Leptomeningeal tuberculosis, 117
Leptomeninges, alteration, 20–23
Leptomeningitis
    purulent, 107–109
    suppurative, 107–109
Leucinosis, 172
Leukemia, 79, 228–229
Leukodystrophies, 146–151
    adrenoleukodystrophy, 150
    globoid cell, 148
    metachromatic, 147–148, 169
    orthochromatic, 149
    simple orthochromatic, 149–150
    sudanophilic, 149
Leukoencephalitis, acute hemorrhagic,
    141–142

Leukoencephalopathy
    of Grinker, 180
    perinatal telencephalic, 175
Leukomalacia, periventricular, 275
Lewy body, 13
Lipidosis, glucocerebroside, 167–169
Lipochrome, 12
Lipofuscin excess, 12
Lipohyalinosis, 56
Lipoma, 234
Liquefaction, 12
Lissencephaly, 265
Lobar atrophy, 155
Louis-Bar disease, 162
Lymphoreticular system tumors, 225–228

Malaria, 140
Maldevelopmental tumors, 230–235
Malformations
    aqueductal, 257–259
    Arnold-Chiari, 262–264
    arteriovenous-vascular, 67–70
    congenital, 253–271
    vascular, 65–67
    venous, 67
Maple syrup urine disease, 172
Marchiafava-Bignami disease, 174
Marinesco body, 13
Medulloblastoma, 202–206
Medulloepithelioma, 206, 214
Melanoma
    metastatic, 250
    neurocutaneous, 241–242
    primary meningeal, 242
Membranous cytoplasmic bodies, 167
Meningeal hemorrhage, 89–92
Meningeal sarcomatosis, 221–224
Meningioangiomatosis, 241
Meningiomas, 214–221
    angioblastic, 220–221
    malignant, 214–221
Meningiomatosis, 241
Meningitis (see also Leptomeningitis)
    aseptic, 131
    carcinomatous, 252
    tuberculous, 117
Meningocele, 254
Meningoencephalocele, 253–254
Meningofacial angiomatosis, 241
Meningomyelocele, 254
Mesenchymal tissue tumors, 220
Mesial temporal lobe sclerosis, 53
Metachromatic leukodystrophy, 147–148,
    169
Metastatic neoplasms, 247–252
Micrencephaly, 266–267
Microaneurysms
    false, 56–57
    true, 56
Microcephaly, 266–267
Microglia, alterations of, 19–20
Microglial nodule, 20
Microglioma, 227
Micropolygyria, 266

Mineralization, 172
Monster neuron, 13
Monstrocellular sarcoma, 224
Motor neuron disease, 163–165
Mucormycosis, 125
Mucosulfatidosis, 170
Multi-infarct dementia, 156–158
Multilocular cystic encephalomalacia, 274–275
Multinucleated neuron, 13
Multiple myeloma, 228
Muscular atrophy
    infantile spinal, 164–165
    peroneal, 165
    progressive spinal, 164
Myelin sheath, alterations of, 14–15
Myelinoclastic diseases, 141
Myelinolysis, central pontine, 174
Myelitis, subacute necrotic of Foix-Alajouanine, 70
Myelocystocele, 254
Myelopathy
    compressive, 104–105
    necrotizing, 178
    subacute necrotic, 178
Myeloschisis, 254
Myoclonus epilepsy, 162–163
Myopathy, carcinomatous, 179

Nasal glioma, 234
Neoplasms, central nervous system, 242–247
Neoplastic lesions, 183–202
Nerve cell change, ischemic, 12
Nerve cell tumors, 206–207
Nerve injuries, peripheral, 105
Nerve sheath tumors, 214
Neurilemoma, 208–211
Neurinoma, 208–211
Neuritis, hypertrophic interstitial, 165
Neuroastrocytoma, 206
Neuroaxonal dystrophy, 14
Neuroblastoma, cerebral, 206
Neurocutaneous pigmentation, 241
Neuroepithelioma, 214
Neurofibroma, 208–211
Neurofibromatosis, multiple, 237–241
Neurofibrosarcoma, 214
Neurohypophysis, granular cell tumor of, 234
Neurologic deficits, reversible ischemic, 49
Neuromelanosis, 242
Neuroma, 208
    amputation, 105
    traumatic, 105
Neuromyelitis optica, 145–146
Neuronal atrophy, 14
Neuronal heterotopia, 265
Neuronophagia, 20
Neurons
    acute cell disease, 12
    acute swelling, 12
    alteration of, 9–13
    binucleated, 13
    multinucleated, 13

Neurons—continued
    monster, 13
    simple atrophy of, 12
Neuropathy
    hypertrophic interstitial, 165
    peripheral, paraneoplastic, 178
Niemann-Pick disease, 170
Nocardiosis, 125

Oligodendroglia
    acute swelling of, 15–16
    alterations of, 15–16
Oligodendroglioma, 196
Olivopontocerebellar atrophy, 162
Onion-bulb hypertrophy of Schwann cells, 15
Optic atrophy, 163
Orthochromatic leukodystrophy, 149

Pachygyria, 265
Palisades, 204
Palsy, progressive supranuclear, 159
Panarteritis nodosa, 72–74
Panencephalitis, subacute sclerosing, 132–133
Papilloma of the choroid plexus, 200–201
Paraganglioma, 246–247
Paralysis agitans, 158–159
Paraneoplastic syndromes, 178–179
Paresis, general, 122
Parkinson-dementia complex of Guam, 159
Parkinson's disease, 158–159
Pelizaeus-Merzbacher disease, 150
Pellagra, 174
Periarteritis nodosa, 72–74
Perinatal central nervous system damage, 275–279
Perinatal infections, 275–276
Perinatal telencephalic leukoencephalopathy, 175
Peripheral chromatolysis, 9–12
Peripheral nerve injuries, 105
Peroneal muscular atrophy, 165
Phakomatoses, 235–237
Phenylketonuria, 172
Phycomycosis, 125
Pick cell, 155
Pick's argentophilic inclusion, 13
Pick's disease, 155
Pigment metabolism disorders, 173
Pigmentary retinal degeneration, 163
Pilocytic astrocytoma, 187
Piloid astrocytoma, 187
Pineal gland
    alterations of, 23
    calcification, 23
Pinealoblastoma, 208
Pinealocytoma, 208
Pituitary adenoma, 242–246
Plaques fibromyeliques, 273
Poisoning
    carbon monoxide, 179
    lead, 180
    organic mercury, 180–182
Polar spongioblastoma, 192, 206

Poliomyelitis, 130–131
Polymicrogyria, 266
Polyneuropathy, nutritional, 173–174
Pompe's disease, 171
Porphyria, 173
Porencephaly, 268
Postencephalitic parkinsonism, 159
Primary irritation, 9
Primary meningeal melanoma, 242
Primitive neuroectodermal tumors, 206
Progressive multifocal leukoencephalopathy, 136
Proliferation disorders, 266
Psammoma bodies, 220
Pseudo-Hurler's syndrome, 158
Pseudohypoparathyroidism, 172
Pseudorosettes, 197, 204
Purpura, thrombotic thrombocytopenic, 76
Purulent leptomeningitis, 107–109

Radiation necrosis, 182
Rathke pouch cleft cyst, 235
Recklinghausen's disease, 237–241
Refsum's disease, 170
Respirator brain, 55
Retinitis pigmentosa, 163
Retrograde degeneration, 12
Reye's syndrome, 179
Rheumatoid arthritis, 75
Rickettsial infections, 138
Rocky Mountain spotted fever, 138
Rosenthal fibers, 150–151

Saccular aneurysms, 62–63
Sandhoff's disease, 168
Sanfilippo's disease, 170
Sarcoidosis, 118
Sarcomas, 221–225
    arachnoid, of cerebellum, 225
    circumscribed, of cerebellum, 225
    fibrosarcoma, 221–224
    giant cell fibrosarcoma, 225
    meningeal sarcomatosis, 221–224
    mixed, 224
    monstrocellular, 225
    neurogenic, 214
    xanthosarcoma, 221
Sarcomatosis, meningeal, 221–224
Satellitosis, 16
Schilder's disease, 146
Schistosomiasis, 140
Schizencephaly, 268
Schwann cells, onion-bulb hypertrophy of, 15
Schwannoma, 208–211, 214, 241
Schwannosis, 241
Scleroderma, 74–75
Sclerosis
    acute multiple, 143–145
    amyotrophic lateral, 163–164
    arteriolar, 29, 55–56
    Canavan's spongy, 151
    cell, 12
    hippocampal, 53
    mesial temporal lobe, 53

Sclerosis—*continued*
   multiple, 143–145
   progressive systemic, 74–75
   transitional, 146
   tuberous, 235–237
Scrub typhus, 138
Selective vulnerability, 52
Senile plaques, 153–154
Septic aneurysm, 111
Septic embolism, 111
Septic infarct, 111
Septum pellucidum
   agenesis of, 268
   hypoplasia of, 268
Shy-Drager syndrome, 162
Simchowicz's granular vacuolar
   degeneration, 13
Simple atrophy of neuron, 12
Simple contusion, 101
Simple orthochromatic leukodystrophy,
   149–150
Skull fracture, 87–89
Sphingolipidoses, 170
Sphingomyelinosis, 170
Spina bifida, 254
Spinal arterial system, 46
Spinal cord injuries, 100–104
Spinocerebellar degeneration, 160–163
Spongioblastoma, polar, 192, 206
Spongy degeneration of nervous system,
   151
Stab wounds, 101
Stagnation anoxia, 25
Stagnation thrombus, 29
Stains
   astrocyte, 5
   axon, 4
   Bodian, 4–5
   Cajal's gold sublimate method, 6–7
   connective tissue, 7
   cresyl violet, 3
   Del Rio Hortega method, 7
   elastic-van Gieson, 7
   fat, 7
   hematoxylin and eosin, 2
   Holzer, 6
   Luxol Fast Blue, 3–4

Stains—*continued*
   Mallory's phosphotungstic
     acid-hematoxylin, 6
   myelin, 3
   neurofibrillary, 4
   Nissl, 3
   periodic acid-Schiff, 7
   reticulin, 7
   trichrome, 7
Steele-Richardson-Olszewski syndrome,
   159
Storage diseases, 170
Sturge-Weber disease, 241
Sturge-Weber-Dimitri disease, 241
Subacute combined degeneration of spinal
   cord, 174–175
Subacute necrotic myelopathy, 178
Subacute necrotizing encephalopathy, 171
Subacute sclerosing panencephalitis, 132–
   133
Subarachnoid hemorrhage, 64, 89–92, 275
Subclavian steal syndrome, 42–43
Subcortical arteriosclerotic
   encephalopathy, 57
Subdural abscess, 107
Subdural hemorrhage, 89, 275
Sudanophilic leukodystrophy, 149
Sulfatidoses, 169–170
Suppurative leptomeningitis, 107–109
Swelling, acute, of neuron, 12
Syphilis
   congenital, 123
   meningovascular, 122
Syphilitic optic atrophy, 123
Syringobulbia, 261
Syringomyelia, 259–261
Systemic lupus erythematosus, 72

Tabes dorsalis, 123
Tay-Sachs disease, 167
Telangiectasia, capillary, 65–67
Telencephalic leukoencephalopathy, 175
Temporal arteritis, 75
Temporal profile, 46
Teratomas, 232
Thrombosis
   arterial, 29, 50

Thrombosis—*continued*
   dural sinus, 76–79
   vein, 76–79
Thrombotic thrombocytopenic purpura, 76
Thrombus, stagnation, 29
Torpedo formation, 14
Toxoplasmosis, 138–140, 276
Transient ischemic attacks, 49
Transitional sclerosis, 146
Transsynaptic degeneration, 12
Traumatic hematomyelia, 102–103
Traumatic hemorrhages, 96
Traumatic neuroma, 105
Trisomy 21, 270–271
Tuberculoma, 113–117
Tuberculosis, leptomeningeal, 117
Tuberculous meningitis, 117
Tuberous sclerosis, 235
Typhus
   epidemic, 138
   scrub, 138
Typhus nodule, 138
Tyrosinosis, 172

Ulegyria, 273

Van Bogaert-Bertrand disease, 151
Varix, 67
Vascular complications, posttraumatic,
   100
Vascular malformations, 65–70
Vein of Galen, 67–70
Venous malformations, 67
Venous thrombosis, 76–79
Vertebral-basilar system, 41–46
Viral infections, 131–138

Wallerian degeneration, 13–14
Walnut kernel brain, 274
Werdnig-Hoffmann disease, 164–165
Wernicke's encephalopathy, 174
Wilson's disease, 172

Xanthomatous tumors, 221
Xanthosarcoma, 221

Zebra bodies, 170–171